Aesthetic and Functional Female Genital Surgery

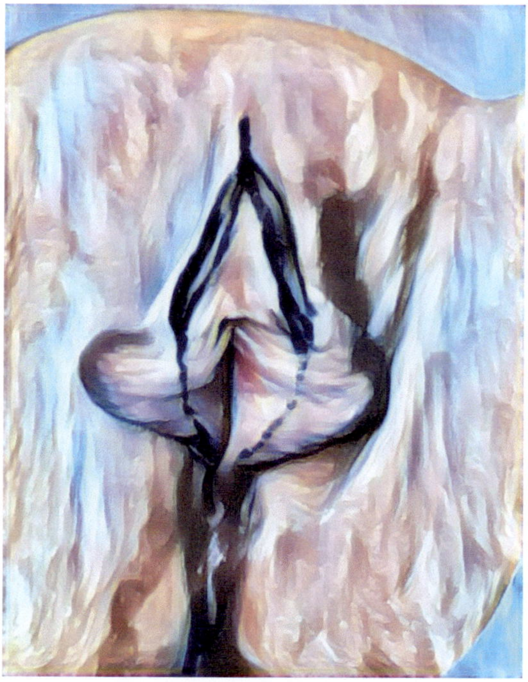

Art of Female Genital Aesthetics

The surgeon performing the aesthetic operation should act like a psychologist during the consultations and as an artist while performing the surgical art, remembering that each patient is different from the others.

Dr. Süleyman Eserdağ

Süleyman Eserdağ

Aesthetic and Functional Female Genital Surgery

Second Edition

Springer

Süleyman Eserdağ
Gynecology
Hera Clinics Istanbul
Istanbul, Turkey

ISBN 978-3-031-16021-9 ISBN 978-3-031-16019-6 (eBook)
https://doi.org/10.1007/978-3-031-16019-6

This Springer imprint is published by the registered company Springer Nature Switzerland AG
The registered company address is: Gewerbestrasse 11, 6330 Cham, Switzerland

Your bonus with the purchase of this book

With the purchase of this book, you can use our "SN Flashcards" app to access questions free of charge in order to test your learning and check your understanding of the contents of the book. To use the app, please follow the instructions below:

1. Go to **https://flashcards.springernature.com/login**
2. Create a user account by entering your e-mail address, assigning a password and inserting the coupon code here below.

MOREMEDIA

Your personal "SN Flashcards" app code DDD3D-70AFD-FF708-1E11E-15BAD

If the code is missing or does not work, please send an e-mail with the subject "**SN Flashcards**" and the book title to **customerservice@springernature.com**.

I devote this book to;

My first mentor, my life teacher, my dear mother Alime Eserdağ (1941–2018),

Altruistic, modest, and unique my dear father Ünal Eserdağ,

My biggest supporter in my academic career and my love Dr. Şenay Eserdağ,

My life energy sources, my dear sons; Can Batu and Batuhan.

Foreword

Asking new questions, new possibilities, looking at old problems from a new angle, requires creative imagination and marks a real breakthrough in science. (Albert Einstein)

It is an honor for me, to be able to write a few introductory words in this wonderful book. It is common for doctors to look in a book perhaps for the chapter that we are interested in consulting, because obviously we do not have time for more. However, this story may be very familiar to many readers. At the beginning of this millennium, I remember how in my daily medical practice hundreds of women year after year complained of problems related to well-being and the quality of sexual life. Curiously, I felt limited by not being able to offer them any valid alternative that could at least alleviate them and thus obtain some benefit for them in this regard. Perhaps this was the trigger that made me twist the course of my professional career as a gynecologist and I began my journey towards what we now know as *"Functional and Aesthetic, Regenerative Gynecology."*

Definitely the book that you are about to enjoy is in my opinion one of the most important written works of this new specialty in this century. It complies in each of its chapters with the proposed educational objectives. In a clear and complete way, it not only shows each of the procedures but also allows us the integration of concepts to be able to apply them all in our daily practice.

When the term *"Aesthetic Gynecology"* was introduced in 1996, it only applied to surgical corrections in the genital area. As in all evolution in medicine, it began, with the passing of the years, to emerge innovators that contributed new techniques not only surgical but also (as in my personal case with the laser) minimally invasive and non-invasive procedures to be applied in the office. After 25 years of evolution, a large number of procedures have been developed with not only aesthetic but also regenerative and functional purposes in gynecology, which gave rise to this new specialty.

Today we are living in an unprecedented time, rather exceptional, that will go down in history and that will mark a before and after (due to a pandemic), where the demand for wellness procedures increased in an incredible way. The desire to be well to improve the biological state prevailed over any other desire in the area of health. In the same way, the demand for procedures in Aesthetic, Regenerative and Functional Gynecology is growing almost exponentially. This means that gynecologists have to supply ourselves with information and we must incorporate new tools to be able to face this growing demand. In this sense, I want to emphasize that this work fills that empty space that we as women's health professionals have.

Regarding the author of this marvel of a book, I just have to say that beyond his vast experience in Aesthetic Gynecology, he is one of the few doctors (if not the only one) in the world who, from the humility that only great people have, has the immense generosity of transmitting absolutely all the information and more as well. Has accumulated experiences, and more than a thousand procedures in the specialty, so as to be able to write and transmit all that world of knowledge that will enrich us for the benefit of our patients. I invite you then to walk the path of Regenerative and Functional Aesthetic Gynecology with the help of Dr. Suleyman Eserdag who will show us how exciting and innovative this concept can mean for our clinical practice. Through each of its pages and each of its chapters, the reader will have a different and attractive feeling, which will go beyond the information they can find in it. I am referring to the passion and motivation that you will find between the lines.

Finally, as a gynecologist dedicated one hundred percent to Regenerative and Functional Aesthetic Gynecology, I would like to convey a message to you and at the same time share a concern with the reader. My message is simple: aging and deterioration is a continuous process that can have consequences on the quality of life. The concern that I want to share with you is that we must be proactive, that is, take action before the symptoms of deterioration occur. For that we have today an innumerable amount of techniques that you will be able to discover in this beautiful written work. I invite you then to enjoy its pages.

OB/GYN & Antiaging Medicine
Mendoza, Argentina

Adrian Gaspar

Foreword

The field of female cosmetic genital surgery and non-surgical genital treatments has had a long and controversial past. More recently, it has found grudging acceptance in the fields of gynecology, urogynecology, urology, plastic and cosmetic surgery, and dermatology.

We owe much of the progress to men and women who were willing to face the bows and arrows from their parent organizations and traditionally minded colleagues. These forerunners include Marco Pelosi II, Marco Pelosi III, David Matlock, Michael Goodman, Adrian Gaspar, Otto Placik, Troy Hailparn, Christine Hamori, Heather Furnas, Sejal Desai, Charles Runels, Alexander Bader, Amr Seifeldin, Joao Brito Jaenisch, Clara Santos, Annebelle Ahererra, and Suleyman Eserdag. We owe much to these pioneers to ease the path for others interested in bravely moving forward and helping women worldwide. Pioneers get arrows, settlers get land. For Turkey and Europe, the Middle East, and Asia, Suleyman Eserdag has proven himself to be a formidable leader and educator.

I heard about Suleyman Eserdag from my professional circles, an admittedly tight group of pelvic surgeons, almost a decade ago. His reputation in Turkey as a young and renowned gynecologic surgeon was growing. I first met Suleyman at the International Society of Pelviperineology (ISPP) meeting in Istanbul in the summer of 2015 where I had the privilege of introducing ThermiVa radiofrequency treatments to the edges of Europe. Legends of pelvic reconstructive surgery and founders of ISPP, Peter Petros and Bruce Farnsworth, wanted me to present my office labiaplasty and vaginoplasty techniques as well as my extensive work in transvaginal prolapse repairs. I had the privilege of meeting outstanding Turkish surgeons and Suleyman stood out. Within a year (2016), he was in Laguna Beach, California, side by side with me as we dove into the brand-new world of non-surgical aesthetic gynecology using energy and biologics for the benefit of suffering women. 2015 was the birth year of the exponential growth of energy for gynecologic use with the advent of vaginal lasers and radiofrequency treatments. Adrian Gaspar from Argentina shepherded the tremendous growth and interest in vaginal lasers while I pursued radiofrequency indications. Because of Charles Runels primarily, it was also the birth year of PRP treatments getting worldwide notice. Charles had fought for many years before that to bring his message out but 2015 was the breakout year. He spoke at my very last Congress on Aesthetic Vulvovaginal Surgery (CAVS) meeting in Orlando,

Florida, in September 2015 and the interest in his O-Shot procedure went ballistic. Suleyman was in the middle of all this outburst of creative energy and recognized that for this field to succeed surgical skill had to be at the forefront. So, we tackled labial and vaginal surgery with intensity in my office setting and planted the seed that would blossom into ISAGSS two years later. I shared all my trade secrets in No IV In-Office Awake Genital Surgery. I shared my skills in Hybrid/Venus/Rim Labia Minoraplasty, Medial Curvilinear Labia Majoraplasty, Lateral and Vertical Clitoral Hood reduction, RF Feathering and Resurfacing of labial edges and anal skin tags, Perineoplasty, and full depth Vaginoplasty. I shared my secrets on my office setup and equipment, modifications of Pudendal and Levator Blocks, and use of Lone Star 3715 APS Retractor to allow safe and solo in-office surgeries. I made sure Suleyman would be an expert in ThermiVa and the O-Shot as we did case after case. I knew Suleyman would bring these life-changing procedures to Europe and the world and help thousands of women in the future. I was very proud of my esteemed graduate and encouraged his professional development. He has proven to be a consummate professional and renowned educator and for this I am very grateful. I feel a sense of relief that the surgical techniques I shared with Suleyman will survive and be taught to others.

Now, seven years after we first met, Suleyman has brought together his experience and skills in his book *"Aesthetic and Functional Female Genital Surgery"* now with recent updates. This textbook clearly shows his love and passion for this emerging field and will be a tremendous core source of knowledge. His personalized modifications and approach show a depth of experience from someone in the trenches, working daily to perfect his craft, and not from someone sitting inside an ivory tower having medical students and residents writing chapters from inexperience. I recommend this collection of written insight without reservation with his recent updates a further advance of this field. It is the perfect partner for my own online and onsite training programs that have spanned several decades. I recommend his book to all my grads.

Alinsod Institute for Aesthetic Vulvovaginal Surgery
South Coast Urogynecology,
Laguna Beach, CA, USA

Red M. Alinsod

Preface

With the new millennium, the increase in internet use and the rapid spread of social and digital media have caused significant changes in societies. The desire of women to feel better, the increasing popularity of general antiaging treatments, especially the visual comparison of races in social media, development of energy-based new technologies, and the incredible increase in social awareness are just a few of the factors that accelerate the popularity of female genital operations. The aesthetic operations of the genital area include a range of surgical and non-surgical procedures with a high level of patient satisfaction for cosmetic, reconstructive, and regenerative purposes, providing excellent results when done with the suitable technique and individualized methods. However, when these procedures are done without sufficient knowledge and experience, they can lead to irreversible results in terms of both aesthetic and functional aspects as well as serious legal problems. For this reason, *training is essential before starting practice*. However, this field is not included in the residency training programs of most universities today. Some associations, organizations, or individuals working with special status are trying to fill this gap. International Society of Aesthetic Genital Surgery and Sexology (*ISAGSS*), which I established in 2017 and still continues to provide hands-on training under my leadership in different parts of the world, uniquely combines aesthetic genital surgery with sexual well-being.

Another important issue is that scientific evidence-based data on genital aesthetic procedures are still insufficient. For this reason, energy-based technologies used in applications and treatments become the target of organizations such as *WHO, FDA*, and *ACOG* from time to time. I hope that as the evidence-based data on genital aesthetic operations increase, this field will soon reach a much stronger position in the scientific arena.

For the physician who intends to work in the field of genital aesthetics, it is essential to have the ability to empathize with his/her patient, not to compromise on ethical principles, and to draw his/her own boundaries with the motto "*first, do no harm.*' The operation demands and expectations of the patients can be quite different from each other. *There is no one-size-fits-all in cosmetic surgeries.* The technique to be used in the operation in line with the experience of the physician should be applied according to the patient's wishes and the condition of the tissue.

As stated in the ACOG declaration published in 2020, some sexual dysfunctions can also be corrected by functional genital surgeries. However, for this, the physician must have sufficient training in the fields of sexual dysfunction and psychiatric disorders, and when necessary, should not hesitate to ask for consultation from different disciplines.

The book *"Aesthetic and Functional Female Genital Surgery"* is blended with nearly 20 years of knowledge and experience in the field of genital area aesthetics, techniques from the most up-to-date literature, and a multidisciplinary perspective. The work, which is the product of the coronavirus pandemic period in 2020, consists of 23 separate sections, and the images in its content were selected from more than 20,000 photographs from over a 20-year-period in this field. Procedures not yet included in the literature, e.g., labia minora asymmetry classification, Venus vaginal aesthetics with Eserdag concept, neolabiaplasty (re-labium formation), inverted-U hoodoplasty, hat trimming in hoodoplasty, Juicy Vagina Syndrome, rooster comb appearance in perineum, painful hymen as a cause of superficial dyspareunia, square mattress suturing in labiaplasty, office labiaplasty, majoraplasty with adipose tissue reduction, and teardrop incision in majoraplasty, as well as procedures of my techniques such as the Inverted-Y plasty procedure in clitoral hoodoplasty operations and primary repair of hymen with vestibulo-introital tightening technique (VITT) in the literature are also discussed in detail.

The book includes basic to advanced methods of aesthetic, reconstructive, and regenerative surgeries and non-surgical applications related to female genital organs and has been enriched with consent forms in the last part. Before you start reading, I recommend that you test yourself with the aesthetic genital surgery MCQ in the Flashcards, or at least take a look. After you finish reading the book, you can return to the exam questions.

My aim is that the physicians who have devoted themselves to this field and whose number is increasing rapidly every year can gain knowledge from the most basic level to advanced techniques in *this happy journey*. I hope that this work, in which I generously share all the methods I apply to my patients, will be beneficial for the global medical community.

Istanbul, Turkey — Süleyman Eserdağ

Contents

About the Author

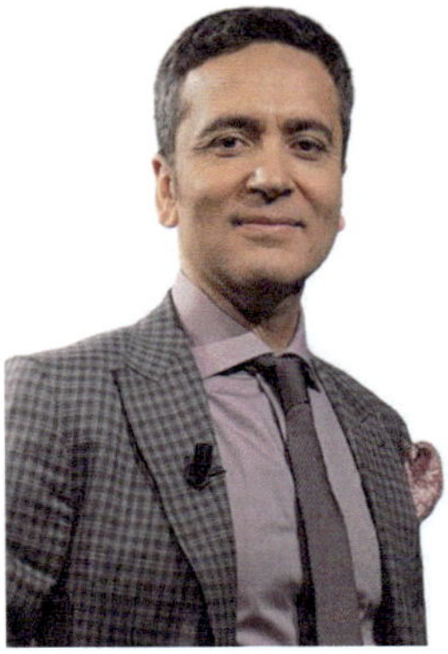

Süleyman Eserdag The author was born in Turkey in 1969 and after completing his primary and secondary education, he graduated from Izmir Science High School in 1986. After graduating from the Medical School of Dokuz Eylül University, he began residency program in Ankara Zekai Tahir Burak Women's Health Educational and Research Hospital, the largest educational maternity hospital in Turkey. He completed his residency education in 1997 and became a gynecologist and obstetrician. Later, he worked as a Gynecology and Obstetrics Specialist and also a Chief Physician at the Kazan State Hospital, which was his first place of appointment. In 2002, he was re-appointed to Zekai Tahir Burak Women's Health Education and Research Hospital and worked in the perinatology, menopause, in vitro fertilization, and infertility clinics of this hospital. In this period, he opened his first clinic named "HERA Clinic" in Ankara. In 2008, he resigned from the hospital and started working full-time in his office.

He, in 2014, passed the board exam organized by the European Society for Sexual Medicine (ESSM) and the European Federation of Sexology (EFS) to become Turkey's one of the first "Fellow of European Committee of Sexual Medicine" (FECSM) gynecologists.

In 2015, he established the HERA Vaginismus Treatment, Education and Research Association, the first national non-governmental organization in the field of vaginismus. He trained physicians and health professionals within the scope of this association.

He has received training from many leaders in the field during his vaginismus and genital aesthetics journey that started in the early 2000s. Prof Adam Ostrzenski (Florida/USA-2011), ECAMS

(Athens/Greece-2015), and Dr. Red Alinsod (California/USA-2016) are some of the mentors or organizations that he received training from.

He was accepted as a senior faculty member at ECAMS (European College of Aesthetic Medicine and Surgery) based in Ireland in 2015. Between 2015 and 2017, he gave hands-on genital aesthetics courses in Istanbul and Vienna. In 2017, he left this faculty and established an international association called ISAGSS (International Society of Aesthetic Genital Surgery and Sexology). In this association within the scope, Turkey, Northern Cyprus, India, Pakistan, UAE, Azerbaijan, Philippines and Indonesia in as many countries, has provided more than 1000 physicians one-to-one training. In addition, he organized the International Reconstructive Aesthetic Genital Surgery and Sexology (RAGSS) congresses in Istanbul in 2018 and 2019.

In 2020, he published the book Sexual Medicine and Genital Aesthetics, which he shared the editorship with two colleagues. This book is the first book published in Turkey in the field of sexual medicine and genital aesthetics.

In 2021, he published the first edition of this book Female Aesthetic and Functional Genital Surgery, both in Turkish and in English.

Inverted-Y plasty procedure in clitoral hoodoplasty operations and vestibulo-introital tightening technique (VITT) in hymenoplasty have been introduced into the literature by Dr. Eserdag. Many national and international studies of him on vaginismus and dyspareunia have also been published in peer-reviewed journals.

He established four private clinics in Istanbul, Ankara, and İzmir under the roof of "HERA Clinic." Now, he is the director of these clinics and accepts the patients in his private clinic in Istanbul. At the same time, he continues giving lectures and trainings within the scope of the ISAGSS and has been invited to many national and international congresses. He is married and father of two boys.

Part I

Introduction and General Instructions

1 Introduction to the Art of Aesthetic and Functional Female Genital Operations

The ladder of the peak of civilization is art.
Mustafa Kemal Atatürk, Founder of the Republic of Turkey

The interest of women in their genital areas, the social meanings they attribute to this region, and the genital practices applied have continued from the time of the Pharaohs to the present. Traditional genital area decorations, painting, tattoos, piercing-like jewelry, procedures to reduce or enlarge tissues, and operations such as genital circumcision are just some of these practices.

When we come to today, the widespread use of the internet, the increase in pornographic video and visual sharing, the rapidly developing social media culture, the increase of our social interest in the visual, and our visual comparison race have increased the interest in genital operations, especially since the early 2000s. In addition, associating bad marriages with sexuality, the increase in the expectations of couples in sexual intercourse, the desire of women to feel better psychologically and sexually, and the increase in antiaging treatments are among the reasons for patients to prefer *"designer vagina"* operations. The development of correct surgical techniques, different suture options, the comfort provided by various anesthesia methods, the physicians who have developed themselves in this field, and the training given by some associations are among the other important factors that enable the development of Aesthetic Genital Surgery (AGS).

The widespread use of genital shaving—a religious requirement in Muslim societies—in Western societies has been one of the factors that has increased the importance of the genital area by eliminating the *"vulvar camouflage."* The emergence of genital fashion trends in the form of Brazilian waxes and Hollywood waxes in Western society are also signs of increased interest in vulva visuality.

Concerns include *"Are genital aesthetic surgeries necessary, should they be performed, are they medically indicated, or can they cause permanent medical damage by causing injuries in the female genitals?"* mainly from ACOG (American College of Obstetricians and Gynecologists), RCOG (Royal College of Obstetricians and Gynaecologists), SOGC (Society of Obstetricians and Gynaecologists of Canada), FDA (American Food and Drug Association), and feminist organizations that think they will turn women into sexual objects. However, despite all the criticism, *Pandora's box* has been once opened, and AGS operations in almost all regions of the world are a rapidly increasing trend with intense patient demands. However, AGS operations, which are not included in plastic surgery or gynecology and obstetrics residency training, resulted in many

S. Eserdağ, *Aesthetic and Functional Female Genital Surgery*,
https://doi.org/10.1007/978-3-031-16019-6_1

complications and malpractice suits when physicians without training, only personal intuitions, attempted these surgeries.

Although there are some associations and organizations that provide training in this field today, the adequacy and quality of the training provided is a matter of debate. It is necessary to include these trainings in residency trainings in branches such as gynecology, plastic surgery, urology, and dermatology. However, considering that it is not easy to include such training programs in the existing curriculum, for now the only solution seems to be special certificate programs.

If we consider that all aesthetic operations are included in the "agreement for work" principles in our laws, the surgeon should:

- be trained in the basic principles of aesthetic surgery, genital aesthetic surgical techniques, energy-based treatments such as laser, radiofrequency, regenerative applications, and sexology before applying,
- select the patients meeting the right indications,
- plan operations well from the start, and
- obtain consent forms after giving detailed information before the operation.

1.1 Etymology and Terminology

The word aesthetics comes from the word *"aisthetikos"* in the ancient Greek language. It has meanings such as aesthetic, sensitive, sensual, related to perception. It is used synonymously with "cosmetics."

Genital aesthetic operations include some surgical and non-surgical applications and are called by different names: vulvovaginal plastic surgery, genitoplasty, cosmetic gynecology, cosmetoplastic gynecology, women's cosmetic plastic genital surgery, aesthetic genital surgery, etc.

Although the term "vaginal rejuvenation" is used for vaginal rejuvenation, vaginoplasty, and perineoplasty, the boundaries of this term have not been defined. It is generally regarded as an *"umbrella term"* that includes all aesthetic and functional procedures performed for optimal correction and repair of the vagina and its neighboring organs [1]. This term is not recommended for use because the name is registered.

"Pudendum" is synonymous with *"pudenda"* and means "external genital organs," especially the vulva. Pudendum, which is derived from the Latin verb *"to be ashamed, shamed part of something"* first appeared in English in the fourteenth century.

Nympha (or nymph) is synonymous with "labium minus pudendi" and means *"bride, young girl, young woman"* in ancient Greek. Nymphs were sometimes beloved by many and dwelt in specific areas related to the natural environment such as mountains, forests, springs. Plural form of nympha is referred to as *"Nymphae"* (labia minora).

"Vulvoplasty" is a general name and defines the surgical procedures to construct, repair, or remodel a vulva. Sometimes, it is also used to define gender-affirming surgery for transgender and nonbinary individuals who are designated male at birth.

Plastic surgery is a specialty in the fields of alteration ("change"), restoration ("architectural renewal, putting together what is broken"), and reconstruction ("replacing and rebuilding what is torn down") of the human body. It includes cosmetic, reconstructive surgery, and newly regenerative categories (Fig. 1.1). Reconstruction aims at the functional restructuring of congenital or acquired defects, while cosmetic (=aesthetic) aims to enhance the appearance. The word plastic is derived from the Greek word *"plastikē"* and is used to mean *"reshaping."* For example, "labiaplasty" means aesthetic operation of the genital labia, "vaginoplasty" means repairing the anterior and/or posterior segments of the vagina, and "hymenoplasty" means repair and reconstruction of the hymen.

Regenerative medicine deals with the process of replacing, engineering, or regenerating human or animal cells, tissues or organs to restore or establish normal function. It has the potential to heal or replace tissues and organs damaged by age, disease, cancer, or trauma and normalize congenital anomalies. Regenerative medicine, an interdisciplinary field that applies engineering and life science principles to promote regenera-

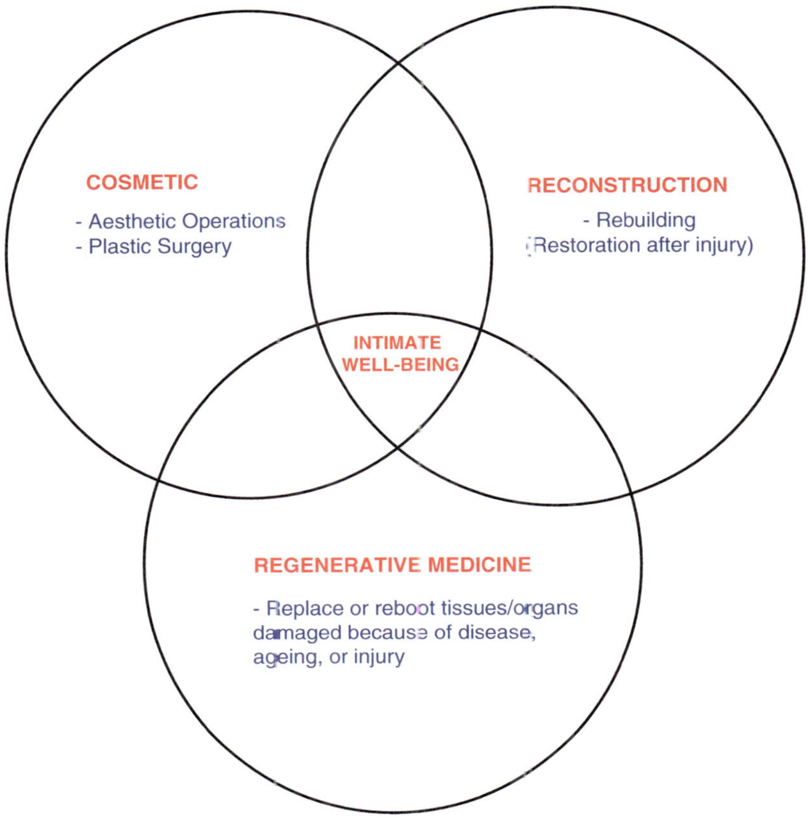

Fig. 1.1 Structures of aesthetic and functional medicine

tion, can potentially restore diseased and injured tissues and whole organs. The treatments with stem cells opened a new gate in cosmetic gynecology and operational practices involving the treatments of vagina atrophy, genitourinary syndrome of menopause, dyspareunia, lichen sclerosus, and lichen planus.

Aesthetic surgery covers the biggest part of plastic surgery. Plastic surgery also includes different subdivisions such as burn surgery, craniofacial surgery, microsurgery, hand surgery, and pediatric plastic surgery. Especially in recent years, the interest of plastic surgeons in genital aesthetic operations has increased. It is important for plastic surgeons interested in this field to be educated about female genital anatomy and physiology.

Genital aesthetic procedures are also known as "cosmetic gynecological operations." Experience in surgeries such as Bartholin's cyst removal, episiotomy repair, colporrhaphy, perineoplasty, and pelvic organ prolapse (POP) surgeries provides advantages to gynecologists regarding genital aesthetic procedures. However, it is important for gynecologists who intend to work in this field to have knowledge about basic aesthetic surgery principles and dermatological diseases.

1.2 Why Do Women Consult a Doctor?

The most common reason patients consult a doctor is aesthetic concerns. This is followed by functional and sexual reasons. Sometimes, hygienic, cultural, and medical indications may be found. These indications can be abbreviated as *5R* in English: "**R**eclaim–**R**estore–**R**evive–**R**econstruct–**R**epair."

The biggest aim of patients who apply to aesthetic clinics is to have a better appearance and to feel more comfortable in terms of psychosocial aspects. In a study, it was observed that women with low body mass index and who were attractive, self-confident, not shy toward the opposite sex, tend to improve their sexual life, and who can easily find jobs and partners are more prone to cosmetic surgery [2].

1.3 Body Perception

Body perception is one of the most important motivational factors that arouse desire for cosmetic surgery. Body perception includes observations, feelings, and thoughts about one's own body. Women with positive body perception are at peace with their own bodies. Physical and psychological factors affect body perception. In one study, women who were looking for cosmetic surgery were quite dissatisfied with their appearance in the preoperative period, while it was observed that their body perception developed positively after the surgery [3].

1.4 Self-Esteem

Self-esteem and body perception are interrelated and are affected by each other in a cause–effect relationship. In a study, it was determined that self-esteem increased after cosmetic surgical procedures. In addition, it was stated that the perspective of the society, self-esteem, and body perception is important in a person's decision to choose cosmetic surgery [4].

The first article on cosmetic gynecological surgeries is a case report published in North America in 1978 [5]. This was followed by the studies conducted by Hodgekinson and Halt in 1984 and Chavis, LaFeria, and Niccolini in 1989 regarding the operation performed for aesthetic and sexual indications [6].

1.5 Genital Area is the Mirror of the Patient

An experienced physician, who carefully evaluates the genital area, has many preliminary thoughts about the patient. A woman with hyperpigmented vulvar skin and a larger-than-normal clitoris is characterized by androgen excess (such as polycystic ovary syndrome and adrenal hyperplasia), a woman whose vulva is larger than normal and whose skin is irritated may have an obsessive compulsive nature due to her habits such as excessive washing of her genital area with soap, a woman with very long genital hair and unhygienic may be depressed, have psychiatric problems, or have a distorted body image as in vaginismus, those who prefer different epilation methods suitable for Brazilian/Hollywood genital waxing fashion or those who have piercings/tattoos in genital area epilation may be fond of aesthetics or sexuality in this area, and those with a larger than normal clitoris and drooping lips (except for structural factors) may have frequent masturbation habits.

Conversely, it should be noted by the physician that there may be problems related to nutritional habits or immune system in those who have frequent vaginal yeast infections and that the partner factors of those who have recurrent purulent discharges despite frequent treatment should also be questioned, and that those with extremely clean vaginas may have frequent vaginal douching habits due to their obsessions. Of course, all these prejudices should always be considered, examining the patients' lifestyle, sociocultural, religious, and economic levels.

Conversely, lesions in the vagina (such as lichen planus and Behçet's) can also manifest in the oral mucosa. Skin problems in the vulva (such as lichen sclerosus, hidradenitis, Fox-Fordyce disease, and psoriasis) may also reflect skin pathologies in different body areas or autoimmune diseases or occur alone. For this reason, an experienced gynecologist or dermatologist should evaluate the patient as a whole and seek a remedy by going down to the root causes rather than treating the tip of the iceberg.

1.6 Aesthetic and Functional Genital Procedures Umbrella

The procedures related to the aesthetic and functional genital area in women include a series of surgical (Table 1.1) and non-surgical (Table 1.2) procedures.

Table 1.1 Surgical procedures

- **Labiaplasty**

Labiaplasty is the reduction and aesthetically correction of the labia minora or labia majora. If specified, labia minoraplasty is aesthetic—plastic operation of labia minora, also known as "*Nymphoplastie,*" especially in French-speaking countries, and labia majoraplasty is attributed to external genital labia

- **Clitoral hoodoplasty**

This is the removal of excess skin tissue on the clitoral hood area, which is also known as "preputium." It is usually performed simultaneously with labiaplasty. Synonymous terms such as clitoral hood reduction, "clitorohoodoplasty", or "clitoral hoodectomy" can be used.

- **Vaginoplasty**

This is a reconstructive surgery to narrow and tighten the vaginal canal surgically. It is also known as "colporrhaphy" or "surgical vaginal rejuvenation". The vaginal mucosa is excised and mostly fascia and muscle repair is performed. Several types can be performed:

  - Posterior colporrhaphy (+/– Levator's plication)
  - Anterior colporrhaphy
  - Lateral colporrhaphy

- **Perineoplasty**

This is also known as perineorrhaphy or perineal aesthetics. In the operation, the introitus and perineal tissue are repaired. In the meantime, episiotomy scars and skin tags in the area are also excised. As a result of perineoplasty, the perineum is slightly raised, while the perineal length is also increased

- **Colpoperineoplasty**

Performing posterior vaginal reconstruction and perineoplasty operations together

- **Hymen procedures**

Hymenoplasty is an aesthetic operation where repair and reconstruction of the hymen are performed. The aim is to restore virginity. It is also called hymenorrhaphy, revirgination, or hymen repair. Conversely, the "hymen protrusion" that manifests itself from the outside can be aesthetically disturbing. In addition, in cases such as vestibulitis and "painful hymen," hymen tissue may be the cause of superficial dyspareunia. In all these cases, hymenectomy operation can also be performed

- **Labia majora reduction (labia majoraplasty)**

The big ("major") genital lip is known as "labium majus." Its Latin plural form is referred to as "labia majora" or "labia majora pudenda." Majoraplasty operations are surgical stretching and reduction of sagging, loosened labia majora. Sometimes fat pad debulking can also be performed

- **Labia majora augmentation**

This is the resurfacing of collapsed labia majora, usually by injection of autologous fat graft. The augmentation process can also be done with HA (hyaluronic acid) injections

Table 1.2 Non-surgical procedures

- **Genital laser treatments**

These are energy-based, non-surgical methods applied to the vulva and vagina. Most common application purposes include:

  - Vaginal rejuvenation, tightening
  - Stress urinary incontinence (SUI) treatments
  - Vulvar and perianal bleaching
  - Vulvar tightening treatments

- **Genital radiofrequency (RF) treatments**

The indication fields are very close to laser treatments. Most common uses are:

  - Vaginal rejuvenation, tightening
  - Stress urinary incontinence (SUI) treatments
  - Vulvar tightening and resurfacing
  - Sexual enhancement treatments

- **G-spot applications**

This is the procedure of HA injection applied to the anterior vagina to increase sexual pleasure. Also known as G-spotplasty or G-shot © operations.

- **O-spot applications**

This is the procedure of platelet-rich plasma (PRP) injection applied to the anterior vaginal wall, vestibulum, and clitoral areas to increase sexual sensitivity. Also known as O-spotplasty or O-shot © operations

- **Genital filler injections**

This is the procedure of applying HA (hyaluronic acid) fillers to the labia majora, perineum, vulvar vestibulum, and vaginal mucosa. It is performed for different cosmetic and functional purposes

- **Regenerative applications**

Regenerative procedures include injections of autologous fat, stem cells, SVF (stromal vascular fraction), exosomes, autologous cytokine rich serum (ACRS), and platelet-rich plasma (PRP) that rejuvenate and regenerate the genital area. They can be applied to all internal and external genital areas. They can be preferred for functional, cosmetic, and antiaging purposes

- **Other non-invasive genital aesthetic procedures**

These include applications such as carboxytherapy, vaginal HIFU (high intensity focused ultrasound), mesotherapy, thread applications to the vagina and vulva, and magnetic chair. The field of genital aesthetic applications is expanding rapidly with new technologies every day

Additionally, AGS functional applications include treatments for diseases such as menopausal genitourinary syndrome, vulvar varicose veins, condyloma, benign tumors, dyspareunia, vulvar vestibulitis, vaginal dryness, sexual desire problems, and lichen sclerosus etc.

1.7 Statistics

According to American Association of Plastic Surgeons (AAPS) statistics, the amount spent annually on all cosmetic procedures in the USA in 2018 is around USD 16.5 billion. In total, 17.7 million cosmetic and 5.8 million reconstructive procedures were applied [7].

The most common cosmetic surgical procedures in the USA in 2018:

1. Breast augmentation (313,000)
2. Liposuction (258,000)
3. Rhinoplasty (213,000)
4. Eyelid surgery (206,000)
5. Tummy tuck (130,000)

The most common non-surgical cosmetic procedures in 2018:

1. Botulinum toxin (7.4 million)
2. Hyaluronic acid (2.6 million)
3. Chemical peels (1.38 million)
4. Hair removal (one million)
5. Microdermabrasion (709,000)

Non-surgical procedures are increasing faster compared to surgical procedures according to the American Society for Aesthetic Plastic Surgery (ASAPS) (Fig. 1.2).

Labiaplasty is the most common genital aesthetic operation in AGS (Table 1.3).

According to the data from American Society for Aesthetic Plastic Surgery (ASAPS), 26.3% of plastic surgeons perform surgical and non-surgical vaginal applications. Between 2012 and 2017, labiaplasty operations (within 5 years) increased by 217.3%. Again, in 2017, a total of 10,787 labiaplasty operations were performed in

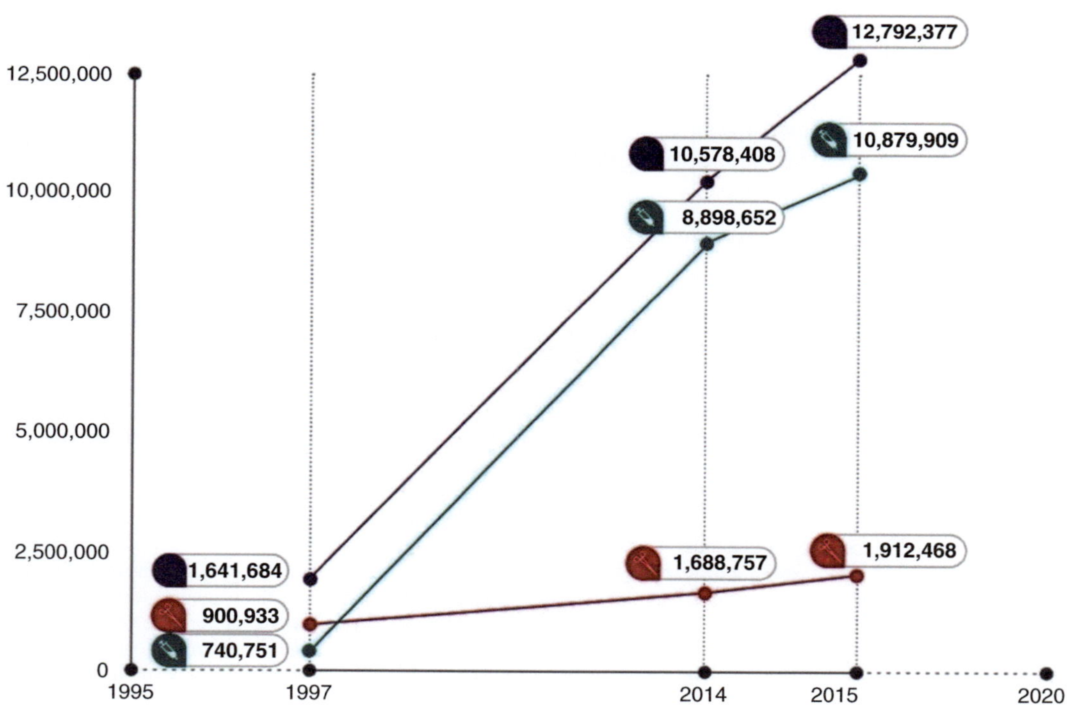

Fig. 1.2 Increase in cosmetic procedures in the USA since 1995. The lower red line shows the number of surgical procedures performed, the green line in the middle shows the number of non-surgical procedures, and the purple line at the top shows the total number of surgical and non-surgical procedures [7]

Table 1.3 Number of labiaplasty and pelvic floor reconstruction operations in the USA in 2017 and 2018 [7]

Year	Labiaplasty	Pelvic floor reconstructions
2017	10,253	1592
2018	10,246	1719

the USA, and labiaplasty ranked 17th among all surgical cosmetic procedures. When we look at the age distribution of patients undergoing labiaplasty, 469 patients (4.3%) were aged 18 and under, 5963 patients (55.3%) between 19 and 34 years, 3685 patients (34.2%) between 35 and 50 years, 603 patients (5.6%) between 51 and 64 years, and 67 patients (0.6%) were over 65 years of age [8].

1.8 AGS Contraindications

AGS is not recommended in the following situations:

- **Pregnancy**
  All elective aesthetic and reconstructive procedures should be avoided during pregnancy.
- **Puerperium period**
  It is recommended to wait at least three months for vaginal tightening and labiaplasty procedures.
- **Active HPV or HSV presence**
  In order to prevent the spread of the infection, it is recommended to first treat the infection and then to perform the operation after recovery.
- **Uncontrolled diabetes mellitus (DM)**
  The operation is not recommended without blood sugar regulation as it will adversely affect wound healing. The situation is the same for patients with impaired glucose tolerance.
- **Morbid obesity (body mass index > 40)**
  Although morbid obesity does not constitute an absolute contraindication, wound healing may be adversely affected. In addition, the risk of developing infection increases slightly due to hygienic reasons.
- **Presence of abnormal scar tissue and keloids**
  This does not constitute an absolute contraindication. Many patients with severe hypertrophic cesarean scars may not develop scars after labiaplasty. High vascularization and lymphatic drainage of the tissue may be a factor in this.
- **Body Dysmorphic Disorder (BDD)**
  This is definitely a situation that should be well evaluated. As stated in the ACOG bulletin in 2020, this group of patients may have dissatisfaction and different emotional changes after surgery. In case of doubt, a psychiatric consultation should be sought before surgery.
- **Psychiatric or serious psychological disturbances**
  Conditions such as depression, anxiety, and obsessive-compulsive disorder (OCD) are important in patient selection. Associating psychological problems with the genital area entirely may lead to an increase in postoperative emotional problems. In addition, cosmetic surgery should not be performed on patients diagnosed with psychosis, bipolar disorder, severe depressive disorder, and eating disorders. Although not every patient who will undergo aesthetic genital surgery requires psychiatric consultation, it is appropriate to request a psychiatric consultation in suspicious cases.

  Some vaginismus patients may also request aesthetic genital operations unnecessarily due to their distorted body image and loss of self-confidence.
- **Mentally disabled**
  All operations for aesthetic purposes are contraindicated in people with mental disabilities.
- **Cancer or suspected cancer**
  Vaginal laser applications should be avoided, especially in those with abnormal cellular cervical and/or vaginal pathology due to effects of HPV. Also, surgical and non-surgical applications are contraindicated in cases of undiagnosed genital cancer or pre-cancer.
- **Over-expecting patients**
  As the patient has the freedom to choose the physician, it is also important that the physician who will perform aesthetic surgery

choose the patient. It is not beneficial for patients with overexpectations as well as those who are overly detailed, indecisive, mentally contradictory, or insecure to undergo plastic surgery. The satisfaction level of such patients after surgery is extremely low. Conversely, many patients do not know exactly what they are looking for, although they consult a physician. Problems with the spouse, cheating, depression, generalized anxiety disorder, or different psychological disorders may underlie this search.

1.9 Patient Selection and Surgery Planning

Patient selection is extremely important in cosmetic genital surgery. At the patient's first visit, the surgeon should ask:

- What kind of complaints she is coming in for,
- What is the primary complaint,
- When did the complaints start,
- Aesthetic and functional expectations regarding the operation,
- Whether she has problems with her marriage or partner relationship,
- Whether the operation is primarily desired by her spouse or herself,
- Whether there are arousal, desire, orgasm, lubrication, and/or pain problems related to sexual life,
- Obstetric and gynecological history,
- Last menstrual period,
- Menstrual cycles,
- Whether there is an incontinence problem,
- Systemic diseases,
- The drugs she uses,
- Drug allergies,
- Whether she has had anesthesia before, and
- Past operations and cosmetic procedures.

While taking anamnesis, the patient's attitudes, general psychology, and symptoms of body dysmorphic disorder should be evaluated.

After the anamnesis, a simple gynecological evaluation should be made for a few minutes in the lithotomy position, accompanied by a female assistant. At the gynecological table, all requests of the patient are listened to and brief information is given about the procedures that can be done on the genital area. It will be easier to demonstrate this information using a mirror given to the patient to hold.

Detailed information about the surgery planned to be performed after the pelvic examination is passed includes:

- Which surgical technique will be applied,
- How long it will take,
- After the explanation, whether it is necessary to stay in the hospital or not, the patient and the physician decide together. In order to facilitate understanding, it would be appropriate to explain what will be done using simple drawings and to show examples from previous surgeries.

After the decision to operate is made, the following should be discussed:

- When and where the surgery will be performed (office/hospital condition),
- What the anesthesia method will be (local/sedation/epidural/pudendal/general),
- What the patient will encounter in the postoperative period,
- What kind of drugs she will need to use,
- How to change medical dressings on her own,
- Detailed explanations are given about toilet, bathroom needs, sports activities, sexual life, and time to return to work or school during the postoperative period.

All physicians working in cosmetic gynecology should be able to analyze the patient's psychology well, have sufficient knowledge in terms of sexual dysfunctions, and should always adopt the principle of *"first, do no harm"* as a principle. The physician must have been trained in genital aesthetic operations and, if he/she will use them, energy-based treatments. In addition, there will be a need for a nurse who is well equipped and trained to assist in plastic/reconstructive surgery.

The physician should not make overly exaggerated discourses, should know his/her own limits, behave honestly with the patient, and never compromise ethical principles.

1.10 Female Circumcision

Female circumcision is a traditional rather than a religious aspect that dates back to the Pharaoh's era, especially in West African countries such as Sudan, Ethiopia, Egypt, and Somalia. Female circumcisions are more often referred to as "Female Genital Mutilation (FGM)" in the literature. Traditionally, it is done by cutting the outer genitalia of young girls between the ages of 6 and 10 years. Girls who are not circumcised in these countries face the risk of social exclusion and labeling. In general, the aim is to protect the chastity of the woman by reducing her sexual desire and the pleasure she will receive during sexual intercourse.

FGM, which is considered a violation of women's human rights, can lead to serious complications such as tetanus, excessive pain, edema, infection, fever, excessive bleeding, shock, chronic pain, organ damage, urinary incontinence, infertility, vaginal delivery difficulties, and obstetric fistula formation if the woman conceives. FGM is usually carried out during childhood, mostly by neighborhood midwives who are not health care professionals, and without any consent.

Its severity (amount of tissue damaged) and health risks are related to the type of mutilation and the amount of tissue cut. According to WHO statements, more than 200 million girls have been circumcised in 30 different countries, led by Sudan, and three million girls are at risk of being circumcised every year [9].

1.11 Types of Genital Mutilation in Women

The WHO defines the practice as "all procedures that involve partial or total removal of the external female genitalia, or other injury to the female genital organs for non-medical reasons." There are four different types of genital mutilation and subtypes defined by the World Health Organization (WHO) in 1997 [10]:

Type I: Partial or total removal of the clitoral glans and/or the prepuce/clitoral hood. When it is important to distinguish between the major variations of Type I FGM, the following subdivisions are used:

- Type Ia. Removal of the prepuce/clitoral hood only.
- Type Ib. Removal of the clitoral glans with the prepuce/clitoral hood.

Type II: Partial or total removal of the clitoral glans and the labia minora with or without removal of the labia majora. When it is important to distinguish between the major variations of Type II FGM, the following subdivisions are used:

- Type IIa: Removal of the labia minora only.
- Type IIb: Partial or total removal of the clitoral glans and the labia minora (prepuce may be affected).
- Type IIc: Partial or total removal of the clitoral glans, the labia minora, and the labia majora (prepuce/clitoral hood may be affected).

Type III: This type is often referred to as "infibulation" and involves narrowing of the vaginal opening with the creation of a covering seal. The seal is formed by cutting and repositioning the labia minora or labia majora. The covering of the vaginal opening is done with or without removal of the prepuce and glans (Type I FGM). When it is important to distinguish between variations of Type III FGM, the following subdivisions are used:

- Type IIIa: Removal and repositioning of the labia minora.
- Type IIIb: Removal and repositioning of the labia majora.

Type IV: All other harmful procedures to the female genitalia for non-medical purposes, for example, pricking, piercing, incising, scraping, and cauterization.

"*Deinfibulation*" refers to the practice of cutting open the sealed vaginal opening of a woman who has been infibulated (Type III). This is often done to allow sexual intercourse or to facilitate childbirth and is often necessary for improving the woman's health and well-being.

Reconstructive surgery of Type III genital mutilation (34 yrs) is shown in Fig. 1.3.

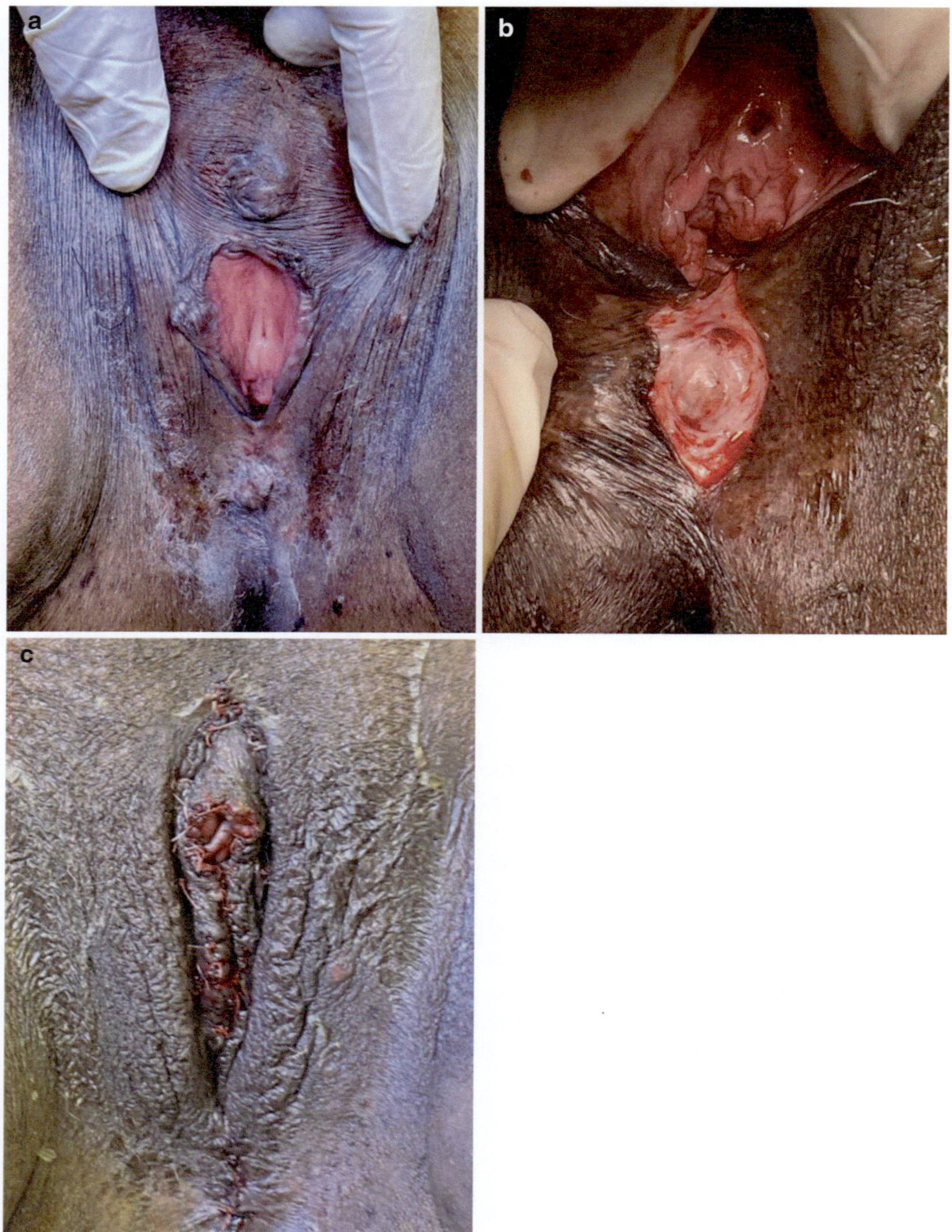

Fig. 1.3 Reconstruction of Type III genital mutilation (**a**). Separation of merged sides of both labia minora and majora, extirpation of the perineal inclusion cyst, perineal repair, revision of the labia minora and preputium, and liberation of the glans clitoridis (**b**). After the procedure (**c**)

In this context, female circumcision is quite different from genital aesthetic operations because:

- It is not recommended to perform genital aesthetic operations for aesthetic purposes under 18 years of age. Mutilations are usually performed in childhood, such as between the ages of 6 and 10 years.
- The purpose of genital aesthetic operations is aesthetic and functional correction. However, genital mutilation procedures are performed with the idea of preventing sexual pleasure.
- Genital aesthetic operations are performed in office or hospital conditions under aseptic conditions. Female circumcisions are usually performed at home, in the presence of neighborhood midwives, and without sterile conditions.
- Written and verbal consent is taken from patients before genital aesthetic operations. There is no consent requirement for mutilation.

1.12 History of Female Circumcision

It is accepted that the Prophet Abraham was circumcised at the age of eighty, that his children were also circumcised, and that the circumcision of men and women began at that time.

> *Prophet Abraham, who lives in Palestine and is married to Sarah (Sara in Arabic), has no children. Sarah offers her black slave Hajar to her husband Abraham and asks her to have a child. However, when Hajar becomes pregnant, Sarah becomes jealous of her and demands that her three limbs be amputated. Being worried about this situation, Abraham orders Hajar to pierce her ears and be circumcised. However, Sarah's anger does not end afterwards. For this reason, Abraham takes Hajar, takes the newborn child Ishmael (Isma'il) to Mecca and leaves them there. Mecca, which was a town that nobody visited at that time, quickly gained popularity with the rebuilding of the Kaaba by Hajar and Abraham who later came to her aid* [11].

The pictures on some papyri and the circumcision scenes on the wall of Karnak Shrine in Luxor are evidence of the prevalence of circumcision in ancient Egypt. Today, approximately 200 million women are circumcised in approximately 30 countries in western, eastern, and north-eastern Africa, in parts of the Middle East and Asia, and within some immigrant communities in Europe, North America, and Australia. In Sudan and Somalia, which are the leading countries for FGM, around 97% of girls are circumcised. Apart from Africa, girls are also circumcised in some parts of Yemen, Northern Iraq, Arabia, India, Pakistan, Malaysia, and in some countries in Asia and Latin America. FGM continues to persist among immigrant populations living in Western Europe, North America, Australia, and New Zealand. The citizens of these countries try to continue their customs in the countries they emigrate to. According to the information I received from my Indonesian colleagues, the ritual is performed by gently scratching the clitoris of girls born in that country with a small syringe needle.

In 2020, the COVID-19 pandemic has negatively and disproportionately affected girls and women, resulting in a shadow pandemic disrupting SDG target 5.3 on the elimination of all harmful practices including FGM. UNFPA estimates an additional two million girls are projected to be at risk of undergoing female genital mutilation by 2030.

Female circumcision is a practice that comes from tradition and is later associated with religion. It is not mentioned in the holy book Qur'an and there is no strong evidence that the Prophet said that girls are to be circumcised. According to the Hanafi sect, circumcision should only be applied to men [12].

Within the framework of "*International Day of Zero Tolerance for Female Genital Mutilation, 6 February*" announced by the United Nations, a wide-ranging global program against female genital mutilation was carried out in 17 African countries by UNICEF and UNFPA. In this context, many advertisements, booklets, and research reports were published against female genital mutilation. Thanks to all these studies, great success has been achieved and female genital mutilation has been prohibited in 24 of 30 countries.

Appendix

With the purchase of this book, you can use our "SN Flashcards" app to access questions free of charge in order to test your learning and check your understanding of the contents of the book.

To use the app, please follow the instructions below:

1. Go to https://flashcards.springernature.com/login
2. Create a user account by entering your e-mail address and assigning a password.
3. Use the following link to access your SN Flashcards set: ▶ https://sn.pub/tvlq7Q

If the link is missing or does not work, please send an e-mail with the subject "SN Flashcards" and the book title to customerservice@springernature.com.

References

1. Karcher C, Sadick N. Vaginal rejuvenation using energy-based devices. Int J Womens Dermatol. 2016;2(3):85–8.
2. Nikolić J, Janjić Z, Marinković M, Petrović J, Bozić T. Psychosocial characteristics and motivational factors in woman seeking cosmetic breast augmentation surgery. Vojnosanit Pregl. 2013;70(10):940–6.
3. Sarwer DB, Wadden TA, Pertschuk MJ, Whitaker LA. Body image dissatisfaction and body dysmorphic disorder in 100 cosmetic surgery patients. Plast Reconstr Surg. 1998;101(6):1644–9.
4. von Soest T, Kvalem IL, Wichstrøm L. Predictors of cosmetic surgery and its effects on psychological factors and mental health: a population-based follow-up study among Norwegian females. Psychol Med. 2012;42(3):617–26.
5. Honoré LH, O'Hara KE. Benign enlargement of the labia minora: report of two cases. Eur J Obstet Gynecol Reprod Biol. 1978;8(2):61–4.
6. Goodman M. Female genital plastic/cosmetic surgery. J Sex Med. 2013;10(8):2125–6.
7. https://www.plasticsurgery.org/documents/News/Statistics/2018/plastic-surgery-statistics-full-report-2018.pdf
8. https://www.surgery.org/sites/default/files/ASAPS-Stats2017.pdf. Accessed 20 May 2020.
9. https://www.who.int/health-topics/female-genital-mutilation#tab=tab_1. Accessed 19 May 2020.
10. https://www.who.int/news-room/fact-sheets/detail/female-genital-mutilation. Accessed 18 May 2020.
11. Nebi Bozkurt S. İslam Ansiklopedisi. c. 38. İstanbul: Türkiye Diyanet Vakfı İslam Araştırmalar Merkezi; 2010.
12. Eryiğit Bader A. Sünnet Olma ve Kadın Sünneti. Eskiyeni. 2018;(37): 81–107.

2 Should Aesthetic Genital Operations Be Done?

> *Before practicing surgery one should gain knowledge of anatomy and the function of organs so that he will understand their shape, connections and borders. He should become thoroughly familiar with nerves, muscles, bones, arteries and veins. If one does not comprehend the anatomy and physiology one can commit a mistake which will result in the death of the patient.*
>
> *(Al-Zahrawi, the greatest surgeon of middle ages, "father of modern surgery")*

In this section, the opinions on genital aesthetic operations of some important obstetrics and gynecology associations, especially the American College of Obstetricians and Gynecologists (ACOG), the American Food and Drug Administration (FDA) warning, the World Health Organization (WHO) definition of health, Patient Rights, Patient Perspective, and Legal Aspects are discussed.

2.1 ACOG Declarations

For the first time in 2007, ACOG made a statement about genital aesthetic operations and declared some warnings (Nr 378). Despite the genital aesthetic operation techniques and developing new technologies, the same declaration was reaffirmed exactly 10 years later, in 2017.

According to the ACOG declaration in the bulletin Nr 378, "It is misleading to give patients the impression that vaginal rejuvenation, G-spot amplification, hymenoplasty, designer vaginoplasty or similar operations are *accepted and routine* procedures. These patients who are disturbed by their genital appearance or sexual problems may be further traumatized by unproven surgical procedures" [1].

In addition, the physician is obliged to discuss the following issues with his/her patient:

- Reason for requesting cosmetic gynecological surgery.
- Whether there are any physical signs or symptoms that warrant surgical intervention.
- Female genital organs may have various appearances.
- There is insufficient data on the efficacy and safety of gynecological cosmetic operations.
- Possible complications such as infection, change of sensation, dyspareunia, adhesions, and scarring in gynecological cosmetic operations.

Despite all these warnings, ACOG did not completely close the door to AGS operations completely and allowed operations with certain indications. Among the medical indications approved by ACOG, deinfibulation (female circumcision correction) and labiaplasty operations are included due to labial hypertrophy and asym-

S. Eserdağ, *Aesthetic and Functional Female Genital Surgery*,
https://doi.org/10.1007/978-3-031-16019-6_2

metry. Although labiaplasty can be performed for both the inner and outer labia, this is not clearly stated in this ACOG declaration. Conversely, according to ACOG's declaration Nr 378, sexual dysfunctions cannot be corrected by aesthetic operations, and sexual function can worsen with cosmetic gynecological operations that have not been proven effective. Behind ACOG's cautious approach to aesthetic genital operations is the scarcity of evidence-based scientific data in this field. Additionally, the fact that this bulletin, published by ACOG, was written by academicians who are not in the ACOG association and who do not have practice in cosmetic gynecology has been another criticism.

ACOG published a new bulletin on elective female genital cosmetic surgery in January 2020. This bulletin numbered 795 replaced the declaration numbered 378 published in 2007. In this declaration, it is stated that sexual dysfunctions can be improved by genital surgeries, but for this, it is important that the physician is educated about sexual dysfunctions and psychiatric disorders [2].

According to ACOG's declaration in 2020 (Nr 795):

- Female genital cosmetic procedures include procedures such as labiaplasty, clitoral hood reduction, hymenoplasty, labia majora augmentation, vaginoplasty, and G-spot amplification.
- Patients should be made aware that surgery or procedures to alter sexual appearance or function (excluding procedures performed for clinical indications, such as clinically diagnosed female sexual dysfunction, pain with intercourse, interference in athletic activities, previous obstetric or straddle injury, reversing female genital cutting, vaginal prolapse, incontinence, or gender affirmation surgery) are not medically indicated, pose substantial risk, and their safety and effectiveness have not been established.
- Women should be informed about the lack of high-quality data that support the effectiveness of genital cosmetic surgical procedures and counseled about their potential complications, including pain, bleeding, infection, scarring, adhesions, altered sensation, dyspareunia, and need for reoperation.
- Obstetrician–gynecologists should have sufficient training to recognize women with sexual function disorders as well as those with depression, anxiety, and other psychiatric conditions. Individuals should be assessed, if indicated, for body dysmorphic disorder. In women who have suspected psychological concerns, a referral for evaluation should occur before considering surgery.
- In responding to a patient's concern about the appearance of her external genitalia, the obstetrician–gynecologist can reassure her that the size, shape, and color of the external genitalia vary considerably from woman to woman. These variations are further modified by pubertal maturity, aging, anatomic changes resulting from childbirth, and atrophic changes associated with menopause or hypoestrogenism, or both.
- As for all procedures, obstetrician–gynecologists who perform genital cosmetic surgical procedures should inform prospective patients about their experience and surgical outcomes.
- Advertisements in any media must be accurate and not misleading or deceptive. Rebranding existing surgical procedures (many of which are similar to, if not the same as, the traditional anterior and posterior colporrhaphy) and marketing them as new cosmetic vaginal procedures is misleading.
- Obstetrician–gynecologists who perform cosmetic procedures should be adequately trained, experienced, and clinically competent to perform the procedure. Extensive familiarity with appearance and function, as well as the ability to manage complications, is expected from obstetrician–gynecologists who perform these procedures.

Similarly, The Society of Obstetricians and Gynaecologists of Canada (SOGC) advises that physicians who will perform cosmetic procedures related to the vagina and vulva should be trained in gynecological and/or plastic surgery in terms of cosmetic surgery of the external genital system.

2.2 FDA Warning

On July 30, 2018, the FDA warned some laser and radiofrequency companies manufacturing energy-based technology (EBT), health care providers, and the patients who use it. They also provided additional information in November of the same year [3].

Here is the declaration:

We are aware that certain device manufacturers may be marketing their energy-based medical device for vaginal "rejuvenation" and/or cosmetic vaginal procedures. The safety and effectiveness of energy-based medical devices to perform these procedures has not been established.

Vaginal "rejuvenation" is an ill-defined term; however, it is sometimes used to describe non-surgical procedures intended to treat vaginal symptoms and/or conditions including, but not limited to:

- Vaginal laxity,
- Vaginal atrophy, dryness, or itching,
- Pain during sexual intercourse,
- Pain during urination,
- Decreased sexual sensation.

To date, we have not cleared or approved for marketing any energy-based devices to treat these symptoms or conditions, or any symptoms related to menopause, urinary incontinence, or sexual function. The treatment of these symptoms or conditions by applying energy-based therapies to the vagina may lead to serious adverse events, including vaginal burns, scarring, pain during sexual intercourse, and recurring/chronic pain.

Healthcare providers should discuss the benefits and risks of all available treatment options for vaginal symptoms with their patients. If any patients experience adverse effects from procedures that involved the use of energy-based devices to perform vaginal "rejuvenation," cosmetic procedures, or treat genitourinary symptoms of menopause, sexual dysfunction, or urinary incontinence, it should be reported.

Behind all these warnings from the FDA and ACOG, despite the rapidly developing technologies and the number of surgeries, there are still insufficient scientific evidence-based data. Conversely, the fact that many pioneering physicians in this field act in partnership with technology-producing companies or have direct commercial partnerships with these companies is also a source of trust.

2.3 FDA Warning and a Review on Laser and Other Energy-Based Technologies

(This article is an excerpt from an article I shared on my social media)

On July 30, 2018, the FDA (US Food and Drug Administration) issued a warning about laser and energy technology devices. Our colleagues expressed their concerns in some physician groups on this issue. I would like to share my thoughts on the subject with you.

First of all, laser and RF devices are technologies that have been used in cosmetic dermatology for years. These devices have been transferred to the treatment of the genital area since the early 2000s. Laser is used in cosmetic dermatology in many areas such as acne, wart, and flesh mole treatment and facial rejuvenation. RF has a place especially in facial and décolleté rejuvenation, regional obesity, and many physical therapy applications. We, gynecologists, met with the production of the vaginal probes of these devices with a delay (about 10 years ago). In fact, medical laser and RF technologies are extremely old. They already have FDA approvals for genital wart treatment and hemostasis.

The laser is obtained with energy-concentrated light waves of the same wavelength without scattering. Lasers can be liquid, solid, or gaseous, depending on the medium used. For example,

CO_2 lasers work on the principle of transferring the intense energy light beam produced by gas (CO_2) medium to the tissue. Each laser has an affinity for a chromophore. CO_2 and erbium: YAG lasers have affinity for water molecule, and when they encounter water in the tissue, they generate heat with a thermal effect. Lasers targeting the melanin chromophore lighten color, and those that reach the oxyhemoglobin chromophore are effective in the treatment of varicose veins.

In radiofrequency, the mechanism is different. With a wavelength of a certain frequency (at the frequencies of radio-TV signal waves where the name comes from), the electric current meets the water in the tissue and generates heat. The effect is again thermal.

In laser and RF, the mechanism is actually similar: *"reversible injury."* As a result of these slight injuries, an inflammatory process begins in the tissue, many cytokines such as TGF-Beta come into play, fibroblasts migrate to the area for repair, and as a result, collagen and elastic connective tissue synthesis starts again.

The term "rejuvenation" mostly used in laser and RF means *"the restoration of a youthful appearance to something."* The same term is used for other parts of the body, such as facial, hand, neck rejuvenation, etc. The terms intravaginal laser tightening or laser narrowing are wrong. With the reversible injury we have provided, the repair process begins, which is different from tightening.

Tissue penetration in lasers is very low (energy accumulates in the lamina propria), and the temperature produced is high (60–65 °C). In radiofrequency, the penetration is higher (subcutaneous tissue), but the energy is lower (40–46 °C). Both procedures are performed while the patient is awake, and the areas other than the perineum and introitus (vaginal entrance) are quite pain free. Since the patient is awake, there is no risk of burning during the procedure. In fact, the temperature given by the thermosensor apparatus at the probe tip of the RF device is constantly controlled, preventing exceeding the limit. Some RF devices even stop directly when the tissue temperature reaches a point.

Competitions between laser and RF companies are great. In our clinics we use both laser and RF. That's why we can evaulate it objectively.

No major problems such as severe burns, scar tissue development, or fibrosis have been encountered in more than 7500 laser and radiofrequency applications performed in our clinic so far. Moreover, there are no major complications mentioned in the literature. It is an unclear on what basis the FDA refers to when talking about side effects related to devices. They are completely non-invasive procedures and have slight differences between the indications.

On the other hand, while laser is slightly ablative, RF has no ablative effect. For this reason, even sexual intercourse can be recommended immediately after RF operation. The duration of sexual abstinence for laser is seven days.

Laser and genital RF can be used in areas such as stress urinary incontinence, vaginal dryness, lichen sclerosus, and menopausal atrophy (thinning of the genital area skin), except for vaginal rejuvenation. They are also used for cosmetic purposes for majora rejuvenation. Laser can be used for anogenital bleaching and cutting in labiaplasty operations. With the increased fibroblastic activity, the vaginal tightening effect becomes noticeable by the patient who undergoes the procedure and by her partner after an average of three weeks.

On the other hand, the decisions made by the FDA should also be questioned. For example, the FDA-approved synthetic meshes in 2001 for vaginal mesh applications. In 2008, they highlighted the complications of mesh erosion, pain, and urinary complaints. They talked about the risks of dyspareunia. In 2016, they changed their mind on the 2001 decision and included meshes in the high-risk group and warned the manufacturers about this issue. On April 16, 2019, the FDA asked all manufacturers to stop their sales and distribution of mesh for cystocele (anterior wall prolapse). We will see what kind of declarations will come later.

Half of women aged 60 and older are incontinent. It is a big social problem. Up to the age of 80, 12% of women are operated on due to POP (pelvic organ prolapse).

We are faced with the fact that many defects and recurrence rates of surgical methods and surgical techniques are high. The risk of dyspareunia in midsling mesh operations is 16%, and permanent hip and groin pain in 12%. This is why constant modifications of the technique are being developed.

Non-invasive laser and RF treatments can be performed easily under office conditions in obese, diabetic, and incontinent cases with poor general health. Anesthesia is not applied, and the procedure takes about 20 minutes. It is indicated in cases of SUI without POP or mild POP. If we set out with the quote of Dr. Victor Gomel *"Surgery is the incompetence of medicine,"* can we save some of the incontinence patients from surgery with these simple applications? It is necessary to think about it very carefully.

Genital aesthetics and technology uses are generally performed in private centers. University and training hospitals act more slowly and conservatively in this regard, which is why there are not enough RCT (randomized controlled trial) data. Most of the studies done are case studies. Behind the decisions made by the FDA commission, there are facts such as the scarcity of evidence-based scientific data and the fact that most of the studies in this area were commissioned by companies in the style of white papers.

It would be a great injustice to close the doors to new technologies so early. Similar mistakes were made by the Women's Health Initiative (WHI) study. All postmenopausal treatments were terminated due to an incorrectly designed study and news in the press. I hope the same will not happen to genital laser, radiofrequency, and other genital technologies.

2.4 World Health Organization (WHO) Definition of "Health"

Health is not just *"not having any disease."* WHO defines health as a state of complete *physical, mental (emotional),* and *social* well-being and not merely the absence of disease or infirmity. According to the Encyclopedia Britannica, health is the extent of an individual's continuing physical, emotional, mental, and social ability to cope with his/her environment. As described in these definitions, the mental and social dimensions of health should also be taken into consideration as well as physical. Therefore, most of the aesthetic medical procedures, although not for therapeutic purposes, are the methods of realizing the right to health, which includes one of the basic human rights, the mental well-being of the person. In this context, most of the aesthetic and reconstructive operations for the genital area are performed *"to be healthy."* For example, in most labiaplasty operations, which are frequently requested by patients, in addition to aesthetic concerns, there are physical problems such as frequent vaginal infections, urine flowing in different directions in the toilet, and irritation due to friction while wearing jeans. The number of women who see themselves as socially flawed or even disabled, who cannot flirt with their boyfriends, cannot marry out of shame, and cannot concentrate on the relationship due to being ashamed of their bodies when they are with their partners during intercourse is quite high. Some patients also face emotional problems such as self-deficiency, inability to feel like a woman, and lack of self-esteem. Therefore, is it enough to focus solely on physical diseases of an anatomical region, when this region has such great effects on a person's social life and psychology? Similar situations apply to women who experience postpartum vaginal enlargement and age-related insensitivity.

2.5 Patient Rights

The first written declaration on patients' rights is the declaration accepted at the 34th Congress of the World Medical Association (VMA), which was held in Lisbon in 1981. According to this declaration, the patient has the right to choose freely and change his/her physician and hospital or health service institution, regardless of whether they are based in the private or public sector.

In the declaration of European Consultation on the Rights of Patients, held in Amsterdam on 28–30 March 1994 under the auspices of the WHO Regional Office for Europe (WHO/

EURO), patient rights are gathered under six main headings:

1. Human rights and values in health care
2. Information
3. Consent
4. Confidentiality and Privacy
5. Care and Treatment
6. Application

Considered from the patient's point of view, everyone has, of their own free will:

- The right to choose the health system.
- The right to choose the type of treatment and procedure.
- The right to choose or refuse procedures with informed consent [4].

2.6 Patient Perspective

From a patient perspective, how can we ignore the following facts below?

2.6.1 Self-Esteem Issues

Some women desire to change their physical appearance in order to feel better and increase their self-esteem. They may perceive the appearance of their external genitalia as an embarrassing defect or *"stigma."* In fact, the main reasons given for all aesthetic operations such as mammoplasty, rhinoplasty, abdominoplasty, and liposuction are almost similar: increased self-esteem, feeling better psychologically.

2.6.2 Being Ashamed, Avoiding Mutual Relations

Some women may experience emotional stress due to their anatomical features and appearance of their genital areas. Being ashamed or avoiding marriage or even dating relationships are common behaviors. I came across many examples on this subject:

A 24-year-old patient who came to my clinic for labial revision said she hated the tissues she thought of as excess in her genital area. Since she was unaware of plastic surgery in this area, she told me that, when she was 16, she cut her labia with a bread knife and rubbed olive oil and sat on it to stop the bleeding. Eight years later she applied to me for the revision of her irregular labia.

Another patient of mine who applied for a labiaplasty operation had a chromosome test after she was doing a research on the internet for her hypertrophic labial appearance, with the thought that she might be a "hermaphrodite male" and contacted me with her test result.

Another 42-year-old patient, who was very successful in her business life, started crying immediately after a mild sedation anesthesia and shared her true story with me. My patient emotionally stated that she had postponed this operation because she was afraid of this surgery, of which she had been thinking for years, but that she hated her own femininity because of the abnormality in her inner labia, that she could not get close to any man, that is why she was still virgin and even could not think of getting married. When she came for a follow-up two months after the operation, I encountered a completely different person whose self-esteem was enhanced incredibly.

2.6.3 Hygienic Problems

Some women may have hygienic problems due to the anatomical features of their external genitalia, and they have frequent genital infections as well as sweating of the genital area, bad odor, and frequent fungal infections. Smegma accumulation on the inner labia after sports is an especially important hygienic problem.

2.6.4 Protrusion while Wearing Trousers

Some women may experience social problems such as avoiding wearing tight tights, pants, bikinis, etc. The inability to wear a bikini due to the external appearance of the external genitalia and avoiding social environments are common avoidance behaviors. Conversely, the labia majora's stance in trousers or tights split on both sides is the appearance known as "camel toe." Some women especially desire this look, while others are quite dissatisfied and embarrassed with it. Today, different silicone pads that are attached to underwear that either look like camel toe or oppositely hide camel toe have been produced.

Many congenital and acquired pathologies can cause aesthetic and functional problems in women as shown in Figs. 2.1, 2.2, 2.3, 2.4, 2.5, 2.6, 2.7, 2.8, 2.9, 2.10, 2.11, 2.12 and 2.13.

2.6.5 Anatomical Defects and Dermatologic Pathologies

Congenital or acquired anatomical defects and skin pathologies bring along many functional problems and aesthetic concerns.

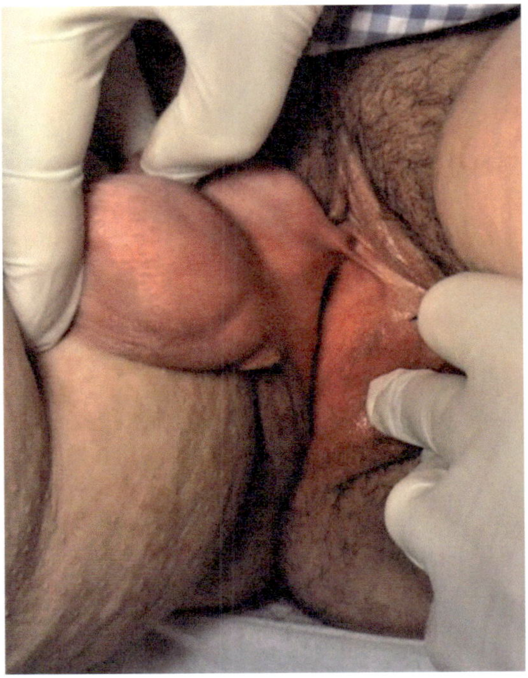

Fig. 2.1 Right labial cyst (18 years old)

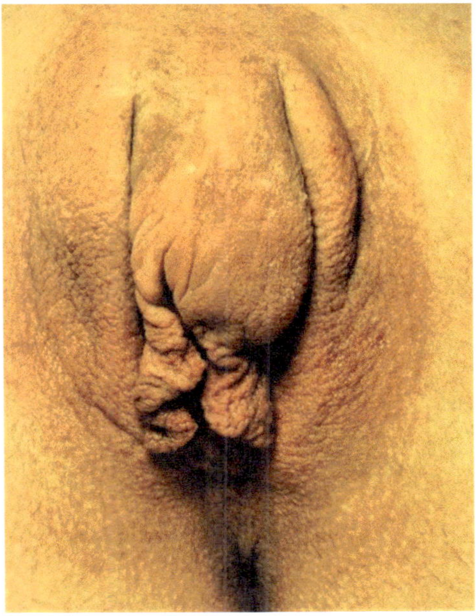

Fig. 2.2 Clitoral hood tumor (19 years old)

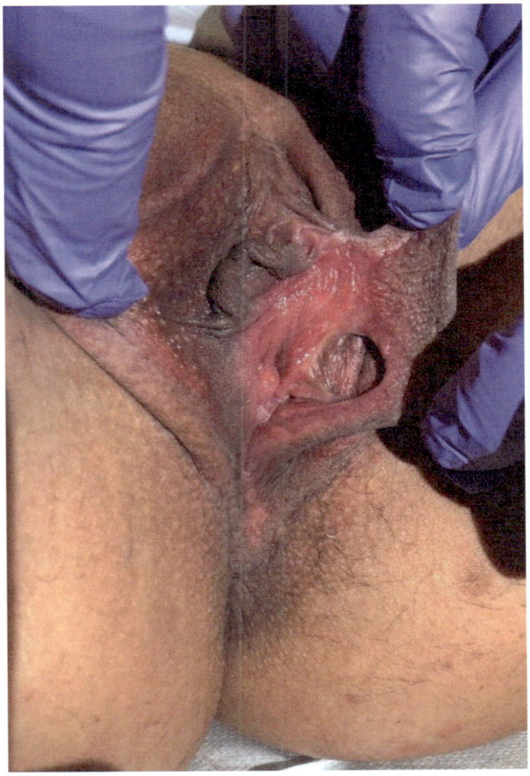

Fig. 2.3 Labial perforation because of silver nitrate placed due to Bartholin's cyst

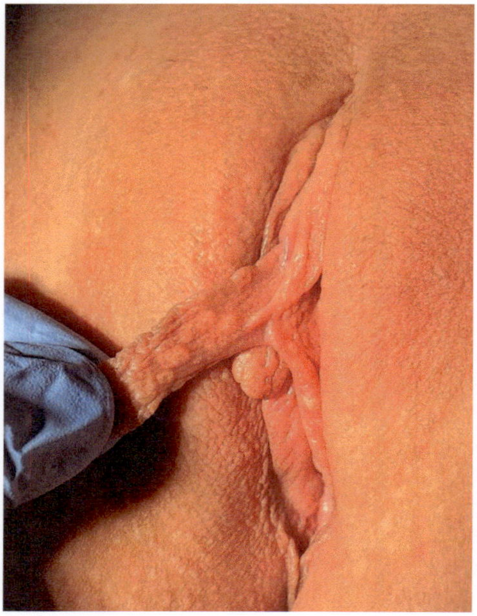

Fig. 2.4 Separation of the left labium due to falling off a bicycle

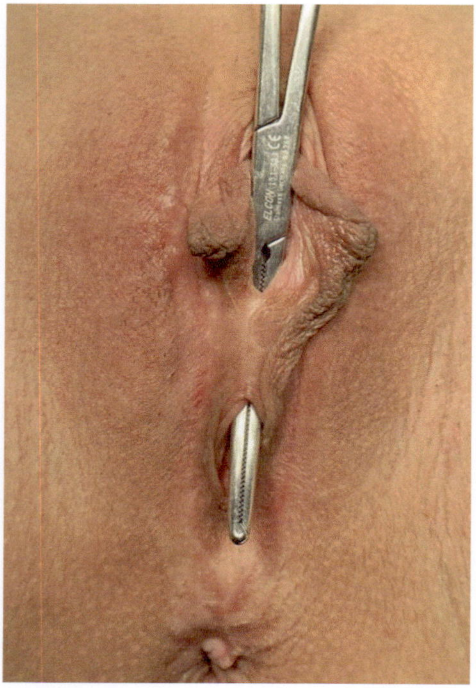

Fig. 2.5 Labial fusion. This patient (39 years) who had vaginismus treatments unnecessarily by many different centers, and applied to our clinic due to inability of sexual penetration. In her anamnesis, she describes a vulvar infection during childhood

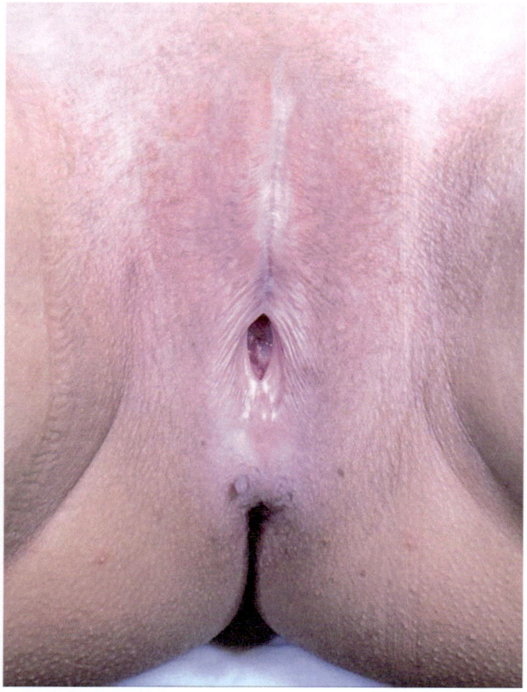

Fig. 2.6 Severe labial fusion caused by lichen sclerosus disease in a patient (26 years). Genital adhesions can obliterate the vaginal entrance and cause permanent deformations. In these cases, surgery is inevitable

2.6.6 Vulvar Irritation

Some women may experience difficulties due to irritation and strain while wearing tight pants, riding a horse, cycling, and using tampons.

2.6.7 Functional Problems Due to Vaginal Relaxation

Some women may experience problems such as the feeling of looseness during sexual intercourse, urinary incontinence problems, and decreased sexual pleasure, especially after childbirth or due to age-related vaginal relaxation. Vaginal enlargement and gaping can be source of distress for male partners and can cause hygienic problems. Genetic predisposition, poor quality collagen structure, aging, menopause, pregnancy, birth(s), smoking, alcohol consumption, and chronic irritations negatively affect both the appearance and the function of the genital area.

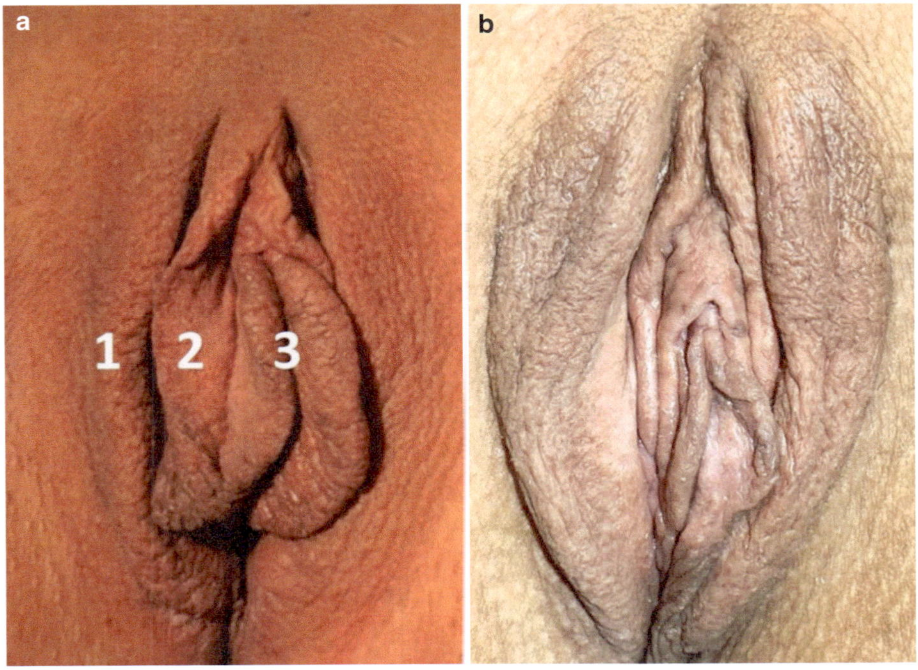

Fig. 2.7 Multilayered labia forms. Labia can have two layers ("double labia") (**a**), three layers ("triple labia") (**b**), and sometimes more. The smegma that is collected between the folds causes hygienic problems. Conversely, the abundance of anatomical variations of labia necessitates the application of different surgical techniques

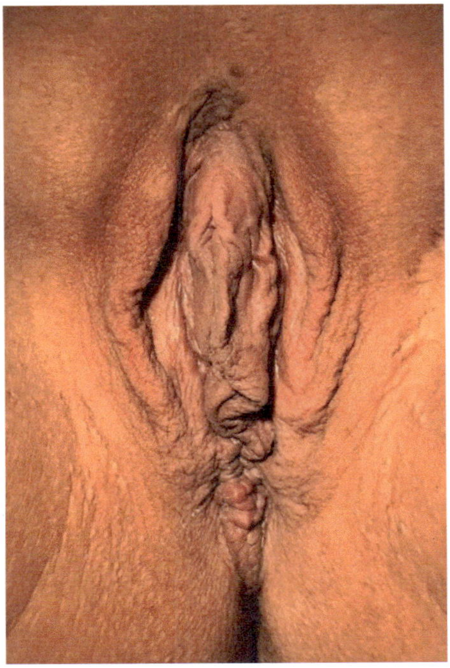

Fig. 2.8 Severe vulvar laxity (32 years old). It can develop especially due to rapidly weight gain and loss periods and bad collagen structure

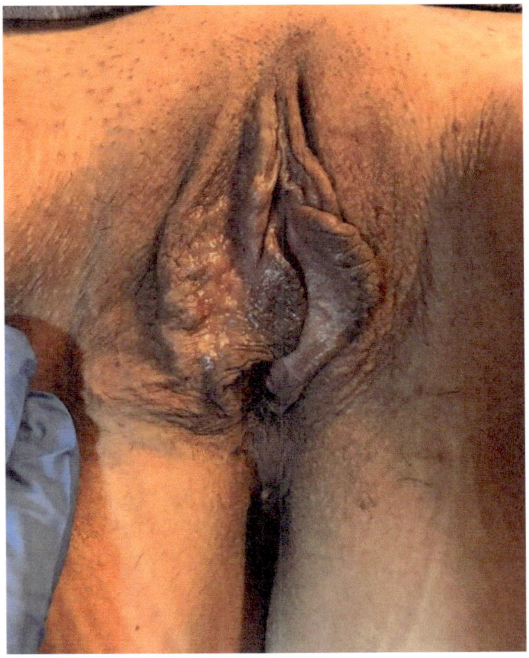

Fig. 2.9 Vulvar varicosities. They can persist, especially after birth, and cause complaints of pain, swelling, thrombosis, and dyspareunia

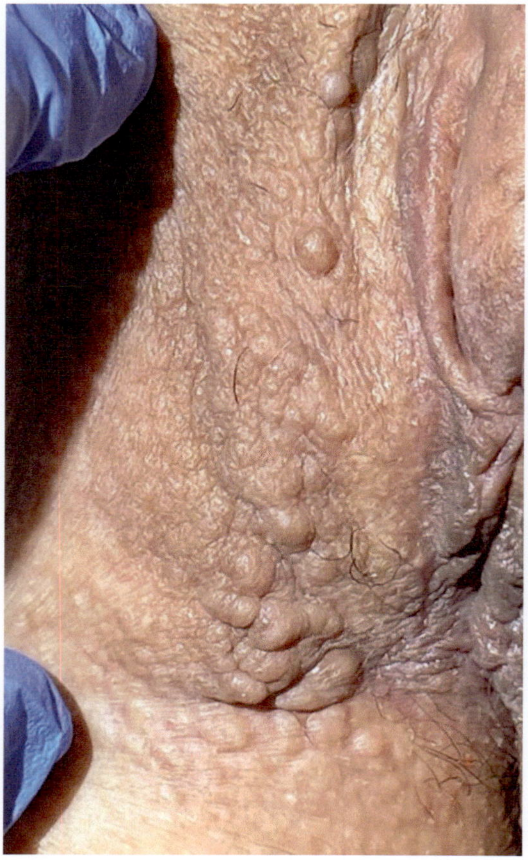

Fig. 2.10 Fox–Fordyce disease. A rare, chronic skin disorder characterized by pruritic follicular papules as a result of apocrine sweat retention due to keratinous obstruction and rupture of apocrine ducts

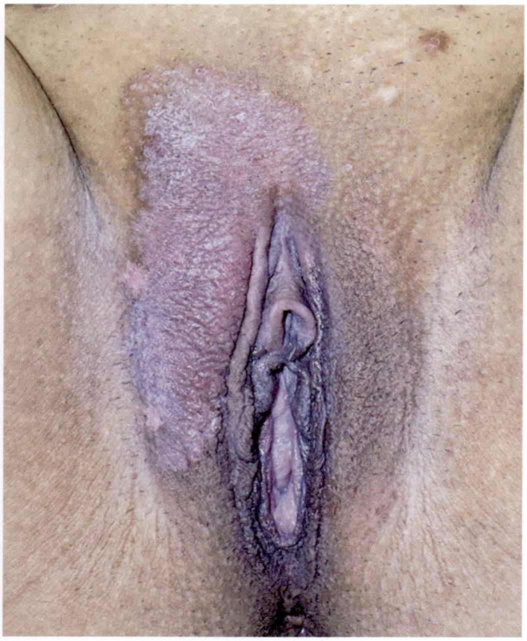

Fig. 2.11 Hyperplastic vulval dystrophy. A chronic inflammatory skin pathology affecting the vulva. It is characterized by thickened, hyperkeratotic lesions on the surface of the vulva with frequent evidence of scratching

With aesthetic genital surgeries, such undesired complaints are reduced, positive changes occur in people's lives, and self-esteem is restored.

2.6.8 Dyspareunia

Some women may experience functional problems such as the feeling of pain due to stretching of labia during intercourse or force themselves to strain during urination due to large and long genital labia.

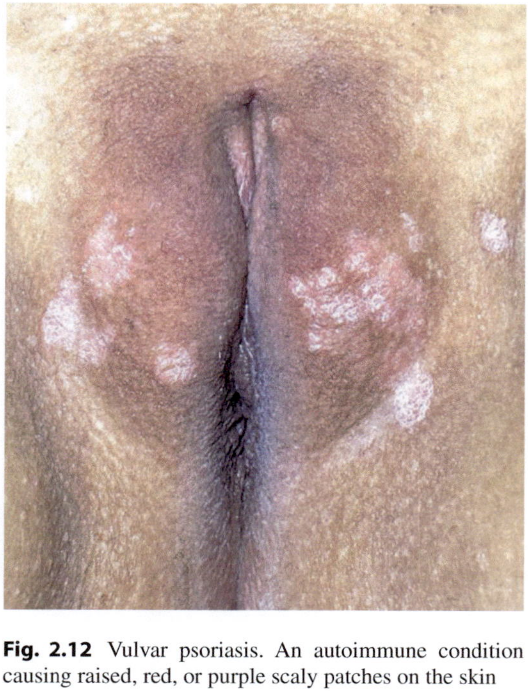

Fig. 2.12 Vulvar psoriasis. An autoimmune condition causing raised, red, or purple scaly patches on the skin

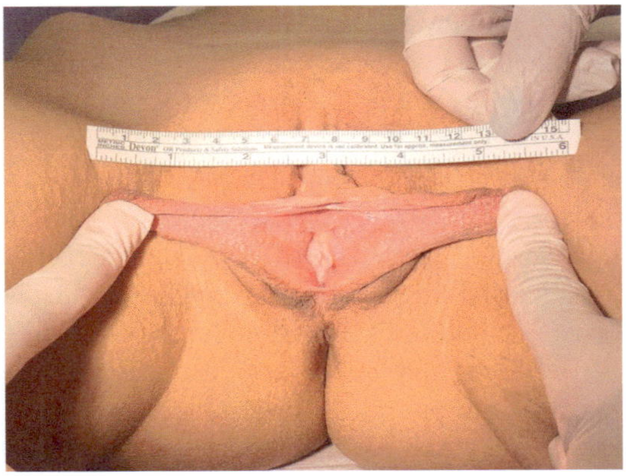

Fig. 2.13 Severe labial hypertrophy. The labia are almost 8 cm long, and the primary complaint of this patient is dyspareunia

2.7 An Example of Legal Aspects: *"Artwork Contract"* in Turkey

Legal surgical applications for aesthetic purposes are medical applications aimed at correcting the appearance disorders that have occurred spontaneously or as a result of a congenital or subsequent factor or to make the person look more beautiful even though there is no such deformity. Treatment/surgery can be done for beautification and functional reasons, sometimes for both purposes.

The surgeon performing the aesthetic operation is obliged to pay more attention and care due to the nature of the job. The most important feature that distinguishes aesthetic surgery operations from other surgical operations is that these operations directly change the external appearance of the person. Since the aesthetic appearance is of great importance in aesthetic surgeries, the responsibility of the surgeon who will perform the surgery also increases; the surgeon is expected to *"produce an artwork"* like an artist, in a way, by demonstrating the manual skill in addition to the responsibility imposed by other surgeons.

There is no special regulation in Turkish law for aesthetic surgeries. Aesthetic surgeries are considered within the scope of the "artwork contract" because they are surgical applications in the appearance of the human. In other words, the surgeon who performs aesthetic operation is expected to produce an artwork as in general artwork contracts. This is a contract in which the contractor undertakes to create an artwork and the employer undertakes to pay a price in return. One of the sides to the contract, the one who performs the surgical application (Contractor) agrees to create the work, and the other side (Employer) agrees to pay a price in return.

The physician has other responsibilities besides making the work:

- Making a diagnosis and choosing and applying the most appropriate treatment
- Performing the work personally
- Informing the patient (informed consent)
- Loyalty and care
- Recording (archiving)
- Maintaining confidentiality

The work produced by the physician should be regarded as a successful result, especially within the framework of medical science and aesthetic surgery rules.

The only responsibility of the patient is to pay for the service she received.

Corrections of existing defects in the tissue, that is, reconstruction surgeries, are also covered within the scope of the work. One of the most important issues here is that the work made can be noticed compared to its previous state.

In accordance with the physician's obligation to inform, the physician is obliged to inform the patient about the form, shape, scope, possible side effects, alternative solutions, possible results, and complications of the surgical intervention and obtain the patient's written consent. It is worth highlighting here, *the patient's consent must be taken by the physician himself/herself*. In case of any conflict, the burden of proof belongs to the physician, and the physician must prove that he/she informed the patient about the surgical intervention.

If additional aesthetic pathologies are seen during the operation, it is best not to touch them. It is recommended that no unspoken or undiscussed procedure should be performed, not even a skin tag be removed, while the patient is under general anesthesia or sedation. The surgery(ies) to be performed should have been discussed during preoperative consultations, and informed consent should be obtained while the patient is conscious.

The aesthetic surgeon is under obligation to perform the aesthetic surgery requested by the patient in accordance with the terms of the contract and create the artwork (result) the patient demands. The patient who suffers damage as a result of surgical intervention can file a material-moral compensation case against her physician and other responsible persons [5].

2.8 Aesthetic Treatment Contracts and Legal Qualifications

In order for the intervention to the body integrity for health purposes to be legal and to be considered as medical, there are four basic elements that must exist:

- There should be a medical necessity for medical intervention (indication stipulation),
- Medical intervention must be done in accordance with the law (legal requirement),
- It must be done by the authorized persons in accordance with the law (authorization condition),
- The patient must consent to the medical intervention to be performed (consent stipulation).

Medical interventions that do not have these elements are against the law.

During the treatment phase, the physician has the right to freely choose the treatment method to be applied but is also under the obligation to act as required by medical science. It is not correct to apply methods that are not medically accepted, that have not been sufficiently tested, or that are not fully concluded to be beneficial.

Just as beautification operations are subject to stricter conditions than therapeutic operations, their responsibilities for physician are also heavier. According to general medical rules, physicians should use their medical knowledge for the benefit of their patients and act with a sense of responsibility within the scope of legal rules to achieve the goal. Awareness of responsibility is a strong assurance for both the physician and the patient. As a result of this assurance, a "consent relationship" occurs. With consent, the risk is assumed and work is done in accordance with the benefit and will of the patient. In case of conflict between the physician and the patient, the patient's file and all documents are examined, and it is checked whether the patient's benefit is properly observed by the physician [6].

2.9 Medical Ethical Aspect

Four medical ethical principles should never be compromised in any medical practice [7].

2.9.1 Autonomy

Autonomy is the right to make one's own decision. However, when making this decision, it is imperative that the person does not have mental illness, BDD, anxiety, or depression. In addition, she should not have decided on the operation due to the force of a third person. During the decision phase, the patient should know all the risks with full transparency, and the physician should not mislead her.

2.9.2 First, Do No Harm (Non-maleficence)

Also known as non-maleficence or "*Primum non nocere,*" this is one of the most important principles of medicine since Hippocrates.

2.9.3 Benefit (Beneficence)

The surgery to be performed by the physician should benefit the patient. For this, the physician must be experienced and choose the most appropriate operation method for his/her patient.

2.9.4 Being Fair (Justice)

Facilities should be used to meet the needs of the general population. In this context, most aesthetic operations can be classified as a luxury for society [8].

Appendix

With the purchase of this book, you can use our "SN Flashcards" app to access questions free of charge in order to test your learning and check your understanding of the contents of the book.

To use the app, please follow the instructions below:

1. Go to https://flashcards.springernature.com/login
2. Create a user account by entering your e-mail address and assigning a password.
3. Use the following link to access your SN Flashcards set: ▶ https://sn.pub/tvlq7Q

If the link is missing or does not work, please send an e-mail with the subject "SN Flashcards" and the book title to customerservice@springernature.com.

References

1. Committee on Gynecologic Practice, American College of Obstetricians and Gynecologists. ACOG Committee Opinion No. 378: vaginal "rejuvenation" and cosmetic vaginal procedures. Obstet Gynecol. 2007;110(3):737–8.
2. Elective Female Genital Cosmetic Surgery. ACOG Committee opinion, number 795. Obstet Gynecol. 2020;135(1):e36–42.
3. https://www.fda.gov/medical-devices/safety-communications/fda-warns-against-use-energy-based-devices-perform-vaginal-rejuvenation-or-vaginal-cosmetic
4. https://www.who.int/genomics/public/eu_declaration1994.pdf
5. Güzelleştirme PH. Amaçlı Estetik Ameliyatlardan Kaynaklanan Hukukî Sorumluluk. Dokuz Eylül Üniversitesi Hukuk Fakültesi Dergisi. 2006;1:177–239.
6. Arıncı A. US Estetik Amaçlı Tıbbi Müdahalelerde Hekimin Hukuki Sorumlulukları ve Eser Sözleşmesi. Turk J Plast Surg. 2017;25(2):84–93.
7. Gillon R. Medical ethics: four principles plus attention to scope. BMJ. 1994;309(6948):184–8.
8. Paarlberg KM, Weijenborg PT. Request for operative reduction of the labia minora; a proposal for a practical guideline for gynecologists. J Psychosom Obstet Gynaecol. 2008 Dec;29(4):230–4.

3 Ideal Vulva Concept and Anatomic Structures

Where the spirit does not work with the hand, there is no art. Nature is the source of all true knowledge. She has her own logic, her own laws, she has no effect without cause nor invention without necessity.

Leonardo da Vinci

As with the whole body, there are great differences between countries and cultures in the aesthetic perception of the genital area. For example, wide labia minora shaped like *"butterfly wings"* are found more attractive in Japanese society. In the Khoikhoi (Hottentot apron) tribe living in southwest Africa, it is a living tradition for girls starting at the age of five years to have their labia stretched up to 10 cm by their aunt or other female relative. Traditionally, the *"sexually attractive looking"* elongated labia that are extended in this way are called "Sinus pudoris" or "Macronympha." This practice formerly fell into the category of Type IV female genital mutilation. In 2008, the WHO reclassified the practice as a body modification due to a perceived lack of harm and a reported much more positive perception of women's sexuality by those who practice it.

However, other than these exceptional cases, the expectations of society about the external genital area are the same around the world. Especially in Western society, it is a general expectation that the inner labia be as small as possible and located inside the outer labia, and having some other features (Fig. 3.1).

The vulva (Pudendum), which is the female external genital area, includes the following anatomical structures (Fig. 3.2):

- Mons Pubis (Mons Veneris, Pubic Mound, Mons Venus)
- Labium Majus Pudendi (*Plural:* labia majora, outer/bigger genital lips)
- Labium Minus Pudendi (*Plural:* labia minora, inner/smaller genital lips)
- Clitoris and Clitoral Hood (Preputium)
- Frenulum (*Plural:* frenula)
- Vestibulum Vagina
- Bulbus Vestibuli
- Hymen
- Glandula Vestibularis Major (Bartholin's glands)
- Glandula Vestibularis Minores (Skene's glands)

S. Eserdağ, *Aesthetic and Functional Female Genital Surgery*,
https://doi.org/10.1007/978-3-031-16019-6_3

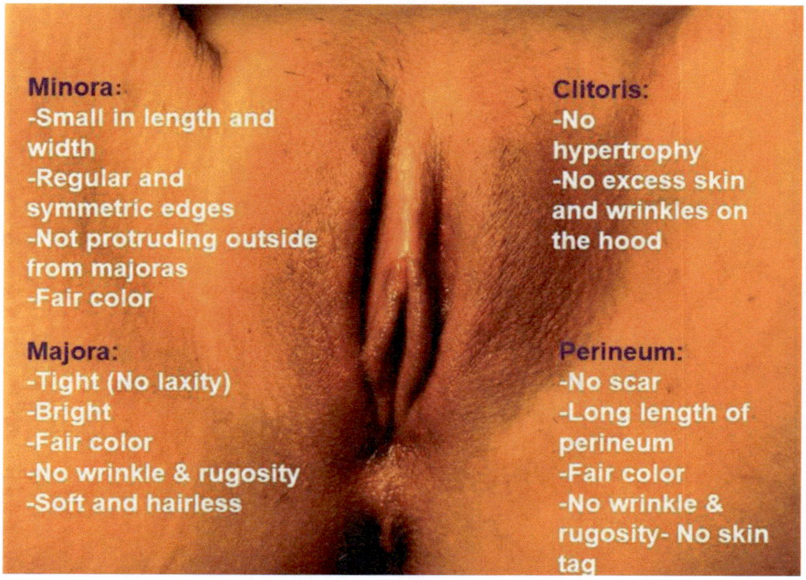

Fig. 3.1 "Ideal vulva concept" according to Western society

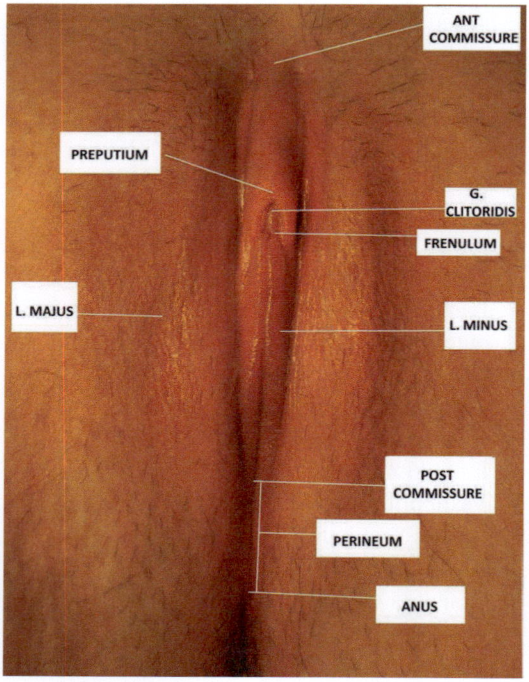

Fig. 3.2 External genitalia

3.1 Reasons for Applying to a Physician for AGS

Patients can apply to the physician for different aesthetic and functional reasons. If we divide it into parts:

- Labia minora: Hypertrophy, asymmetry, wrinkles, discoloration
- Labia majora: Atrophy, hypertrophy, discoloration, looseness, wrinkles, collapse
- Perineum: Presence of scar tissue, tears, skin tags, discoloration
- Clitoris: Embedded clitoral glans, hypertrophy, excess skin folds in the clitoral hood
- Vagina: Loosening, enlargement, gaping, pelvic organ prolapse (POP), congenital and subsequent vaginal strictures, hymenal tags, loss of sensation

3.2 Anatomical Structures and their Place in Cosmetic Gynecology

3.2.1 Mons Pubis (Mons Veneris)

This is the triangular shaped area located in the anterior part of the pubic bone. It consists of hairy skin and underlying fat tissue. Adipose tissue in the mons pubis increases with puberty and weight gain and decreases during menopause. The hairs (pubes) decrease with menopause. The fibers of the lig. Suspensorium clitoridis and lig. Teres uteri are found in adipose tissue in the mons pubis.

Some women desire mons pubis reduction because of the discomfort they feel due to the excess skin or fat tissues. Mons pubis reduction can be done by conventional manual lipoaspiration, energy-based liposuction methods, or mini-abdominoplasty operation. Mons pubis reduction is also known as "monsplasty operation."

3.3 Labium Majus Pudendi

The labia majora are the continuing segment of the mons pubis. Two skin folds meet at the midline posterior fourchette. It is 7–12 cm from the clitoral hood to the fourchette. It consists mostly of adipose tissue and thin smooth muscle tissue. It is covered with hairs. Round ligaments end in this area. It is rich in sebaceous glands, apocrine glands, and sweat glands. It has lateral and medial parts. The hair density on the medial part decreases. The cleft between the two labia majora is known as the "pudendal cleft" or "rima pudendi." The function of the labia majora is to protect the urethral and vaginal openings against mechanical impacts (cushion function).

Aesthetic problems such as excessive fullness of this area, laxity, excess wrinkles, collapse, and dark color can occur. Within AGS operations, augmentation, reduction, tightening, and bleaching operations are performed for the labia majora.

The dartos layer located in the subcutaneous tissue of the labia majora is an area rich in smooth muscle and connective tissue (Fig.3.3). Deeper is the fibrous tunic (elastic sac). During labia majora augmentation, HA (hyaluronic acid) injection is placed into this gap between dartos and the fibrous tunic, namely the "interfascial area."

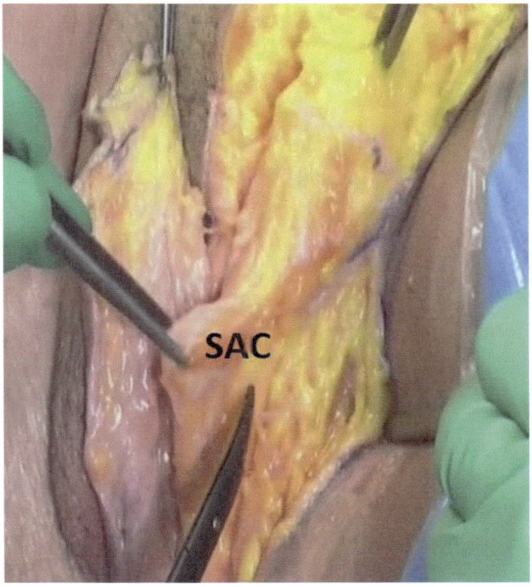

Fig. 3.3 Elastic sac in the labia majora in a cadaver study

The labia majora are separated from the labia minora by a deep sulcus (interlabial sulcus). The skin of the medial area toward the labia minora is devoid of hair.

3.4 Labium Minus Pudendi

Labia minora are hairless skin folds located medial to the labia majora. They do not contain adipose tissue, and they are highly vascularized and sensitive. They are rich in skin and mucous sebaceous glands. They are lined with squamous epithelium. The labia minora merge with the medial skin tissue posteriorly, and this area is named "fourchette," "posterior commissure," or "frenulum labiorum pudendi."

The labium minus is divided into two segments upward. The superior part merges with the opposite side and forms the "clitoral hood" or "preputium" (prepuce) that surrounds the glans clitoridis. The inferior part adheres to the lower

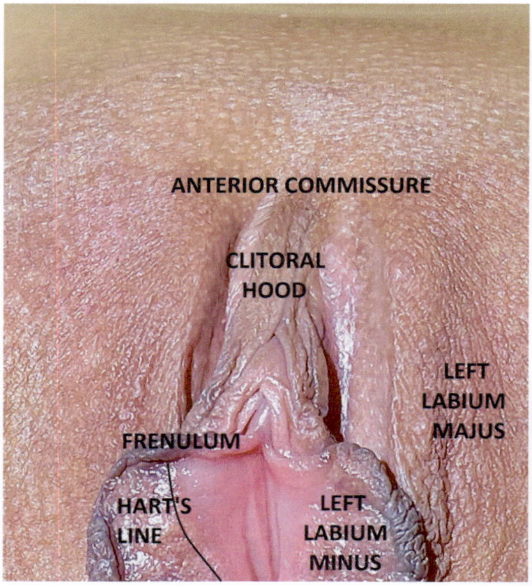

Fig. 3.4 Clitoral hood (prepuce). It is formed by the combination of the superior segments of the labia minora

part of the glans clitoridis as a thin mucosal fold and is named "frenulum" (Fig. 3.4).

Sensory innervation of the labia minora is provided by the perineal and posterior labial branches of the pudendal nerve.

The width of the labium minus is between 0.7 and 5 cm, and the length of it from the glans clitoris to the fourchette is between 2 and 10 cm. The functions are to regulate the flow of urine during urination and to protect the vagina from drying out.

The Hart's line separates the keratinized epithelium of the labia minora from the non-keratinized epithelium of the vulvar vestibulum. This demarcation line is also the border between the labia minora that develops embryologically from the ectoderm and the vestibule that develops from the endoderm. Labiaplasty incisions in the trimming method are generally made over this Hart's line or a bit lateral of it. Labiaplasty, which is applied especially in cases of labial hypertrophy (Fig. 3.5) and/or asymmetry, is the most frequently requested genital aesthetic operation by patients and performed by physicians. Clitoral hood hypertrophy and frenula hypertrophy can also be seen in the vulvar region in addition to labial hypertrophy (Fig. 3.6).

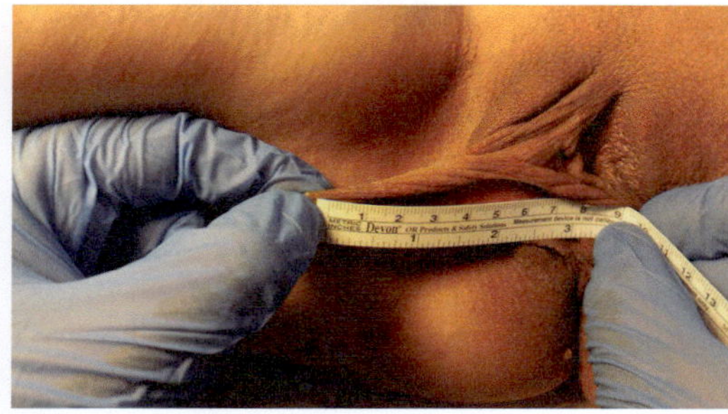

Fig. 3.5 Severe labial hypertrophy

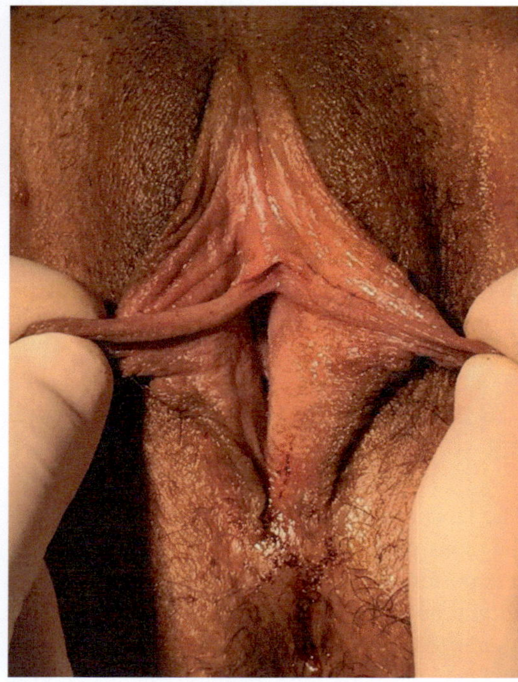

Fig. 3.6 Frenula hypertrophy. In this case, frenulaplasty operation should be combined with labiaplasty

Labial reconstruction and plastic operations can also be performed due to tears due to traffic accidents or bicycle injuries as well as removal of deformations after vaginal birth or Bartholin's cyst removal.

3.4.1 Labial Blood Circulation

Blood flow to the labia minora and majora is provided by the posterior labial artery and the

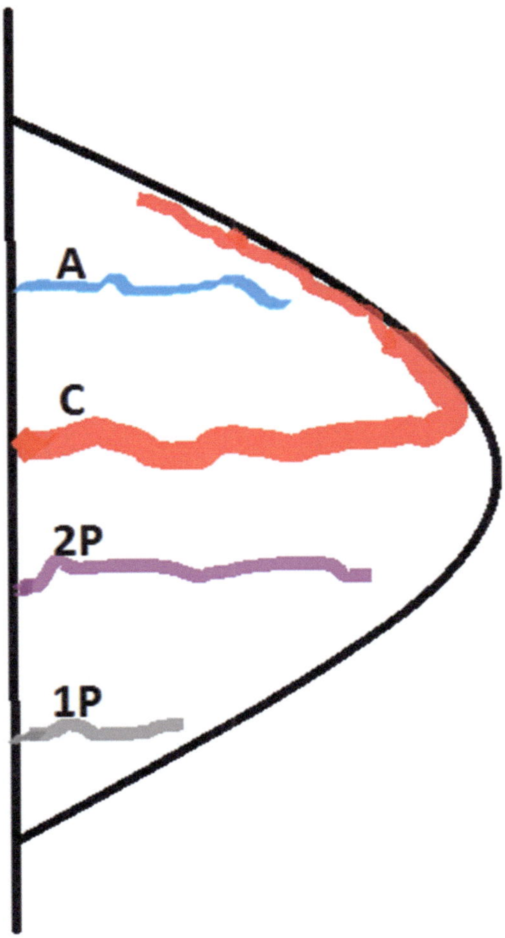

Fig. 3.7 Labial blood circulation. A: anterior artery, C: central artery, 2P: second posterior artery, 1P: First posterior artery

perineal artery, which are branches of the internal pudendal artery. In addition, the internal pudendal artery branches into the dorsal artery of the clitoris. Georgiou et al. detailed the arterial circulation in the labia in a cadaver study [1] (Fig. 3.7). In their study, they also confirmed the connection between the anterior system of the external pudendal artery and the posterior system of the internal pudendal artery. They also underlined that the safest labiaplasty method is curvilinear excision in labia where blood flow is very intense.

Another point that should not be forgotten is that vascularization is more in hypertrophic organs. *"The larger the organ, the greater the vascularization and the risk of associated excessive bleeding."*

Knowing the anatomy of the labial blood circulation is important in order to prevent wound dehiscence due to avascularization, especially in labiaplasty operations performed with the wedge technique.

3.4.2 Labial Morphology

The Banwell classification can be used to describe the morphology of labia minora before labiaplasty operations [2]. According to this classification system, the labium is divided into three separate sections with horizontal lines, with the upper line on the glans clitoris and the lower line on the posterior commissure. In the horizontal regions that are formed, the furthest lateral point of the labium is classified as Type 1 if at the top, Type 2 in the middle, and Type 3 in the lower 1/3 (Fig. 3.8). Wrinkles and hyperpigmentation are also noted.

Banwell also classified the labia in three categories as low, medium, and high "perineal elevation" (take off) according to the distance of the posterior end parts of the labia to the perineum (Figs. 3.9 and 3.10).

3.4.3 Labial and Clitoral Dominance

Another issue is the anatomical harmony of the clitoral–labial complex with each other. The structure where the clitoral hood is in the foreground is called "clitoral dominance" and the structure where the labia are in the foreground is called "labial dominance."

Generally, in cases of labial asymmetry, the skin folds on the larger labium extend far beyond

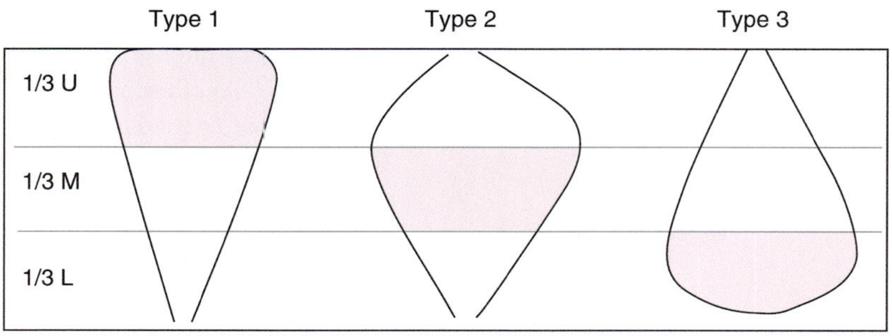

Fig. 3.8 Labial morphology (Banwell classification)

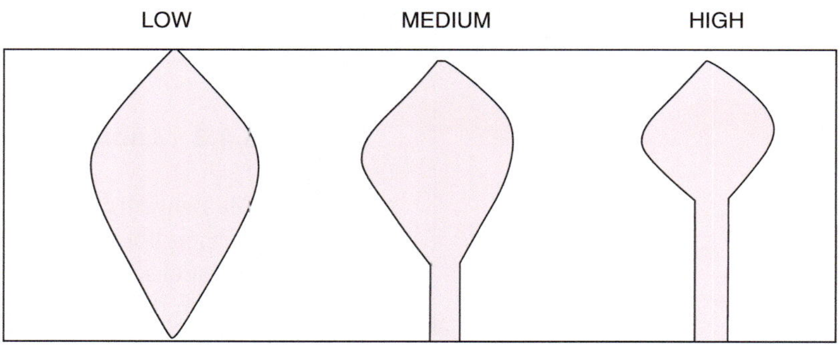

Fig. 3.9 Perineal take off

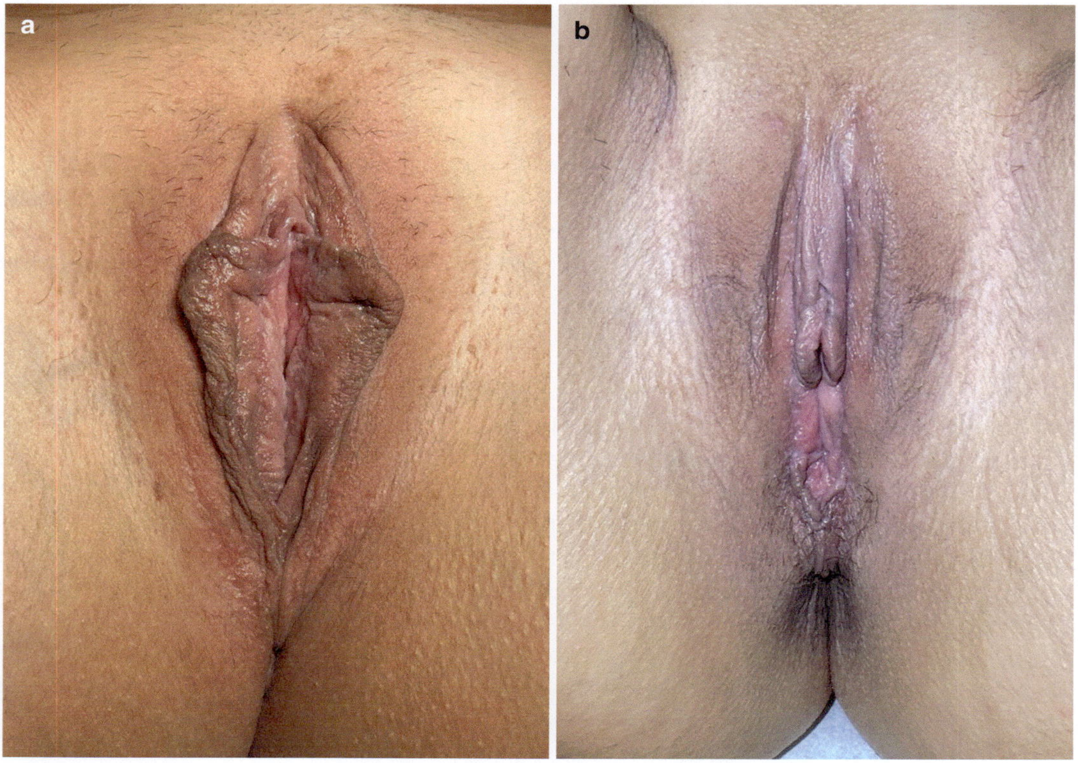

Fig. 3.10 Perineal take off. Low perineal take off (**a**) and high perineal take off (**b**)

the clitoral hood, creating asymmetry on the clitoral hood (Fig. 3.11).

According to the Banwell classification, both labial width and perineal elevation should be categorized separately.

3.4.4 Labial Asymmetry

Labial asymmetry can be characterized by one of the labia being bigger, located more superior, or based more frontal, deformed, or hyperpigmented compared to the other (Figs. 3.12 and 3.13).

It develops due to environmental factors, mechanical traumas, irritations, and genetic factors. It has an incidence much higher than expected. According to my experience, more than 90% of women have an easily noticeable labial asymmetry. For many women, this is unimportant or they are unaware. In these cases, this does not present a problem. However, in some women, as with hypertrophic labia, asymmetry may cause negative psychological and social effects. The woman may see herself as handicapped or have a serious lack of self-esteem, and this condition can affect her quality of life. In this case, labiaplasty operation will be inevitable.

The new classification system developed by us for labial asymmetries is described in Chap. 9.

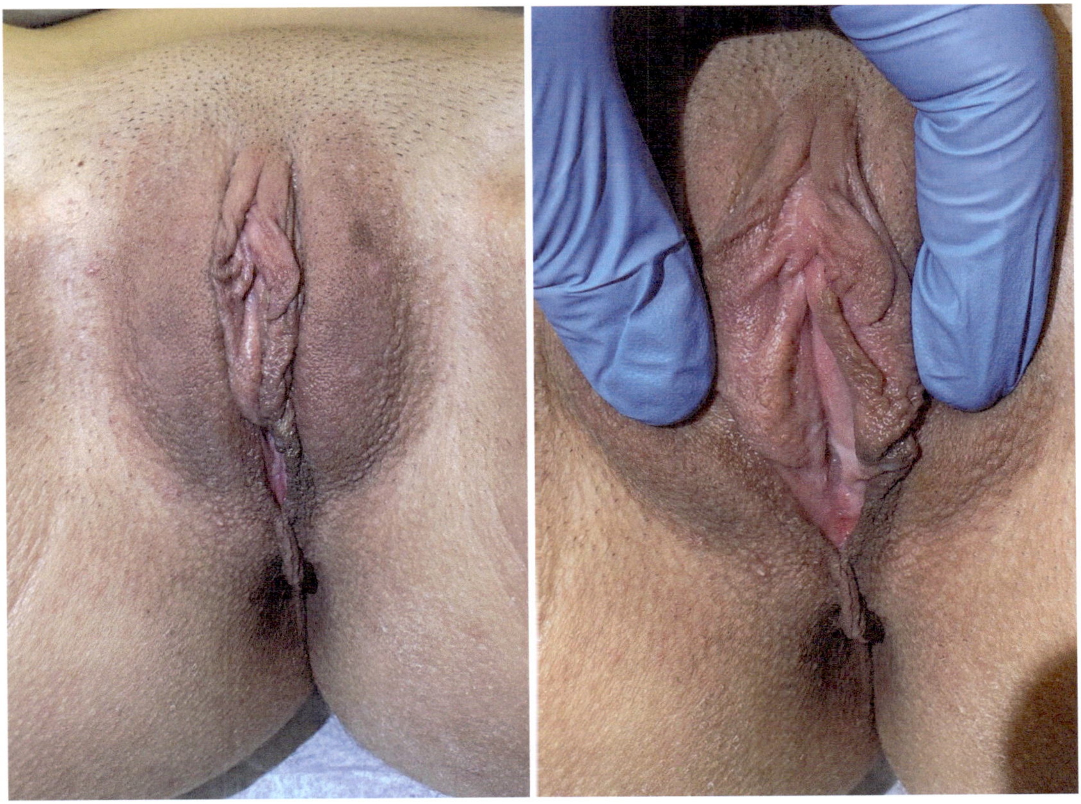

Fig. 3.11 A patient with hood dominance and frenula hypertrophy. Hypertrophic frenula mimic labia minora

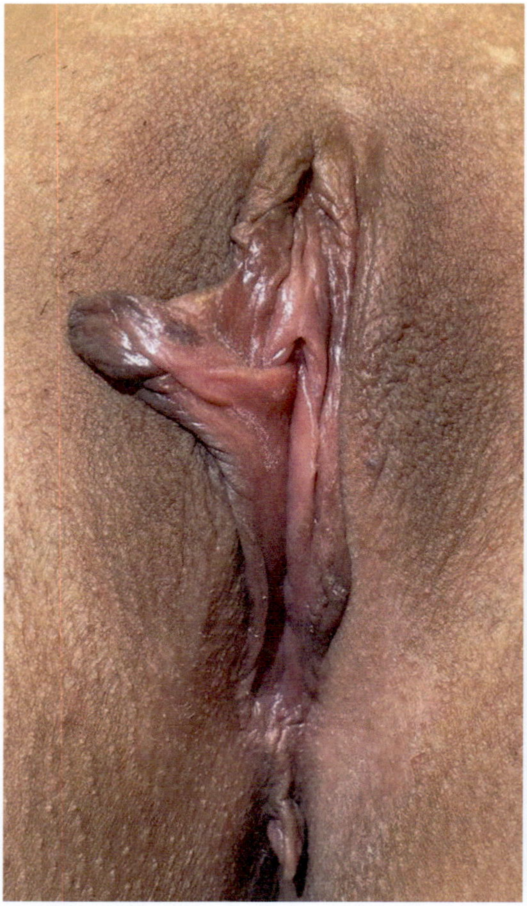

Fig. 3.12 Combined labial asymmetry. The right labium is more hypertrophic than the left, higher (more superior), and the base is more frontal

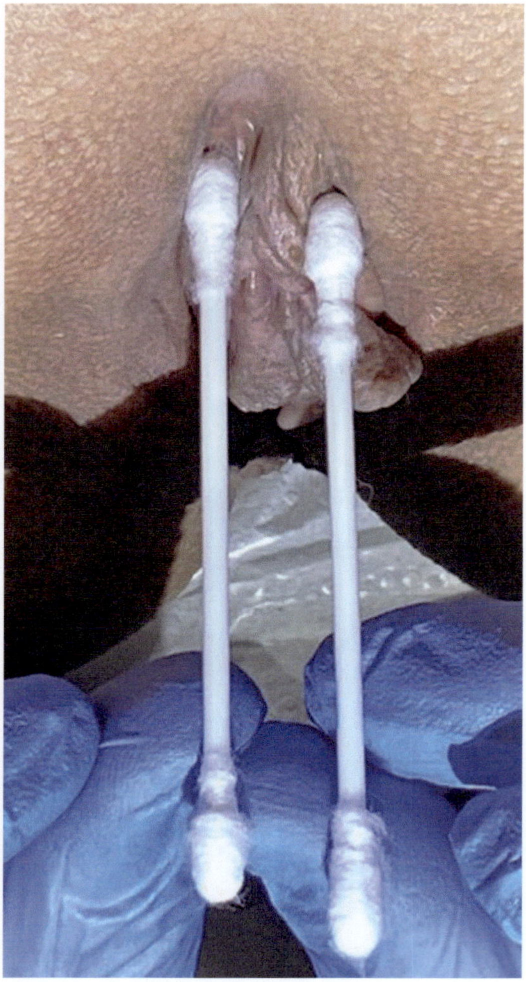

Fig. 3.13 Labial asymmetry. Demonstrating the base of the left labium is located more frontal

3.4.5 Labial Protrusion

Labial protrusion is when the labia minora protrude beyond the majora. In the classification made by Motakef et al., labial protrusion was divided into three separate classes according to the degree of protrusion of the lateral edge of the labia minora from the majora [3]. In this simple classification, protrusion is defined as class 1 (0–2 cm), class 2 (2–4 cm), or class 3 (over 4 cm).

3.5 Vulvar Vestibulum

This is the area covered by mucosa at the entrance of the vagina. The vestibulum is rich in nerves and vessels. Its borders are the hymen in distal, Hart's line at laterals, frenula anteriorly, and the fourchette posteriorly.

The vulvar vestibulum is the opening area of the numerous Skene's glands (paraurethral, minor vestibular glands) around the urethral orifice and the Bartholin's glands (major vestibular glands) at 5 to 7 o'clock. Thus, the glands provide lubrication of the vaginal entrance.

The pit area between the hymen and the fourchette is known as the "navicular fossa" and it is a part of the vulvar vestibulum.

Vulvar vestibulitis syndrome (VVS, vulvar vestibulitis, vestibulodynia) is generally an inflammatory reaction of the vulvar vestibulum that causes very sharp and superficial pain, especially during sexual intercourse (Fig. 3.14). Unlike vaginismus, the pain felt is of organic origin. Vulvar vestibulitis is one of the most important causes of superficial dyspareunia in women, but it is often either undiagnosed or mistaken for vaginismus.

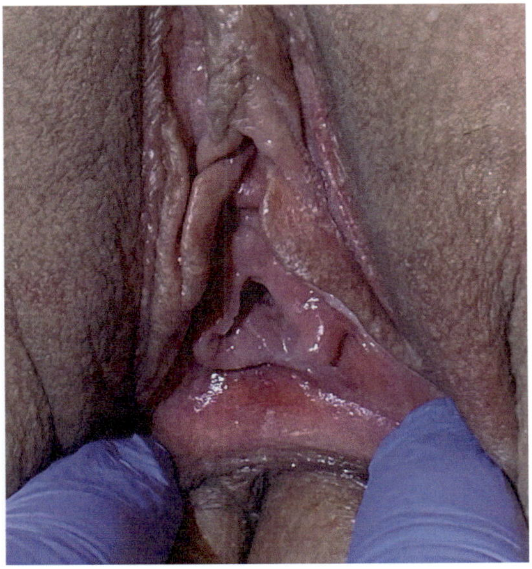

Fig. 3.14 Vulvar vestibulitis. There is hyperemia at 6 o'clock. Often, no hyperemia is detected in the gynecological examination of these patients, but hypersensitivity is determined by the cotton-tipped test

Most of the vulvar vestibulectomy operations yield very successful results and the dyspareunia problem is often solved. Histopathological examination of the mucosa of the vestibulum removed is also recommended after surgery. HPV-related effects are frequently observed in these patients. According to a study, in the histopathological examinations of 38 patients who were operated on for vulvar vestibulectomy, the researchers found 14 (36.8%) had LGSIL, 21 (55.2%) had vestibulitis-related inflammation, and 3 (7.8%) had lichen simplex chronicus [4].

3.6 Clitoris

Having an erectile structure and being the embryologic homologue of the corpora cavernosa of the penis, the clitoris is the most important organ in female orgasm and sexual pleasure. The clitoris has an inverted-Y shape and is composed of three parts. The only part seen externally is the glans (head). It also consists of the corpus (body, shaft) and two crura inside. The glans and corpus are 2–4 cm, and the crura are 9–11 cm long. The clitoris has erectile structures (corpus cavernosum) adhered to each other in the middle and continues with bilateral crura. Two separate crura of the clitoris extend toward the bilateral perineum on the lower surface of the pubis along the ischiopubic rami. Ultrasonography studies show that clitoral length and diameter increase and blood supply almost doubles during arousal [5].

More than 8000 nerves are involved in the clitoral hood area. The clitoris is innervated by the hypogastric, pelvic, and pudendal nerves. It is also associated with L5-S1, T12-L4, and S2-S4.

"Clitoral hood," "prepuce," and "preputium" are synonymous terms.

3.7 Hymen

This is a thin mucosal fold in the ostium vagina with varying shape, size, and consistency (soft-medium-hard). The hymenal fold is an anatomical border between the external and internal genitalia. Although it is mostly shaped in annular form, there are also different shapes such as semilunar, cribriform, septated, and dentate forms (Fig. 3.15).

There are three basic processes related to hymen within the scope of EGC:

3.7.1 Hymenoplasty

This procedure involves long- and short-term hymen reconstruction operations. The aim is to restore anatomical integrity or ensure bleeding at the first sexual penetration. Long- and short-term hymen reconstruction operations are within the scope of AGS. Hymenoplasty is described in detail in Chap. 15.

3.7.2 Excision of Hymen Protrusions

Prolapsed hymen caruncles may cause aesthetic concerns in some patients. This condition called "hymen protrusion" can be solved by simple surgical excision (Fig. 3.16). "Carunculectomy" operations can also be performed during vaginal tightening operations.

3.7.3 Painful Hymen (Eserdag)

According to our terminology, "painful hymen" describes caruncles that cause pain during contact or sexual intercourse. This condition, which we can define as the *mildest form of vulvar vestibulitis*, is the cause of superficial dyspareunia, and it can lead to sexual desire problems and vaginal dryness over time. It mostly occurs in remaining caruncles after the perforation of thick-based or high-edged hymen in the first intercourse. Painful hymen can be easily diagnosed by cotton-tip test in gynecological examination, and the problem can be solved by simple surgical excision.

We attach great importance to the evaluation of the hymen during gynecological exam-

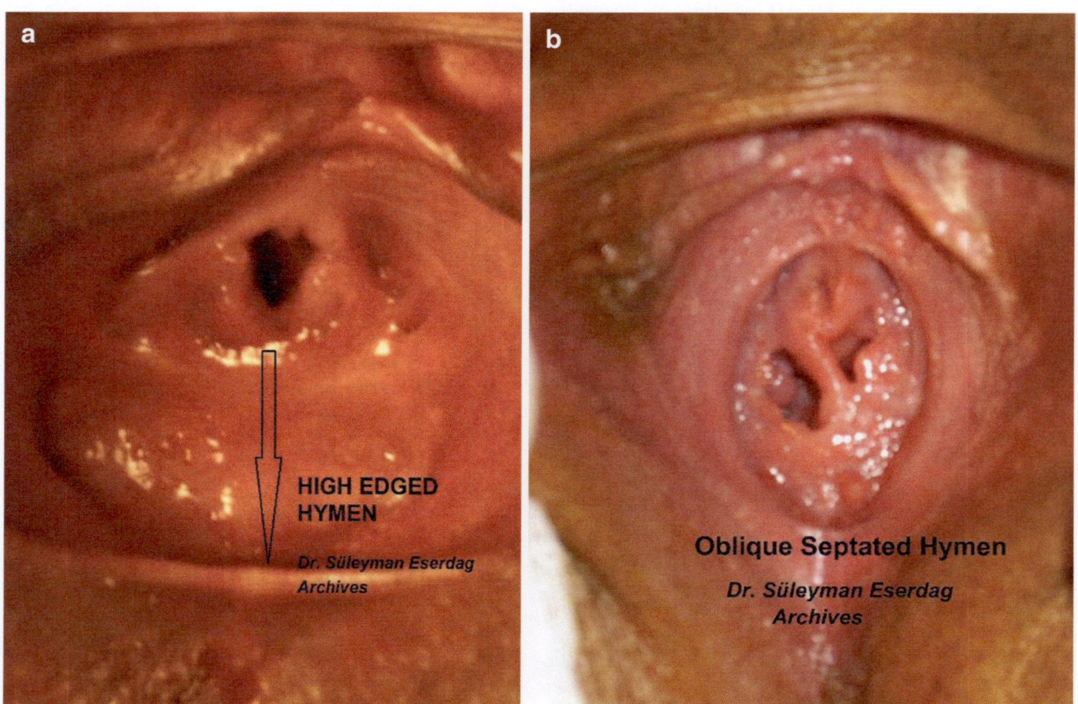

Fig. 3.15 Anatomic variations of hymen. Left—High-edged hymen (semilunar) (**a**), Right—Oblique septated hymen (**b**)

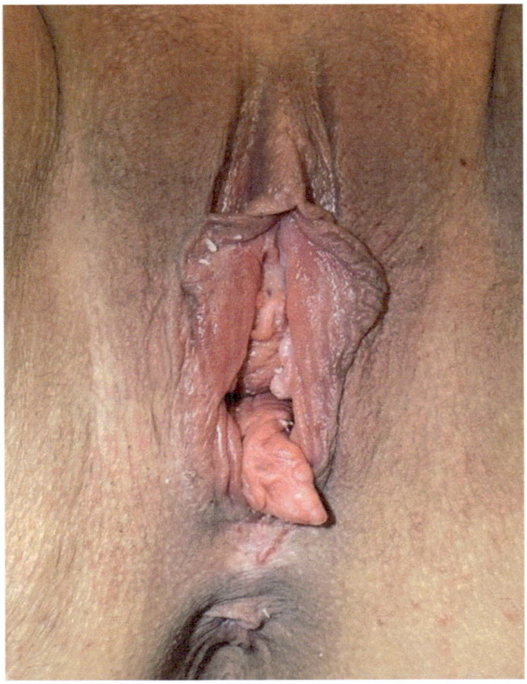

Fig. 3.16 Vaginal gaping and hymenal protrusion

inations of vaginismus and dyspareunia patients. Gynecological exam and diagnosing abnormalities related to the hymen have a predictive value for the treatment of vaginismus patients. In a recent study involving 281 vaginismus patients aged between 18 and 45 years, 48 (17%) of the patients had to undergo hymenotomy or hymenectomy operations. It is also important to combine cognitive behavioral sexual therapies after hymen surgeries [6].

Conversely, the high rates of hymen surgery procedures performed on vaginismus patients may be related to the lower pain threshold values of these patients, in addition to anatomical defects. In another prospective case-control study involving 32 vaginismus patients and 29 healthy women in control group, we showed that the pain threshold values of vaginismus patients were lower, and even these values decreased in higher degree of vaginismus patients [7].

3.8 G-Spot

This is a functional rather than an anatomical organ in the anterior vaginal wall that is thought to be located 1–2 cm proximal to the urethra. It is one of the erogenous zones during sexual pleasure in women, first described by Gräfenberg in 1950. Although there are articles reporting that orgasm is facilitated by direct stimulation of the G-spot, the evidence supporting the claims on this issue is still insufficient. This controversial issue will be discussed in detail in Chap. 19.

3.9 Innervation and Vascularization of the Vulva

The vulva is innervated by the pudendal nerve that originates from the nerve roots in S2-S4 and originates from the Alcock canal located medial to the ischial tuberosities.

The branches of the pudendal nerve are:

- Dorsal nerve of the clitoris
- Perineal nerve
- Inferior rectal nerve

In addition to the pudendal nerve, the posterior cutaneous femoral nerve, ilioinguinal nerve, and genitofemoral nerves also innervate the vulva.

The blood flow of the vulva is provided by branches of the internal pudendal artery (r. labiales posteriores, r. bulbi vestibuli and a. profunda clitoridis, a. dorsalis clitoridis), which is one of the branches of the internal iliac artery.

3.10 Normal Vulva Measurements

The female vulva varies depending on structural, racial, and age-related factors. Anatomical variations in vulva bring along different surgical methods. In general, the definitions in the measurements of the labia made without stretching are given in Table 3.1 and Fig. 3.17.

Table 3.1 Regional lengths in vulva anatomy

Width of labia minora	Length from the infralabial sulcus to the widest part of the labium in external measurement
Length of labia minora	Distance between the inferior end of the glans clitoridis and the lowest part of the labium
Length of labia majora	Distance from anterior commissure to perineal body
Width of clitoris	Transverse width of the clitoral glans
Length of clitoris	Longitudinal length of the clitoral glans
Length of perineum	Distance between the fourchette (posterior commissure of labia minora) and anterior anal edge

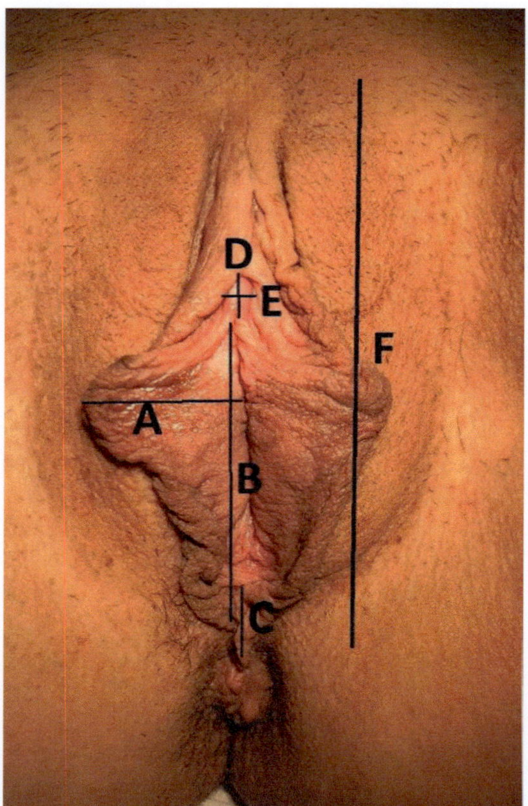

Fig. 3.17 Vulva measurements. (**a**) Labia minora width, (**b**) labia minora length, (**c**) perineal length, (**d**) clitoral glans length, (**e**) clitoral glans width, (**f**) labia majora length

Table 3.2 External genital measurements (whole cohort)

	Mean (in mm)	Standard deviation	Minimum (in mm)	Maximum (in mm)
Width of clitoris	4.62	2.538	1	22
Length of clitoris	6.89	4.965	0.5	34
Distance clitoris-urethra	22.63	7.661	3	65
Introitus opening	27.91	10.36	6	75
Length of perineum	21.34	8.544	3	55
Length of labia majora (right)	79.71	15.25	12	180
Length of labia majora (left)	79.99	15.44	20	180
Length of labia minora (right)	42.1	16.35	6	100
Length of labia minora (left)	42.97	16.29	5	100
Width of labia minora (right)	13.4	7.875	2	61
Width of labia minora (left)	14.15	7.643	1	42

In a study involving 657 women aged 15–84 years in Switzerland, the anatomical structures in the vulvar region were examined and the results are shown in the table below [8] (Table 3.2).

3.11 Vaginal Anatomy and Histology

The vagina is a fibromuscular canal located between the vestibulum and the cervix. In addition to being a sexual organ, it is also a transfer organ. It has an average length of 7.5 cm in the front and 9 cm in the back and narrows toward the distal. It is adjacent anterior to the bladder and urethra, posterior to the rectum and anal canal, lateral to the lig. Latum uteri, and distal to the ureter, vasa uterina, Bartholin's glands, bulbus vestibuli, and bulbospongiosis muscle. There are dead ends between the cervix and the vagina called "fornix" in front, back, and on both sides. The deepest fornix is posterior, located in the lower anterior part of the rectouterine pouch (Douglas) and is covered by the peritoneum from above.

The blood supply to the vagina is from A. vaginalis, a branch of the internal iliac artery (Fig. 3.18). A. vaginalis sends branches to the uterus and also forms the azygos artery of the vagina with branches coming from the A. uterina. Vagina is also supplied from the internal pudendal artery and the vaginal branches of the medial rectal artery. Its veins drain into the uterine and vesical plexuses through the vaginal plexus and then into the internal iliac vein. The neural innervation of the vagina is provided by the uterovaginal plexus, the pelvic plexus, and, in the lower part, by the pudendal nerve.

There are no sebaceous or sweat glands in the vagina. The vagina, which has a transport function during birth and menstruation, is an organ of sexual penetration and pleasure in women. With the parasympathetic effect that occurs by sexual arousal, vasodilatation and lubrication develop.

There are three main sources of lubrication caused by sexual arousal in women:

- Secretions of vestibular glands,
- Transudation depending on vaginal congestion (tumescence), and
- Secretions of endocervical glands.

Vagina is a fibromuscular canal, with a three-layer structure that changes by aging and menopause.

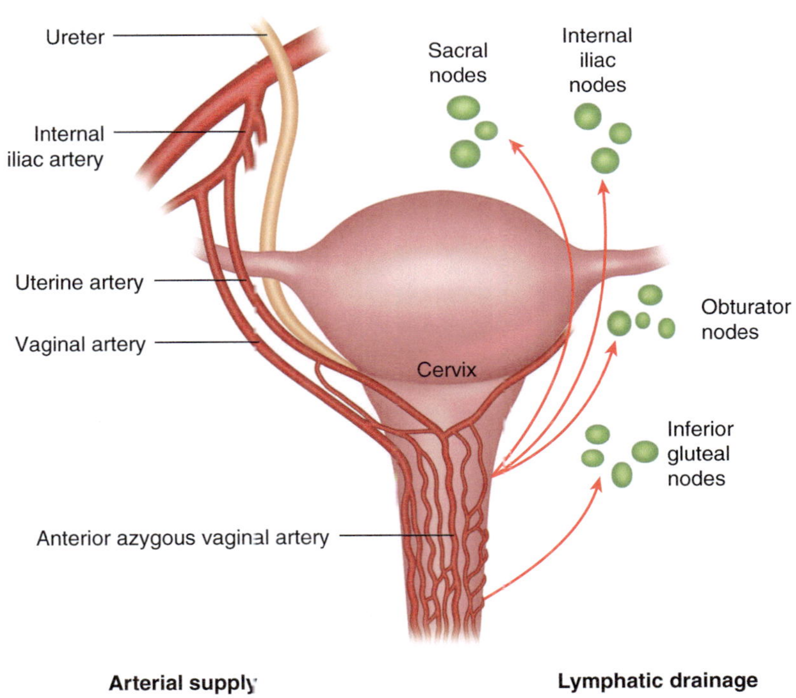

Fig. 3.18 Arterial and lymphatic circulation of the vagina

3.12 Mucosal Layer (Superficial Layer)

It has two layers: "lamina epithelialis" and "lamina propria." Lamina epithelialis consists of nonkeratinized stratified squamous epithelium. The glycogen synthesized in the intermediate layer is then stored in superficial cells. The glycogen released after the most superficial cells are poured into the vaginal lumen constitutes the main food source of lactobacilli. Lactobacilli digest glycogen and convert it to lactic acid, thus keeping vaginal pH acidic. Acidic pH protects the vagina against foreign bacteria and fungal infections.

The multilayered squamous epithelium is separated from the lamina propria by a single layer columnar epithelium called the "basal layer." The task of the basal layer is to constantly renew the multilayer squamous epithelium. The basal layer has a notched structure called "papilla" and is rich in vascular structures (Fig. 3.19). As a result of menopausal atrophy, glycogen stores decrease, pH rises, and the epithelium becomes thinner.

Lamina Propria (LP) consists of dense connective tissue containing collagen and elastin fibrils. It also includes small blood vessels, lymphatic vessels, and the dense plexuses of nerves. Density increases toward the surface. Lamina propria papillae are less common in the anterior vaginal wall, while they are more prominent and deep in the posterior vaginal wall.

Collagen and elastin fibrils are the biomechanical substances of the vagina. While collagen fibrils are responsible for the strength and mechanical resistance of the vaginal wall with their highly rigid structure, elastin fibrils provide the elasticity of the tissue. Although the main collagen in the lamina propria is type 1, it also contains many types of collagen.

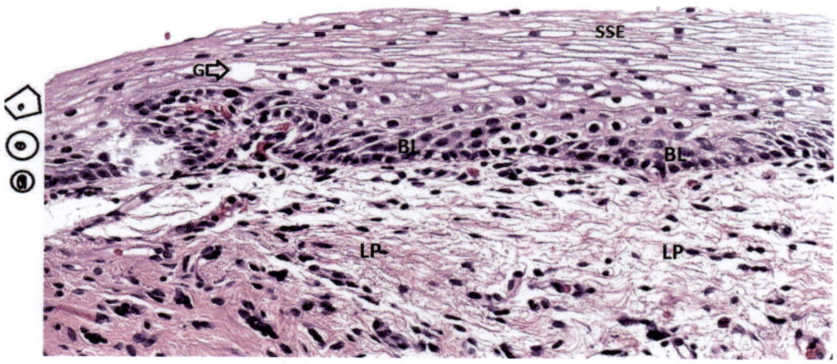

Fig. 3.19 Histology of the epithelial and Lamina Propria (LP) components of the vagina in reproductive ages. Thick stratified squamous epithelium (SSE), papillary protruding structure, glycogen-rich vacuoles (G). The basal layer (BL) consists of a single layer of the columnar epithelium. The visuals on the left side symbolize cell and nucleus shapes (H&Ex100) (Modified from the archive of Zekioğlu Osman with permission)

3.13 Muscular Layer (Second Layer)

The inner part is circular and the outer part is covered with longitudinal smooth muscles. Voluntary bulbospongiosis muscles on the lower side act as a sphincter around the vagina.

3.14 Adventitia Layer (Tunica Fibrosa, Deeper Layer)

The adventitia layer, which limits the muscular layer, is a tissue rich in loose collagen and elastic fibers that support the vaginal wall. Loose connective tissue forms the outer part of the adventitia together with the dense venous plexus network.

The mucosal epithelium exhibits an estrogen-dependent behavior and function throughout the woman's life, even throughout the menstrual cycle. The estrogenic epithelium is rich in glycogen. Glycogen, which is transported to superficial cells after being produced by intermediate cells, is fermented by lactobacilli. The lactic acid formed in this way is important for keeping vaginal pH low.

The cells grow and their nuclei shrink when they move toward the surface of the vaginal mucosa. Vaginal maturation index (VMI) includes Parabasal%/Intermediate%/Superficial% rates. It is read from left to right. For example; A VMI of 0/30/70 indicates estrogenized epithelium with the presence of 0% parabasal cells, 30% intermediate cells, and 70% superficial cells. For the clinician, dysfunctional bleeding is important in evaluating hormonal changes in menopause and prepuberty and in predicting ovulation. It is also frequently used to measure the response to hormonal therapy, especially in menopausal atrophy. As the amount of estrogen increases, the index shifts to the right, that is, the number of superficial cells shed increases [9].

Estrogen functions through α and β estrogen receptors in the vagina, vulva, urethra, and bladder trigone. Important anatomical and physiological changes occur in the urogenital tissue with estrogen withdrawal: the vaginal epithelium becomes pale and thinner, its elasticity decreases, and rugal folds decrease. Also, collagen content and hyalinization decrease, elastin decreases, functions of smooth muscle cells change, connective tissue density increases, and blood vessels decrease. In later periods, blood flow and secretions decrease, vaginal elasticity and flexibility decrease, the tissue becomes more sensitive, vaginal pH increases, and the lactobacilli in flora leave their place to gram-negative rods and gram-positive cocci. Changes in menopausal complaints from person to person may be due to individual differences in genetic regulation and estrogen receptor expression (Table 3.3).

Genetically poor collagen structure, smoking, excessive alcohol intake, malnutrition, aging, menopause, pregnancies, and birth(s) can negatively affect the anatomy and physiology of the vagina. Surgical vaginal tightening and laser vaginal rejuvenation are the most frequently requested procedures within the art of AGS.

Another important structure in the vaginal structure is the rugae. Histologically, the role of the rugae, with a non-keratinized multilayer squamous structure, is to expand the vaginal surface and provide stretching. In addition, they also have a duty to grip the penis during coitus and increase sexual pleasure through friction. Age-related scarcity of rugae may bring along desensitization during sexual intercourse.

Table 3.3 Comparison of estrogenized and non-estrogenized vagina

	Estrogenized vagina	Non-estrogenized vagina
Complaints	No complaints, GSM symptoms are very rare	50% of women have symptoms of GSM during the menopausal period
Physical appearance and examination findings	Pinkish Damp Ruga folds distinct, lively appearance Flexible, elastic, durable No pain sensation with mechanical compression	Pale color Dry Ruga folds are faint, soft, and shiny Flexibility and elasticity are reduced, fragile Pain sensation in mechanical compression (sensitive)
Histology	In the vaginal swab: Dominance of superficial cells with larger, angular, and smaller nuclei VMI has shifted right Papillae are prominent Rich in blood vessels (especially in the papillae area) Lamina propria rich in collagen and elastin fibrils Rich in glycogen	In the vaginal swab: Decreased number of superficial cells, and dominance of smaller and rounded parabasal, and intermediate cells VMI shifted left Papillae are faint Poor blood vessels Lamina propria poor in collagen and elastin fibrils Poor in glycogen
Vaginal Flora and PH	Lactobacilli dominance Vaginal pH 3.5–5	Anaerobic gram-negative rod and gram-positive cocci dominance Vaginal pH > 5

3.15 Pelvic Floor Muscles

The pelvic floor is one of the most important anatomical regions. It is horizontal and supports the pelvic organs in the form of a hammock to prevent POP and incontinence. At the top is the perineal membrane (urogenital sphincter, urogenital diaphragm), below it the pelvic diaphragm muscles, and below that is the endopelvic fascia. While the pelvic diaphragm muscles create active support, bones, ligaments, and endopelvic fascia provide passive support.

Bulbospongiosis, ischiocavernosus, and superficial transverse perineal muscles are located in the upper compartment of the perineal membrane, and the sphincter urethra and deep transverse perineal muscles are located in the deep compartment. The pelvic diaphragm is formed by the levator ani muscle, which consists of the pubococcygeal, ileococcygeal, and puborectal bundles and the coccygeal muscles (Table 3.4 and Fig. 3.20).

Table 3.4 Pelvic floor (Top to bottom)

Superficial Urogenital Diaphragm (Perineal Membrane)

. Superficial Components:

M. Bulbospongiosus

M. Ischiocavernosus

M. Transversus Perinei Superficialis

. Deep Components:

M. Sphincter Urethrae

M. Transversus Perinei Profundus

Pelvic Diaphragm:

M. Levator Ani (Pubococcygeus, Ileoccoccygeus, Puborectalis)

M. Coccygeus

Endopelvic fascia

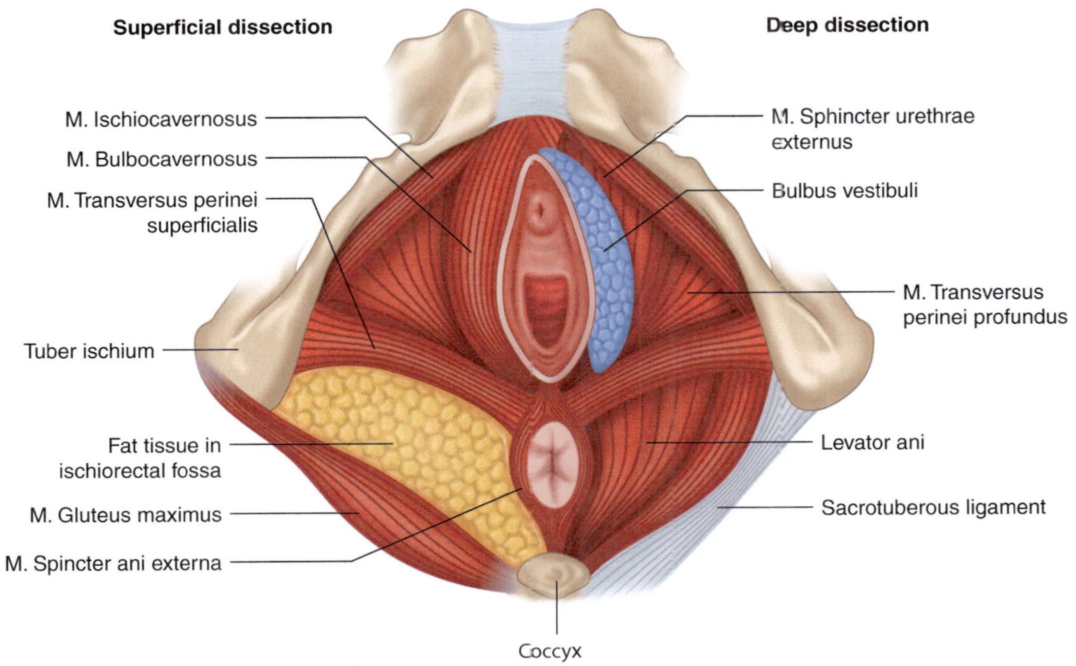

Fig. 3.20 Superficial and deep plane pelvic floor muscles

3.16 Perineal Body

The perineal body is the pyramidal area located between the vagina and the lower part of the rectum. It consists of the following layers (except the inner part):

- Skin and subcutaneous adipose tissue
- Superficial perineal muscles: external anal sphincter muscle, bulbocavernosus muscle (sphincter vaginae), transverse perineal muscles, and ischiocavernosus muscles

Except for the ischiocavernosus muscle, these are attached to a single point in the center of the perineal body. The crossing of the levator ani muscle between the vagina and rectum (deep perineal muscles) creates the apex of the perineal body.

3.17 Derivatives of Embryological Structures

Both urinary and genital systems originate from mesodermal tissue. Sex differentiation consists of a complex process involving many genes, some of which are autosomal. The embryo, which is unisex until the eighth week of gestation, develops male or female sex characteristics after the eighth week. The key to this differentiation is the Y chromosome, which carries the testicular determining factor (TDF) gene on its short arm. If testosterone is not produced by the gonads, the Wolffian duct regresses, and the dominant Müllerian duct differentiates into the fallopian tubes, uterus, and upper third of the vagina. As a result, 5α-reductase type 2, which is located in the genital fold, lacks a substrate to form dihydrotestosterone, and the labia remain open because fusion of the labioscrotal folds cannot occur.

The urogenital sinus (persistent cloaca) is divided into the urinary system and the genital system. The urinary system is divided to form the bladder and urethra, and the genital system to form the vaginal plane and lower two-thirds of the vagina (Table 3.5).

Table 3.5 Embryological origins of the genital organs

Mesonephric duct (Wolffian duct)	Gartner duct, ureter, renal pelvis, collecting tubules
Paramesonephric duct (Müllerian duct)	Fallopian tubes, uterus, upper 1/3 vagina
Urogenital sinus	Bladder, urethra, lower 2/3 subdivision of the vagina, urethral/paraurethral, and vestibular ducts
Sinus tubercle	Hymen
Phallus	Clitoris, glans, vestibular bulb
Urogenital folds	Labia minora
Labioscrotal swelling	Labia majora

Homologous Structures in Men

Labia majora → Scrotum
Labia minora → Penile urethra base
Skene's glands → Prostate
Vestibular bulb (corpus spongiosum) → Corpus spongiosum of penis
Clitoris → corpora cavernosa of penis
Round ligament → Gubernaculum testis
Gartner duct → Vas deferens
Bartholin's glands → Bulbourethral glands

Appendix

With the purchase of this book, you can use our "SN Flashcards" app to access questions free of charge in order to test your learning and check your understanding of the contents of the book.

To use the app, please follow the instructions below:

1. Go to https://flashcards.springernature.com/login
2. Create a user account by entering your e-mail address and assigning a password.
3. Use the following link to access your SN Flashcards set: ▶ https://sn.pub/tvlq7Q

If the link is missing or does not work, please send an e-mail with the subject "SN Flashcards" and the book title to customerservice@springernature.com.

References

1. Georgiou CA, Benatar M, Dumas P, Chignon-Sicard B, Balaguer T, Padovani B, Baqué P. A cadaveric study of the arterial blood supply of the labia minora. Plast Reconstr Surg. 2015;136(1):167–78.
2. Banwell PE. Labiaplasty: anatomy, techniques and new classification. Olympia, London: Clinical Cosmetic and Reconstructive Expo; Oct 2013.
3. Motakef S, Rodriguez-Feliz J, Chung MT, Ingargiola MJ, Wong VW, Patel A. Vaginal labiaplasty: current practices and a simplified classification system for labial protrusion. Plast Reconstr Surg. 2015;135(3):774–88.
4. Eserdag E, S, Kurban D, Kiseli M, Alan M, Alan Y. The histopathological results of vestibulectomy specimens in localized provoked vulvodynia in Turkey. Pan Afr Med J. 2020;24(37):267.
5. Foldes P, Buisson O. The clitoral complex: a dynamic sonographic study. J Sex Med. 2009;6(5):1223–31.
6. Eserdağ S, Anğın AD. Importance of gynecological assessment for the treatment of vaginismus as a predictive value. J Obstet Gynaecol Res. 2020;47(7):2537–43.
7. Eserdag S, Sevinc T, Tarlacı S. Do women with vaginismus have a lower threshold of pain? Eur J Obstet Gynecol Reprod Biol. 2021;258:189–92.
8. Kreklau A, Vâz I, Oehme F, Strub F, Brechbühl R, Christmann C, Günthert A. Measurements of a 'normal vulva' in women aged 15-84: a crosssectional prospective single-Centre study. BJOG. 2018;125(13):1656–61.
9. Weber MA, Limpens J, Roovers JP. Assessment of vaginal atrophy: a review. Int Urogynecol J. 2015;26(1):15–28.

4 Skin Histology and Physiology

There is no state in the world more valuable than a breath of health.

Suleiman the Magnificent

Our skin, the largest organ of our body, has different thicknesses in different parts of our body. Five different tasks of the skin are defined:

1. Protection: It protects the body against pathogens, chemical and thermal stress, and UV light.
2. Thermoregulation: It keeps body temperature in balance through hair and sweat glands. Also, it ensures hydration of the body.
3. Metabolic functions: It provides metabolic functions such as vitamin D production and fat storage.
4. Sense: It provides sensation with pain, heat, pressure, and touch receptors.
5. Sexual attraction and intimacy: It provides an aesthetic appearance. Also, it has a very important place in sexual intimacy. Our skin is accepted as the biggest sexual organ!

4.1 Layers of Skin

The skin has three layers: epidermis, dermis, and hypodermis (Fig. 4.1).

S. Eserdağ, *Aesthetic and Functional Female Genital Surgery*,
https://doi.org/10.1007/978-3-031-16019-6_4

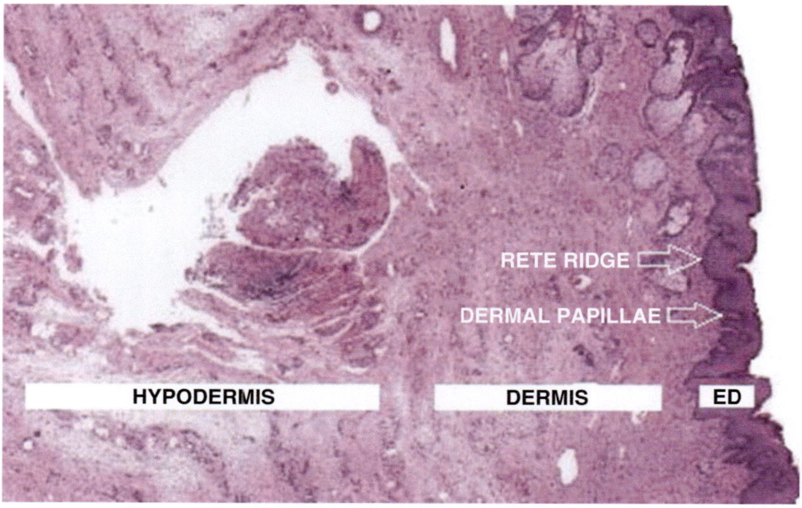

Fig. 4.1 Layers of Skin. ED (epidermis), dermis, and hypodermis (H&Ex100) (with the permission of Zekioğlu Osman)

4.2 Epidermis

The epidermis, the most superficial layer, is the area that is in constant contact with the external environment. It can regenerate itself continuously, produces "keratin," and is lined with multilayered squamous epithelium. The produced keratin both protects the skin from mechanical effects and prevents water loss. Although the thickness of the epidermis varies in all parts of the body, the thickest parts are located on the palms and soles.

The extensions of the epidermis that descend to the dermis are protrusions known as "rete ridge" or "rete peg." Dermal papillae located between the rete protrusions contain sensory receptors, blood vessels, and stem cells.

The epidermis has four separate layers (Fig. 4.2). While the keratinocytes produced by the stratum basale at the bottom migrate upward, they also undergo some structural and functional changes.

The layers of the skin from the bottom to the top:

4.2.1 Stratum Basale (Stratum Germinosum)

The stratum basale, the lowest layer of the epidermis, separates the epidermis from the dermis with a single-layered columnar or cuboidal cell line. It is the only mitotic layer of the epidermis. Stem cells in this area provide the formation of keratinocytes (epidermal skin cells) in all upper layers by mitosis. This is also the layer that contains the melanocytes that produce the skin pigment. Melanin colors the skin and absorbs UV light. Merkel cells located in this area provide sensation against light touch in the form of mechanoreceptors [1].

4.2.2 Stratum Spinosum

Keratinocytes formed in the basal layer migrate to this layer above. Keratinocytes in all layers are connected by "spine" structures called "desmosomes," which give this layer its name. Thus, the

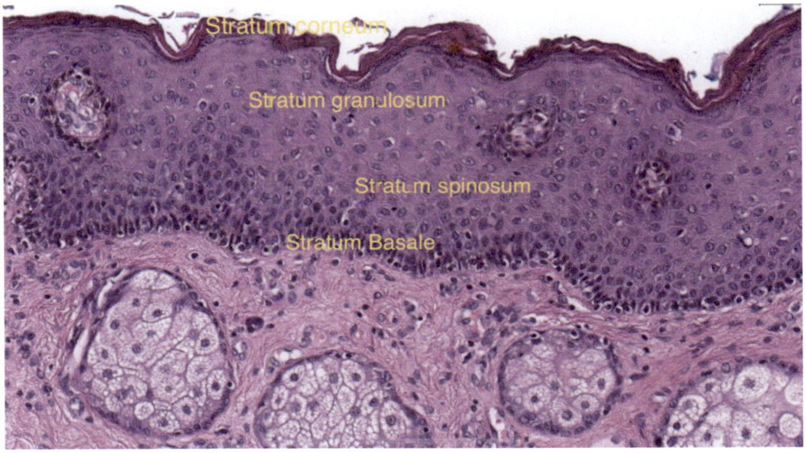

Fig. 4.2 Four separate layers of the epidermis (H&Ex100) (with the permission of Zekioğlu Osman)

stability of the skin is provided. Desmosomes are quite prominent in the stratum spinosum.

4.2.3 Stratum Granulosum

In this layer, keratinocytes appear squamous and contain dark-colored "keratohyalin granules." These protein-containing granules interact with cytokeratin to transform into keratin.

Only on thick skins (palms and soles), there is another thin, transparent layer called stratum lucidum between the stratum granulosum and the stratum corneum.

4.2.4 Stratum Corneum (Keratin Layer)

The stratum corneum, the most superficial layer of the epidermis, consists of keratinized cells that are constantly shed (desquamation) and replaced. The keratinized cells (corneocytes) in this layer are comprised of flat cells that have completely lost their nucleus and cytoplasmic organelles by completing their differentiation program.

The stratum corneum contains "keratin," the final product of keratinocytes. After the cells that die due to apoptosis are shed, the surface will remain covered with keratin. Keratin consists of a combination of cytokeratin and keratohyalin. It also prevents water loss since it is coated with a lipid-rich substance.

Thick or thin skin is mostly related to the thickness of the stratum corneum layer.

The turnover time until the keratinocytes produced from stem cells in humans are shed by desquamation is 40–56 days [2].

The epidermis also contains bone marrow-derived dendritic "Langerhans cells" that play a role in the development of the immune response. Langerhans cells capture the foreign antigen and pass into the lymph circulation and present the antigen to the T cells in the nearest lymph node.

4.3 Dermis (Cutis)

Located under the epidermis, the dermis is the layer of the skin rich in collagen and elastin fibers. It also includes fibroblasts, macrophages, and adipocytes. It is rich in vascular and nervous structures. Sensory cells are also in this area.

The dermis has two different regions, superficial and deep.

4.3.1 Superficial Dermis (Papillary Dermis)

The superficial dermis is also called the "papillary dermis," and it covers 20% of the dermis. This area is rich in loose connective tissue and capillary vessels. Small projections given by the dermis into the epidermis are called "dermal papilla." Since the multilayered squamous epithelium of the epidermis does not allow the presence of blood vessels, the epidermis provides its nutrition from the capillary circulation within the epidermal papillae. In this region, there are also "Meissner's corpuscles," which are touch receptors and unmyelinated free nerve endings sensitive to heat.

4.3.2 Deep Dermis (Reticular Dermis)

The deeper part that constitutes 80% of the dermis is called the "reticular dermis." The reticular dermis is composed of dense irregular collagen and elastin connective tissue. While the main task of collagen is to provide mechanical support against stretching in many directions, elastin is important for the flexibility of the tissue. There are also fibroblasts, macrophages, and fat cells in this region.

Sweat glands are located in both the dermis and the hypodermis. Hair follicles and sweat glands of the skin are important in thermoregulation.

4.4 Hypodermis (Subcutaneous Tissue, Subcutis)

The deepest layer of the skin, the hypodermis, is the layer richer in connective tissue, sweat glands, adipose tissue, and larger blood vessels than the dermis. In adipose tissue, fat-filled cells are known as "adipocytes." The fat tissue in this region is important for both metabolic support and the prevention of heat loss. "Pacinian corpuscles" in the deep dermis and hypodermis provide sensation against deep compression and vibration.

Subcutaneous tissue is the most suitable application area for many drug treatments due to its adipose tissue and blood vessel content. Some medications injected into this area are stored in adipose tissue and gradually pass into the bloodstream.

4.5 Skin Pathologies

Different skin diseases can occur with different pathologies of the skin.

1. Inflammatory dermatoses: Eczema, psoriasis, acne vulgaris, lichen planus, contact dermatitis
2. Bullous dermatoses: Pemphigus Vulgaris, bullous pemphigoid, herpes infections
3. Epithelial tumors: Basal cell cancer, squamous cell cancer, seborrheic keratosis
4. Pigmentation disorders: Vitiligo, albinism, nevus, melanoma
5. Infections: Impetigo, cellulitis, verruca, molluscum contagiosum

Many diseases and metabolic disorders have skin symptoms.

"Parakeratosis" is the presence of nucleated corneocytes in the stratum corneum layer. Although it is normal in some skin areas, it is often considered abnormal. Parakeratosis indicates an increased cell turnover level and can be seen in skin diseases such as psoriasis.

"Hyperkeratosis," which appears in eczema, warts, and calluses, is the thickening of the stratum corneum layer due to an abnormal keratin increase.

4.6 How Does Skin Color Occur?

The color of the skin is under the influence of two separate factors, genetically innate and acquired by accumulation.

4.6.1 Melanocyte Structure

"Melanin," which is the most important component in pigmentation, is a pigment located on the epidermis–dermis border of the skin, secreted by the melanocytes in the basal layer of the epidermis, and has the task of protecting the body by absorbing sunlight in the skin.

"Melanocytes," which secrete melanin pigment, have extensions called dendrites, similar to the arms of the octopus, and their average density is 1000/m^2. Melanocytes provide melanin synthesis using the amino acid L-tyrosine. This is controlled by the tyrosinase enzyme in organelles called melanosomes. "Tyrosinase" enzyme activity is essential for pigmentation. For example, tyrosinase gene mutations lead to albinism.

Melanosomes transported to the end protrusions of melanocytes are phagocytosed by neighboring keratinocytes. Although melanocytes produce melanin, they are pale in color compared to the surrounding basal cells.

Embryologically derived from the neuroectoderm, melanocytes are dendritic cells located in the basal part of the epidermis (Fig. 4.3).

Apart from the skin, melanin pigment is also found in hair, eyes, and parts of the brain. As the amount of sunlight exposure increases, the amount of melanin production increases in direct proportion, and thus the color of the skin becomes darker. Not all melanocytes in the skin are active. They are activated by exposure to the sun.

Fig. 4.3 Melanocyte structure

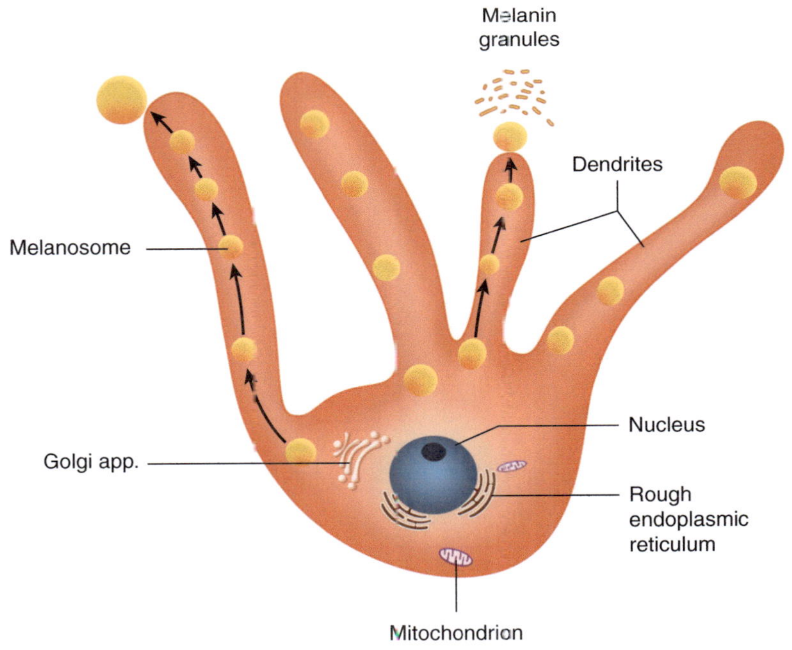

Appendix

With the purchase of this book, you can use our "SN Flashcards" app to access questions free of charge in order to test your learning and check your understanding of the contents of the book.

To use the app, please follow the instructions below:

1. Go to https://flashcards.springernature.com/login
2. Create a user account by entering your e-mail address and assigning a password.
3. Use the following link to access your SN Flashcards set: ▶ https://sn.pub/tvlq7Q

If the link is missing or does not work, please send an e-mail with the subject "SN Flashcards" and the book title to customerservice@springernature.com.

References

1. Khavkin J, Ellis DA. Aging skin: histology, physiology, and pathology. Facial Plast Surg Clin North Am. 2011;19(2):229–34.
2. Halprin KM. Epidermal "turnover time"--a reexamination. Br J Dermatol. 1972;86(1):14–9.

5 Vulvar Lichen Sclerosus

I did what every person had to do: gratefully greet the achievements of the former, correct their mistakes without fear, entrust to future generations the things that seemed to me true.

Biruni

Lichen sclerosus (LS) is a chronic inflammatory disease most commonly involving the anogenital skin and mucosa with a relapsing course and a potential for destruction, functional impairment, atrophy, and malignant changes in both women and men. The lesions are oval with sharp borders and ivory color in the beginning, and with the progressing disease, they may represent signs of atrophy, papules, and plaques. If it is not treated properly, it has 2–6% risk of transformation to malignant squamous cell carcinoma [1, 2].

LS is classified into two types, as genital and extragenital, regarding the affected locations. Despite it is most commonly affecting the genital region (94%), it may occur in the thorax, abdomen, neck, hip, inner thighs, shoulders, axilla, and elbows as extragenital involvement [3]. Vulvar lichen sclerosus (VLS), which is even seen in childhood, is most commonly observed in the fifth decade [1, 4].

The localization of VLS is variable and, according to the literature, it is defined as an "8-shaped" involvement of the vulvar, perineal, and perianal skin. Nevertheless, the lesions may be seen in the perianal region, clitoris, labia majora, labia minora, and introitus as a single area involvement [5]. Although rare, vaginal involvement may also be seen (Fig. 5.1).

S. Eserdağ, *Aesthetic and Functional Female Genital Surgery*,
https://doi.org/10.1007/978-3-031-16019-6_5

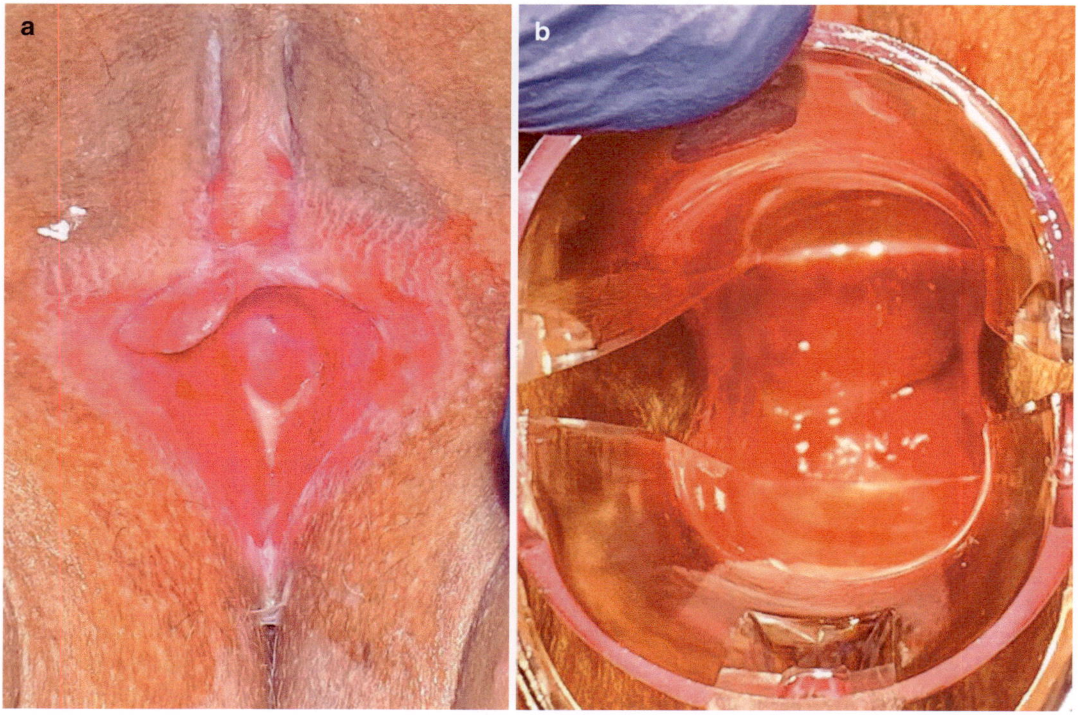

Fig. 5.1 A lichen sclerosus patient with vulvar (**a**) and vaginal (**b**) involvements. Note the evident erythematous appearance of the vaginal walls (**b**)

5.1 Epidemiology

LS was first described by Hallopeau in 1887. The frequency of this mucocutaneous disease in the population is not known due to inadequate diagnosis and low awareness. However, in the literature, it is reported that 10% of the newly diagnosed vulvar dermatoses are VLS [1, 6]. Also, it is diagnosed in 1.7% of patients during routine gynecological examination [4]. It is six times more common in women than in men.

5.2 Symptoms

VLS usually results in symptoms in women between the ages of 50 and 60 years. The most common symptom in adults is itching, which is present in 93% of patients [7]. Complaints such as scratching, cracking, and dryness of the skin and associated pain are also common. In extensive genital involvement, complaints such as dyspareunia, clitoral hyperesthesia, dysuria, vulvar pain, anal pruritis and pain are observed. With the presentation of the disease commonly in menopause, the complaints may be confused as genitourinary syndrome of menopause.

VLS may cause vulvar fusions that may obstruct the outflow of urine and menstrual blood. If the clitoris becomes embedded, it may also lead to problems such as a decrease in sexual pleasure and difficulty in orgasm. Due to the changes in vulva structure, psychological and sexual problems may also be present. Also, it may sometimes be completely asymptomatic and may be incidentally diagnosed during the routine gynecological assessment.

5.3 Etiology

The etiology of VLS is not clearly defined. There are four main reasons that have been evaluated.

5.3.1 Autoimmunity, Molecular Mechanisms, and Genetic Factors

In the pathogenesis of LS, immune dysregulation is primarily emphasized. Family history is present in 30% of the patients [8]. The most common accompanying diseases are autoimmune thyroiditis and vitiligo. Additionally, morphea, alopecia areata, pernicious anemia, diabetes mellitus, psoriasis, and celiac disease are also related to VLS [9–12]. However, all these associations may also be coincidental [11–13]. In patients with LS, despite the presence of the ANA positivity and thyroid autoantibody positivity, there is still little evidence that this disease has an autoimmune origin [14].

Epigenetic changes may lead to functional disruption in the genome unrelated to DNA sequences. These changes may cause differentiation in gene expression and phenotypic changes. Recent studies have shown that the changes in enzyme expression in VLS could be caused by epigenetic changes. Therefore, it is proposed that epigenetic factors may also play a role in the pathogenesis [15]. In patients with Turner syndrome, a high incidence of 17% has been observed [16].

5.3.2 Infections

LS has been related to several infections, some of which are acid-resistant pleomorphic bacilli, viral agents, and spirochetes.

A relationship has been reported between the *Borellia burgdorferi* spirochete that causes acrodermatitis chronica atrophicans and LS [17]. However, this relationship was not confirmed with serology and polymerase chain reaction (PCR).

Viral agents were also analyzed in LS etiology. The major suspected virus is human papillomavirus (HPV). It is observed that children with LS had a higher probability of HPV virus infection [18]. It was found that LS was localized between herpes zoster scars; however, the persistence of varicella-zoster virus DNA was not detected in lesions [19]. The relationship between HCV and autoimmunity is well known. Therefore, a possible relationship between HCV infection and LS was also analyzed. There are case reports in the literature on this issue, and HCV is believed to cause an autoimmune reaction in the development of LS [20].

5.3.3 Hormonal Effects

In women, the highest incidence of LS is seen in the period of lowest estrogen status. The fact that LS is more common before puberty and after menopause proposes a relationship with the hormonal status. However, LS does not have an association with pregnancy, hysterectomy, and hormonal contraceptive methods. Nevertheless, topical hormonal supports have a positive relationship with treatment [21, 22].

5.3.4 Local Factors

The "Koebner phenomenon" was first described for the formation of lesions in the psoriasis disease. It is described as the formation of lesions on the skin following a localized trauma. A flare-up of lesions with the Koebner phenomenon that occurs in LS is also proposed as an etiologic factor [23, 24]. The occurrence of the disease after sunburn, radiotherapy, and vulvectomy was related to these local factors.

5.4 Diagnosis

VLS is usually seen as sclerotic plaques on atrophic, wrinkled skin. The tissue is often whitened, with a thin, crinkled appearance classically appeared such as "cigarette paper". However, it may also present in different clinical forms (Fig. 5.2), such as:

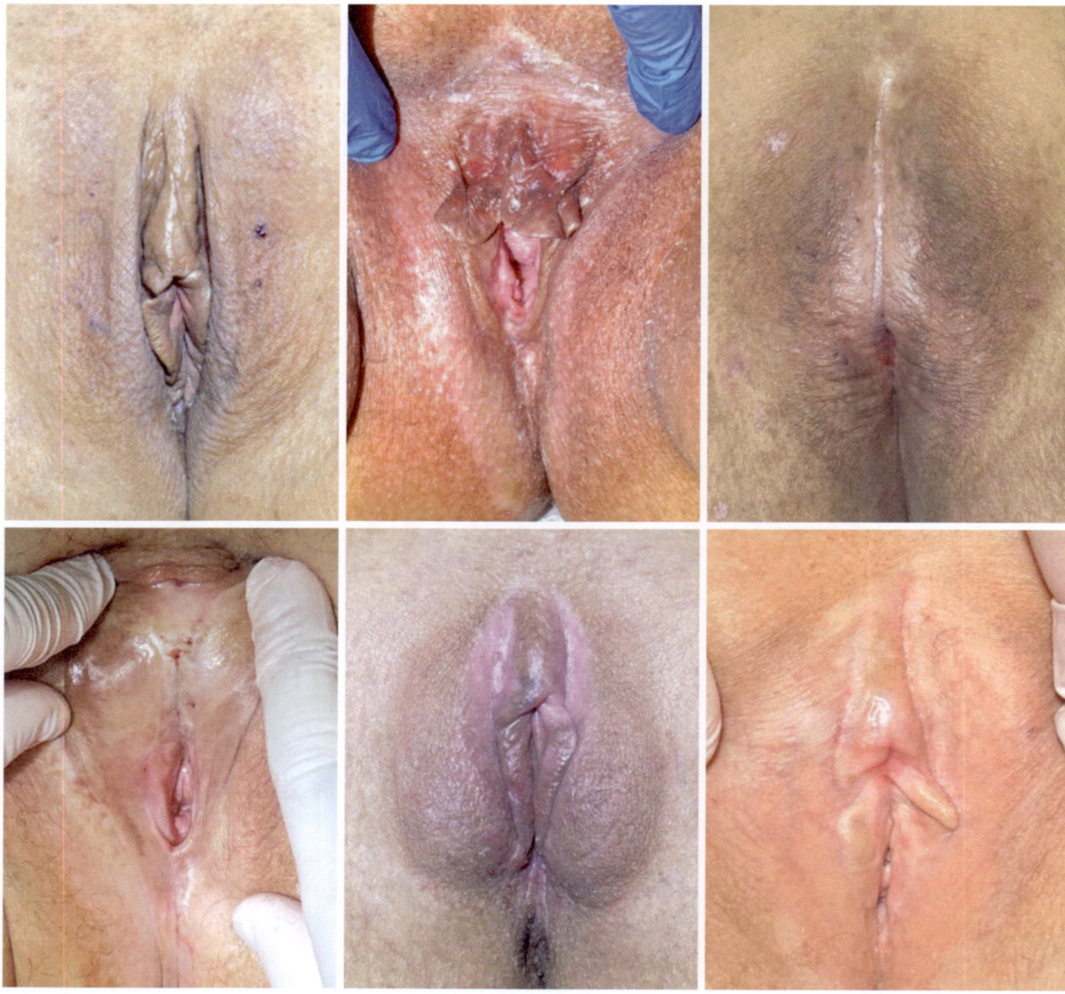

Fig. 5.2 Different clinical forms of the lichen sclerosus disease

- Spotted areas with many white papules and macules
- Thickened hypertrophic plaques
- Plaques restricted in small areas like labial edges or clitoral hood
- Edema in a pale base
- Telangiectasia, purpura, or hemorrhagic area on a pale base
- Angiokeratomas on a pale base
- Fissures and traumatic ulcers
- Erosions
- Fusions (adhesions, especially on hood area, perineum, and vestibulum)
- Water bubbles

- LS accompanied by erythematous-like vulvar psoriasis
- Post-inflammatory hyperpigmentation-like brown hyperpigmentation

In suspected cases for the definitive diagnosis, and exclude the skin malignancy 4-mm Keyes punch biopsy is essential.

5.5 Histopathology

The definitive diagnosis of lichen sclerosus is made by skin biopsy. Biopsy should be taken from the hyperkeratotic area and should be sent for histopathologic examination.

Lichen signs in the histopathologic evaluation are reported as (Fig. 5.3):

- Hyperkeratosis in epithelium
- Hydropic degeneration of basal cells
- Sclerosus of subepithelial collagen
- Atrophic epidermis characterized with loss of rete ridges
- Dermal mononuclear cell infiltration
- Homogenization of collagen on the top of the dermis
- Lichenoid appearance on the dermis

Improvement is observed in histopathological signs as well as the clinic of the disease, following the treatment. The first biopsy before the treatment has significant importance. Serial biopsies are recommended for follow-up of the disease and the response to the treatment [25].

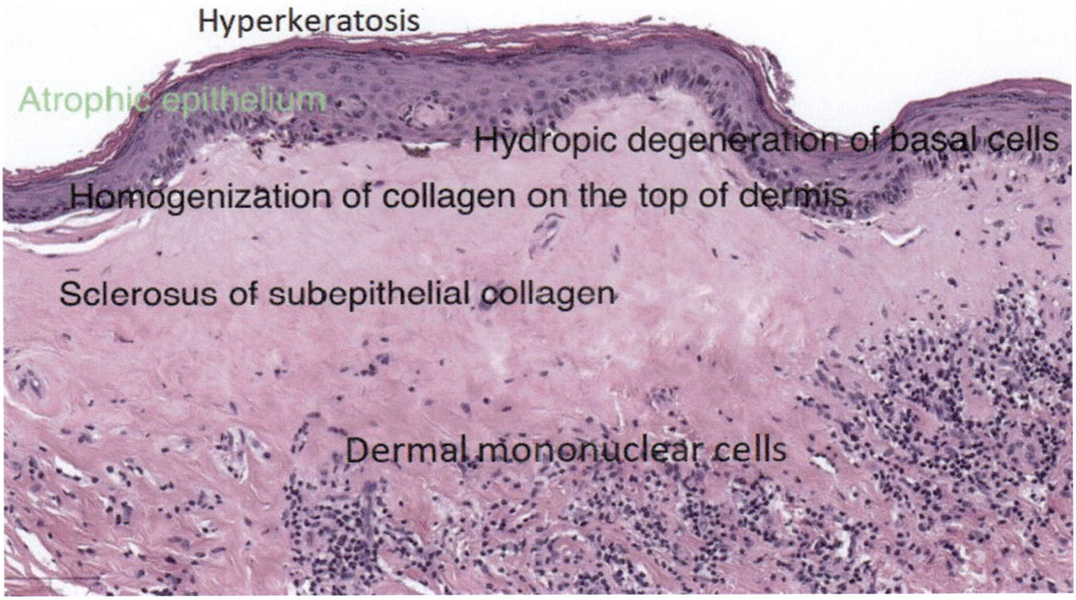

Fig. 5.3 Histopathological structure in lichen sclerosis (H&Exd7100) (With the permission of Zekioğlu Osman)

5.6 Pediatric Vulvar Lichen Sclerosus

The 7–15% of VLS cases are seen in the pediatric age group, and the mean age of diagnosis is five years [3]. In this period, extragenital involvement is extremely rare. The most common VLS symptoms in children are pruritus and pain. Other signs are purpura, bleeding, dysuria, constipation, genital erosions, and extragenital lesions [26].

In the pediatric age group, histopathologic signs and morphologic appearance is similar to adults. Vulva, perineum, and perianal region are involved. The clitoris becomes embedded, labia minora fade, and fissures occur in the perianal region. Therefore, difficulties in urination and constipation are common symptoms.

The progression of pediatric vulvar lichen sclerosus is similar to adults; if untreated, it is progressive and has a risk of permanent damage. Malignant transformation is not reported. However, some studies showed, in older ages, there is an increased risk of detection of HPV viruses with high oncogenic potential [27].

5.7 Differential Diagnosis

LS may have similar signs with all skin diseases that have lichenification symptoms. It is mostly confused with dermatitis in atopic individuals. In addition, it should be differentiated from Paget disease, vitiligo, candidiasis, psoriasis, non-pigmented seborrheic keratosis, genital warts, and vulvar intraepithelial neoplasia. The differentiation from lichen planus is also difficult. Graft-versus-host disease that leaves a scar and mucosal pemphigoid is clinically more common in lichen planus than VLS; however, it also needs to be distinguished in the differential diagnosis [28]. Sometimes, lichen planus and lichen sclerosus may appear simultaneously.

In the perimenopausal transition and postmenopausal course, atrophy in labia minora, narrowing of the vaginal introitus, dryness, and scratches on the skin that occur due to the lack of estrogen may also mimic lichen sclerosus. Therefore, in this patient group, the diagnosis may be delayed.

In lichen disease, local hyperpigmentation areas due to benign melanocytic proliferation may also be observed that may imitate a skin cancer. The malignity in VLS is in form of hyperplasia histopathologically.

LS in the vestibular area shows histological differences from LS of other sites in the vulva, and it is not sensitive to steroid treatment.

5.8 Differences Between Lichen Sclerosis and Other Lichen Diseases

Both LS and lichen planus (LP) are diseases of immunological origin that affect the genital area. The treatment management principles of both are the same. There are minor differences between them. While LP mostly involves mucosal tissues such as the mouth and vagina (Fig. 5.4), LS emerges more often in skin tissue. While high potency topical corticosteroid (TCS) treatments are the first step in LS, these treatments are more difficult in erosive vulvovaginal LP. Topical calcineurin inhibitors and systemic agents are used in second-line treatments. There is insufficient evidence about the effectiveness of systemic treatments in both diseases. The risk of vulvar squamous cell carcinoma is increased in both of them, and it is not known how treatment affects this risk. On the other hand, LS should be distinguished from lichen simplex chronicus (LSC) that is also characterized by severe genital pruritus. However, LSC is a non-scarring vulvar disease. LSC can occur in patients with LS, often superimposed. In these cases, significant thickening of the skin associated with scratching and excoriations may be noted. LSC causes vulvar itching and scratching, often arising from chronic irritation without vulvar architectural changes. Histologic features of it include acanthosis, hyperkeratosis, and inflammatory infiltrates. Recurrence rate is common in LSC, even after complete resolution.

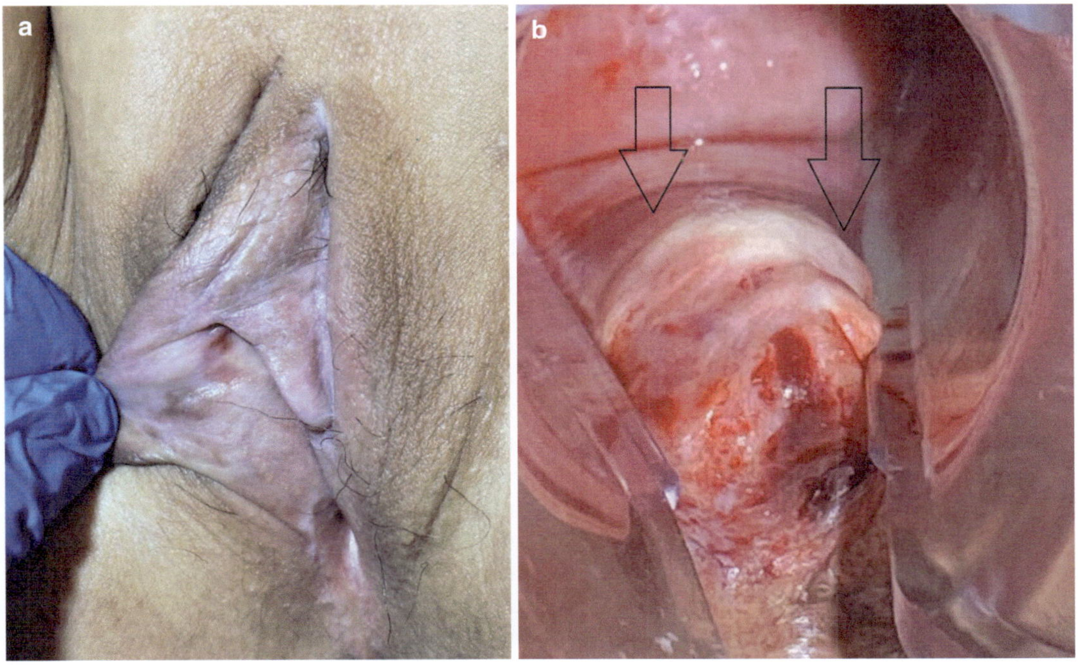

Fig. 5.4 Lichen planus (LP). Vulvar (**a**) and vaginal (**b**) lesions of a patient whose histopathological diagnosis was confirmed LP. Note that the hyperkeratosis is located mostly on the mucosa, not on the skin

5.9 Management

Vulvar lichen sclerosus is a skin disease that decreases the quality of life of the patient. There is not a treatment algorithm that provides a complete cure. Yet, the most commonly accepted management option is *"the patients should be treated depending on the level of the hyperkeratosis"* [7]. The fundamental medical treatment, which is a topical corticosteroid (TCS), is also prescribed according to the level of hyperkeratosis.

5.9.1 Medical Treatments

Medical treatment of VLS is either performed topically or systemically. Usually, topical treatment is recommended.

5.9.2 Topical Treatments

Topical medical treatment for VLS: Lifetime maintenance treatment and intermittent remission treatment are given. The type and dose of TCS should be adjusted according to the severity of hyperkeratosis. Clobetasol propionate 0.05%, the most potent TCS, is the *gold standard* in lichen disease treatment.

When we consider the treatment recommendations according to the severity of the disease [7]:

- *Severe hyperkeratotic disease (very thick white plaque):*

  Ultra-potent TCS (clobetasol propionate 0.05% ointment) twice daily (usually 1–2 weeks) until the itching resolves, followed by once-daily administration for 6 weeks and control at 6 weeks.

- *Hyperkeratotic disease (moderately thick white plaque):*

  Super-potent TCS (e.g., betamethasone dipropionate 0.05% or mometasone furoate 0.1%) twice daily until itching resolves, followed by once-daily administration for 6 weeks and control at 6 weeks.

- *Mild disease with only paleness and little hyperkeratosis:*

  Medium-potent TCS (e.g., triamcinolone acetonide 0.02%, methylprednisolone aceponate 0.1%) once-daily administration, control at 6 weeks. Some of the patients who feel good in the short term can stop their treatment half. These patients should be informed that they should continue their treatment for a while even if their symptoms improve.

5.10 Other Topical Treatments

The topical immunosuppressive treatments, as an alternative to topical immunosuppressive treatments 0.1% tacrolimus (Tacrolin cream™) and pimecrolimus (Elidel cream™) have also come to the fore. Although the success of the treatment is similar to TCS, they may facilitate the development of malignancy with systemic immunosuppression effects [29]. It is reported that good results can be achieved with the vitamin D3 analog topical calcipotriol (Daivonex ointment™), which is used for the treatment of psoriasis.

Despite the insufficient data on topical tretinoin and topical testosterone treatments, it has been reported that there are patients who benefit from the treatment [30, 31]. Topical estrogen therapy should be added to the treatment of patients who do not have a breast cancer risk, especially in the postmenopausal period. Although there is insufficient data that it changes the course of VLS, its effectiveness is proven in the treatment of complaints related to the menopausal genitourinary syndrome that develops due to estrogen deficiency.

5.11 Systemic Treatments

The response of VLS to topical treatments is good. Rarely, systemic treatments are needed in very resistant patients. Oral retinoic acid and hydroxychloroquine treatments can be used together with topical steroids. Methotrexate treatment can also be applied due to its immunomodulatory effect. It is reported that good results can be achieved within 6–8 weeks with an oral treatment of 10 mg once a week after the first test dose of 2.5 mg. However, it cannot be said that a definite cure is provided with these systemic treatments [32]. Oral antibiotics can also be used in infected cases to reduce inflammation.

5.12 Surgical Treatments

VLS may cause functional losses in some patients. Labial fusion, narrowing of the vaginal introitus, and permanent scar formation do not respond to medical treatment. In these cases, the adhesions must be surgically opened for functional improvement.

With surgery, labial adhesions can be opened, the introitus can be expanded, perineal scars can be excised, and the buried clitoris can be re-exposed (Figs. 5.5 and 5.6). Care should be taken, as these patients tend to be bleeding due to deteriorated skin texture.

Topical steroid application is also recommended until recovery after the surgical procedure [33].

Vulvectomy, which was frequently performed in the past, is absolutely contraindicated today.

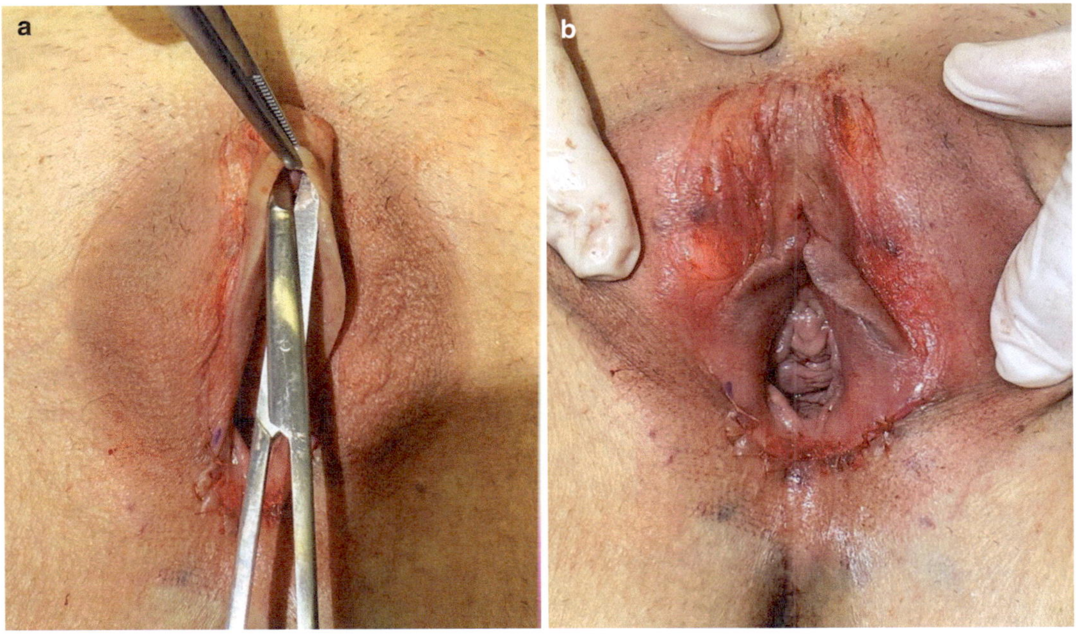

Fig. 5.5 Simple surgery of vulvar lichen sclerosus of a 44-year-old patient who could not have sexual intercourse for five years. She had scar in perineum, buried clitoris, and dens adhesion on clitoral hood and labia minora. The labia minora was freed with blunt dissection, the clitoris was exposed, and the perineal entrance was enlarged by surgical excision (**a**). The image on the right is just after the operation (**b**). Postoperative topical anti-inflammatory treatment was also recommended

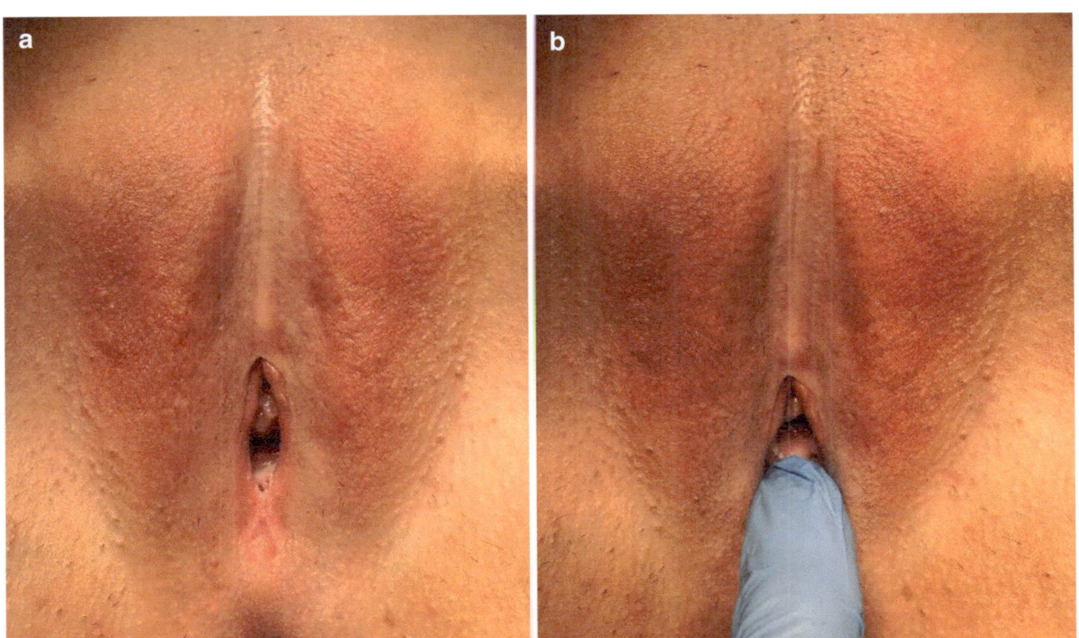

Fig. 5.6 Lichen sclerosus (**a**). Vaginal entrance allows only index finger's insertion (**b**). In this permanent deformity, surgery is essential. Post-op appearance (**c**)

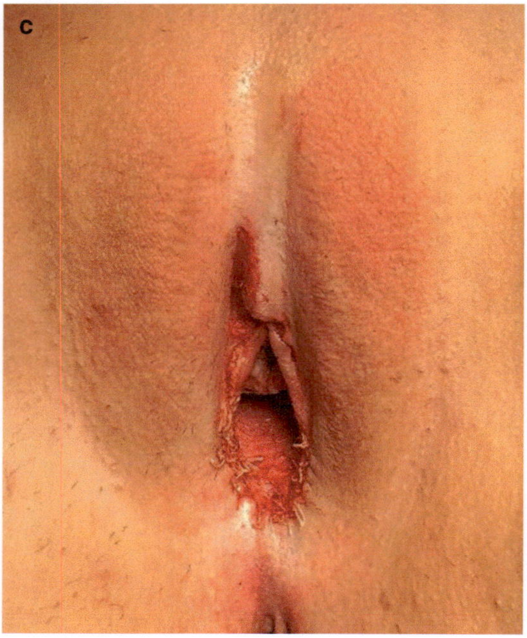

Fig. 5.6 (continued)

5.13 New Approaches in the Treatment of Vulvar Lichen Sclerosus

New treatment methods performed today are promising for VLS. These include platelet-rich plasma (PRP), stem cell therapy, fat graft, and ablative laser applications.

Intralesional PRP injections are performed in the treatment of persistent hyperkeratotic VLS. Although sufficient publications on the effectiveness of the treatment are not yet available, high patient satisfaction has been reported [34]. Similarly, lipo-injection and stem cell therapies have begun to be performed, and good results are achieved [35].

In the hyperkeratotic stage, especially in patients with severe adhesions and dyspareunia, ablative laser treatment is also recommended [36]. Along with these energy modalities, topical treatments, PRP, and stem cell treatments can also be administered in combination. All these treatments are discussed in detail in the relevant chapters of the book. Carboxytherapy (Chap. 22) can be another alternative/additive treatment method; however, it is missing data in the literature.

We propose "sandwich technique" (*Eserdag*) as a new regenerative multimodal approach for the treatment of severe lichen sclerosus, including autologous microfat grafting, SVF, and PRP injections in the same session. In this technique, in accordance with the histologic layers of skin texture, microfat is injected into the hypodermis, SVF is injected into the dermis, and PRP is injected into the all of the layers of the skin. It is aimed to get optimal advantages of regenerative components and reconstruct long-term stability of the tissue (Fig. 5.7).

In photodynamic therapies, phototherapy has also been reported to be effective in the treatment of VLS [37, 38]. Narrowband UVB therapy can provide good results, especially in resistant cases. However, administering phototherapy to the genital area is both difficult and not always practical. There is also a study showing the effectiveness of narrowband UVB therapy in the treatment of extragenital LS [39].

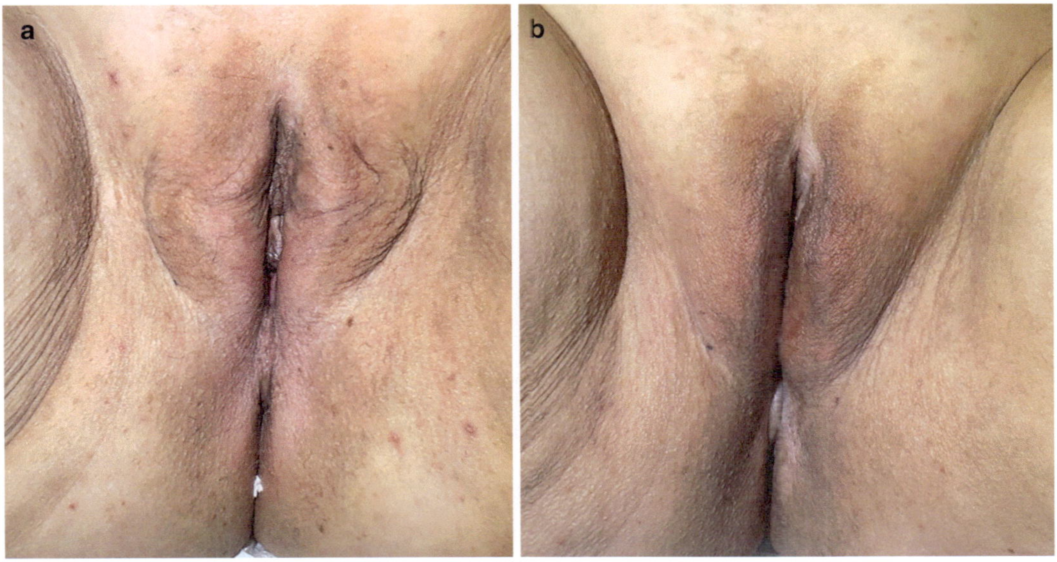

Fig. 5.7 One session of "sandwich technique" has been performed for a lichen sclerosus patient. Before (**a**) and 1 year after (**b**)

5.14 Prognosis

If VLS is not treated, the vulvar architecture completely deteriorates in half of the patients over time, and partial changes occur in the remaining half. Embedding of the clitoris, deletion and cracks in the labia minora, adhesions, wiping and bleeding areas, narrowing of the vaginal introitus, scarring and fissure formation in the perineal area, and malignant transformation (Fig. 5.8) are among the irreversible changes.

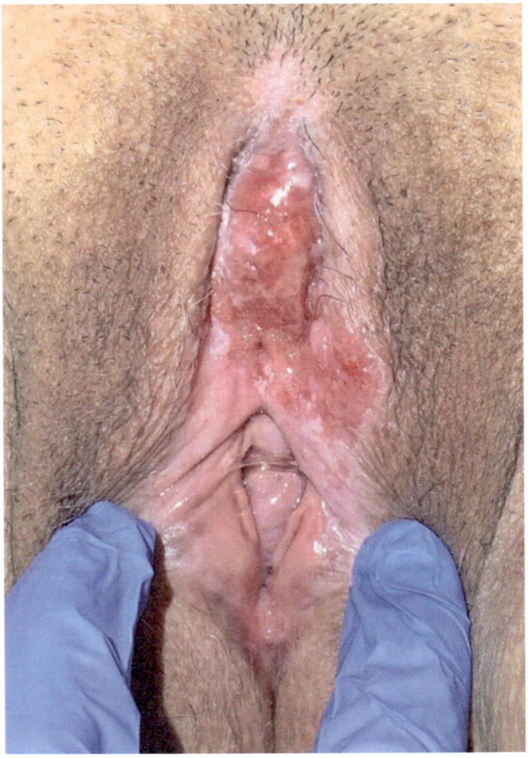

Fig. 5.8 Malignant squamous cell neoplasia transformation in the clitoral hood skin due to chronic lichen sclerosus disease

It is important to inform the patients that vulvar LS is treatable but not curable; once symptoms are controlled, maintenance is essential to prevent severe relapses and progression of disease and to reduce cancer risk. The risk of malignancy is between 2 and 6% in cases that are not treated over their lifetimes or are insufficiently followed up. The risk of transformation is most often for vulvar intraepithelial neoplasia, malignant squamous cell neoplasia of the vulva, and invasive squamous cell carcinoma [1]. For this reason, starting treatment from the moment of the diagnosis, calling patients for regular follow-up, and periodic biopsy controls are among the measures to be taken. Especially if a patient is not responding to treatment, additional biopsies should be considered to rule out differentiated vulvar intraepithelial neoplasia or malignancy that may explain treatment failure and continued itching. With early diagnosis and adequate treatment, the risks of transformation into cancer and scar formation can be reduced.

Appendix

With the purchase of this book, you can use our "SN Flashcards" app to access questions free of charge in order to test your learning and check your understanding of the contents of the book.

To use the app, please follow the instructions below:

1. Go to https://flashcards.springernature.com/login
2. Create a user account by entering your e-mail address and assigning a password.
3. Use the following link to access your SN Flashcards set: ▶ https://sn.pub/tvlq7Q

If the link is missing or does not work, please send an e-mail with the subject "SN Flashcards" and the book title to customerservice@springernature.com.

References

1. Bleeker MC, Visser PJ, Overbeek LI, van Beurden M, Berkhof J. Lichen Sclerosus: incidence and risk of vulvar squamous cell carcinoma. Cancer Epidemiol Biomark Prev. 2016;25(8):1224–30.
2. Dell EA, Miest RYN, Lohse CM, Torgerson RR. Vulvar neoplasms in 275 women with genital lichen sclerosus and impact of treatment: a retrospective chart review. J Eur Acad Dermatol Venereol. 2018;32(9):e363–5.
3. Powell J, Wojnarowska F. Childhood vulvar lichen sclerosus: an increasingly common problem. J Am Acad Dermatol. 2001;44(5):803–6.
4. Goldstein AT, Marinoff SC, Christopher K, Srodon M. Prevalence of vulvar lichen sclerosus in a general gynecology practice. J Reprod Med. 2005;50(7):477–80.
5. Zendell K, Edwards L. Lichen sclerosus with vaginal involvement: report of 2 cases and review of the literature. JAMA Dermatol. 2013;149(10):1199–202.
6. Fischer GO. The commonest causes of symptomatic vulvar disease: a dermatologist's perspective. Australas J Dermatol. 1996;37(1):12–8.
7. Lee A, Bradford J, Fischer G. Long-term Management of Adult Vulvar Lichen Sclerosus: a prospective cohort study of 507 women. JAMA Dermatol. 2015;151(10):1061–7.
8. Cooper SM, Ali I, Baldo M, Wojnarowska F. The association of lichen sclerosus and erosive lichen planus of the vulva with autoimmune disease: a case-control study. Arch Dermatol. 2008;144(11):1432–5.
9. Harrington CI, Dunsmore IR. An investigation into the incidence of auto-immune disorders in patients with lichen sclerosus and atrophicus. Br J Dermatol. 1981;104(5):563–6.
10. Kyriakis KP, Emmanuelides S, Terzoudi S, Palamaras I, Damoulaki E, Evangelou G. Gender and age prevalence distributions of morphea en plaque and anogenital lichen sclerosus. J Eur Acad Dermatol Venereol. 2007;21(6):825–6.
11. Hofer MD, Meeks JJ, Mehdiratta N, Granieri MA, Cashy J, Gonzalez CM. Lichen sclerosus in men is associated with elevated body mass index, diabetes mellitus, coronary artery disease and smoking. World J Urol. 2014;32(1):105–8.
12. Simpkin S, Oakley A. Clinical review of 202 patients with vulval lichen sclerosus: a possible association with psoriasis. Australas J Dermatol. 2007;48(1):28–31.
13. Jacobs L, Gilliam A, Khavari N, Bass D. Association between lichen sclerosus and celiac disease: a report of three pediatric cases. Pediatr Dermatol. 2014;31(6):e128–31.
14. Oyama N, Chan I, Neill SM, Hamada T, South AP, Wessagowit V, Wojnarowska F, D'Cruz D, Hughes GJ, Black MM, McGrath JA. Autoantibodies to extracellular matrix protein 1 in lichen sclerosus. Lancet. 2003;362(9378):118–23.
15. Gambichler T, Terras S, Kreuter A, Skrygan M. Altered global methylation and hydroxymethylation status in vulvar lichen sclerosus: further support for epigenetic mechanisms. Br J Dermatol. 2014;170(3):687–93.
16. Chakhtoura Z, Vigoureux S, Courtillot C, Tejedor I, Touraine P. Vulvar lichen sclerosus is very frequent in women with turner syndrome. J Clin Endocrinol Metab. 2014;99(4):1103–4.
17. Weide B, Walz T, Garbe C. Is morphoea caused by borrelia burgdorferi? A review. Br J Dermatol. 2000;142(4):636–44.
18. Drut RM, Gómez MA, Drut R, Lojo MM. Human papillomavirus is present in some cases of child-

hood penile lichen sclerosus: an in situ hybridization and SP-PCR study. Pediatr Dermatol. 1998;15(2): 85–90.

19. Requena L, Kutzner H, Escalonilla P, Ortiz S, Schaller J, Rohwedder A. Cutaneous reactions at sites of herpes zoster scars: an expanded spectrum. Br J Dermatol. 1998;138(1):161–8.
20. Yashar Y, S, Han KF, Haley JC. Lichen sclerosus-lichen planus overlap in a patient with hepatitis C virus infection. Br J Dermatol. 2004;150(1):168–9.
21. Kohlberger PD, Joura EA, Bancher D, Gitsch G, Breitenecker G, Kieback DG. Evidence of androgen receptor expression in lichen sclerosus: an immunohistochemical study. J Soc Gynecol Investig. 1998;5(6):331–3.
22. Skierlo P, Heise H. Testosteronpropionat-Salbe--ein Therapieversuch beim Lichen sclerosus et atrophicus [Testosterone propionate ointment--a therapeutic trial in lichen sclerosus et atrophicus]. Hautarzt. 1987;38(5):295–7.
23. Miller RA. The Koebner phenomenon. Int J Dermatol. 1982;21(4):192–7.
24. Pock L. Koebner phenomenon in lichen sclerosus et atrophicus. Dermatologica. 1990;181(1):76–7.
25. Dalziel KL, Millard PR, Wojnarowska F. The treatment of vulval lichen sclerosus with a very potent topical steroid (clobetasol propionate 0.05%) cream. Br J Dermatol. 1991;124(5):461–4.
26. Smith SD, Fischer G. Paediatric vulval lichen sclerosus. Australas J Dermatol. 2009;50(4):243–8.
27. Powell J, Strauss S, Gray J, Wojnarowska F. Genital carriage of human papilloma virus (HPV) DNA in prepubertal girls with and without vulval disease. Pediatr Dermatol. 2003;20(3):191–4.
28. Yahiro C, Oka M, Fukunaga A, Fukumoto T, Sakaguchi M, Takahashi Y, Komori T, Ueda T, Nishigori C. Mucosal lichen sclerosus/lichen planus overlap syndrome with cutaneous lesions of lichen sclerosus. Eur J Dermatol. 2016;26(2):204–5.
29. Funaro D, Lovett A, Leroux N, Powell J. A double-blind, randomized prospective study evaluating topical clobetasol propionate 0.05% versus topical tacrolimus 0.1% in patients with vulvar lichen sclerosus. J Am Acad Dermatol. 2014;71(1):84–91.
30. Borghi A, Corazza M, Minghetti S, Virgili A. Topical tretinoin in the treatment of vulvar lichen sclerosus: an advisable option? Eur J Dermatol. 2015;25(5):404–9.
31. Sideri M, Origoni M, Spinaci L, Ferrari A. Topical testosterone in the treatment of vulvar lichen sclerosus. Int J Gynaecol Obstet. 1994;46(1):53–6.
32. Kreuter A, Tigges C, Gaifullina R, Kirschke J, Altmeyer P, Gambichler T. Pulsed high-dose corticosteroids combined with low-dose methotrexate treatment in patients with refractory generalized extragenital lichen sclerosus. Arch Dermatol. 2009;145(11):1303–8.
33. Bradford J, Fischer G. Surgical division of labial adhesions in vulvar lichen sclerosus and lichen planus. J Low Genit Tract Dis. 2013;17(1):48–50.
34. Goldstein AT, King M, Runels C, Gloth M, Pfau R. Intradermal injection of autologous platelet-rich plasma for the treatment of vulvar lichen sclerosus. J Am Acad Dermatol. 2017;76(1):158–60.
35. Boero V, Brambilla M, Sipio E, Liverani CA, Di Martino M, Agnoli B, Libutti G, Cribiù FM, Del Gobbo A, Ragni E, Bolis G. Vulvar lichen sclerosus: a new regenerative approach through fat grafting. Gynecol Oncol. 2015;139(3):471–5.
36. Lee A, Lim A, Fischer G. Fractional carbon dioxide laser in recalcitrant vulval lichen sclerosus. Australas J Dermatol. 2016;57(1):39–43.
37. Criscuolo AA, Schipani C, Cannizzaro MV, Messinese S, Chimenti S, Piccione E, Saraceno R. New therapeutic approaches in the treatment of anogenital lichen sclerosus: does photodynamic therapy represent a novel option? G Ital Dermatol Venereol. 2017;152(2):117–21.
38. Shi S, Miao F, Zhang LL, Zhang GL, Wang PR, Ji J, Wang XJ, Huang Z, Wang HW, Wang XL. Comparison of 5-Aminolevulinic acid photodynamic therapy and clobetasol propionate in treatment of vulvar lichen Sclerosus. Acta Derm Venereol. 2016;96(5):684–8.
39. Colbert RL, Chiang MP, Carlin CS, Fleming M. Progressive extragenital lichen sclerosus successfully treated with narrowband UV-B phototherapy. Arch Dermatol. 2007;143(1):19–20.

Physiology of Wound Healing

6

A true artist is not one who is inspired, but one who inspires others.

Salvador Dali

Wound is the disruption of the normal integrity of the body due to physical damage after trauma, accident, or elective procedure. The word wound can also be expressed with terms such as "erosion," "ulcer," and "fissure." In reality, erosion refers to focal epidermal losses that do not progress to the dermis. Fissure marks epidermal and/or dermal vertical losses in the form of cracks, and ulcers indicate focal losses with dermal and epidermal wounds that tend to become chronic. Wound healing is not limited to the wound area; it includes many highly complex cellular, physiological, and biochemical mechanisms involving all systems [1, 2].

6.1 Phases of Wound Healing

Wound healing takes place in three phases that are intertwined with each other:

1. Hemostasis/inflammation phase
2. Proliferation phase
3. Maturation (remodeling) phase

6.1.1 Hemostasis/Inflammation Phase

The first step of the wound healing cycle is hemostasis. Platelets adhering to collagen in the vessel wall opened after the injury become amorphous, aggregate in this area, and form the temporary clot by activating Thromboxane A2. Later, bleeding is reduced by secreted serotonin and other vasoconstrictor substances. The coagulation cascade begins with coagulation factors such as vascular endothelial damage, platelets, and thromboplastin. Each end-product formed in this cycle activates the next step, and the result is a permanent fibrin plug. Vasoconstriction, which lasts only 5–10 min, is replaced by vasodilation with the activated histamine and complement system. Vasodilation increases vascular permeability and causes the accumulation of intercellular exudate. With the effect of many chemotactic factors, 1 h after injury, polymorphonuclear leukocytes (PNL) and monocytes are collected in the field and activated by environmental factors. While neutrophils fight bacteria in the wound,

S. Eserdağ, *Aesthetic and Functional Female Genital Surgery*,
https://doi.org/10.1007/978-3-031-16019-6_6

monocytes transform into macrophages and secrete various growth factors and cytokines. While macrophages kill and phagocytose bacteria, they also remove dead tissue and leukocytes from the area. Thus, the first 2 days after injury, PNL, and, 72 h later, macrophages are the dominant cells in the region.

Through new vessel formation due to growth factors, both the formation of granulation tissue and the delivery of oxygen and nutrients to the area are provided. T cells provide vasodilation by increasing inflammation while increasing the activities of macrophages. While fibroblasts provide collagen synthesis around new vessels, they ensure that the proteoglycans they produce and collagen are bound together and become more flexible. Also, they keep collagen and other cells together with the fibronectin they produce. The formation of granulation tissue starts on the fifth day on average. It is important to have good oxygenation and nutrition so that this phase can begin. Also, vitamin C is essential for the conversion of proline to hydroxyproline.

The inflammation phase is extremely important for wound healing. However, as in immunodeficiencies, the prolongation of the inflammation phase and failure to proceed to the proliferation phase are the causes of chronic wounds.

6.1.2 Proliferation Phase

In this phase, the wound area is surrounded by fibroblasts, keratinocytes, and endothelial cells. The extracellular matrix (ECM), which contains proteoglycans, hyaluronic acid, collagen, and elastin, replaces the clot by shaping the granulation tissue. Many cytokines and growth factors, including the transforming growth factor β (TGF-β) family, angiogenesis factors, and the interleukin (IL) family, are involved in this phase.

Epithelialization and subsequent contraction develop in this phase. Fibroblasts produce collagen fibers that increase the contraction and tensile strength of the wound. If the tissue loss is too great, regeneration starts from the wound edge. Epithelialization proceeds over the granulation tissue and ends when both epithelia come together. Later, myofibroblasts move in and reduce the size of the wound by providing contraction. After the granulation tissue is formed and epithelialization is complete, the proliferation phase will end.

6.1.3 Maturation (Remodeling) Phase

In this process, which is characterized by the remodeling of collagen fibers, the soft and gelatinous Type III collagen transforms into denser Type I collagen. Some of the contraction develops at this stage. More than normal ECM and immature Type III collagen are degraded. The wound regains 95% of its initial strength after about 6 weeks. The maturation phase can last for years. In this phase, there must be a perfect balance between the apoptosis of existing cells and the production of new cells. Defects that occur can lead to excessive wound healing or chronic wounds.

Excessive wound healing is age-dependent. The risk of its occurrence increases with increasing age. For example, fetal wound healing is in the form of regeneration of normal dermal architecture. Due to anti-inflammatory cytokines in wound healing in fetal skin, the inflammatory response is less and biomechanical stress is lower. Also, fibroblasts produce more ECM, and the amount of hyaluronic acid and Type III collagen in the ECM is greater. Fetal stem cells play an important role in the perfect recovery [3].

6.2 Factors That Negatively Affect Wound Healing

6.2.1 Lack of Oxygenation

The better the blood flow and oxygenation, the faster the recovery. Therefore, a surgical technique that affects the blood circulation the least should be preferred.

6.2.2 Development of Hematoma and Seroma

Wound healing slows down due to the decomposition of wound tips and bacterial contamination.

6.2.3 Development of Infection

Operations performed under aseptic conditions or subclinical infections that are not noticed before the operation disrupt postoperative wound healing. For example, postoperative infection risk increases if bacterial vaginosis is skipped before surgery in patients undergoing labiaplasty. Accordingly, recovery will be delayed.

6.2.4 Surgical Technique Defects

Factors such as the use of thick suture materials, too frequent and tight sutures, suturing by locking, excessive stretching of the tissue especially in flap operations, not being gentle on the tissue, excessive use of devices such as cautery or laser, and prolonged operation time negatively affect wound healing. In choosing the suture material, the materials remaining in the tissue for the least amount of time should be preferred.

6.2.5 Advanced Age

As age increases, recovery slows down relatively. This effect is more obvious especially after the age of 60.

6.2.6 Poor Diet

Vitamin C is important for collagen synthesis and wound contraction. It is recommended to take 1 g/day in the postoperative period. Trace elements such as zinc, copper, and magnesium are also important in wound epithelialization. A diet rich in protein and vitamins should be recommended in the postoperative period for good wound healing.

6.2.7 Smoking and Alcohol Intake

Smoking significantly disrupts the inflammation and proliferation phases. It may cause problems such as wound dehiscence, delayed healing, flap necrosis, and decreased tensile strength of the wound. Passive smoking has a similar effect. In a recent study it has been stated that the labiaplasty patients should be advised strongly not to smoke for 4 weeks preoperatively and postoperatively, because of the wound dehiscence risk. In patients who do not stop smoking preoperatively, the technique can be modified to an edge resection instead of a wedge resection [4].

Alcohol intake disrupts wound healing by affecting the proliferative phase and also increases the possibility of infection. It also harms re-epithelialization, wound closure, collagen production, and angiogenesis.

6.2.8 Poor Postoperative Care

Factors such as poor postoperative wound care and dressings, application of excessive compression to the wound site, non-compliance with hygiene rules, and application of ice compression longer than 3 days can prolong the wound healing process.

6.2.9 Medication Use

Some medications adversely affect wound healing. Isotretinoin-containing drugs, high-dose A vitamins, and cytotoxic drugs are some of them. Nonsteroidal anti-inflammatory drugs (NSAID), which are often prescribed in the postoperative period, selective COX-2 inhibitors, and aspirin are used as pain relievers by inhibiting PGE2 production. The suppression of PGE2, an inflammatory mediating prostaglandin, also occurs with excessive wound scarring and therefore NSAIDs may increase scar formation, especially if they are used during the proliferative phase of healing [5]. Although it is generally thought that they affect wound healing negatively, there are opposing opinions in the literature on this issue.

Steroid-derived drugs also impair the inflammatory response, increase collagen lysis, impair epithelialization, and increase susceptibility to infection. Especially after labiaplasty operations, if antihistamines are not sufficient to treat the problem of itching due to suture allergy and the healing process, non-potent hydrocortisone-derived topical creams can be used for a short time.

6.2.10 Chronic Diseases

Diabetes mellitus, hypertension, connective tissue diseases, rheumatic diseases, autoimmune diseases, thyroid diseases, anemia, and metabolic diseases also delay wound healing. Wound healing is adversely affected in patients with previous radiotherapy, hypoalbuminemia (albumin <3 g/dl), uremia, and some genetic diseases.

6.2.11 Pain

The patient's excessive postoperative pain and a stressful lifestyle can adversely affect the nutrition of the wound site as a result of vasoconstriction due to adrenaline/noradrenaline discharge and may delay healing accordingly.

6.3 Wound Complications

6.3.1 Bleeding

The most common cause of bleeding is due to incomplete hemostasis. Coagulation problems, anticoagulant/antiaggregant drugs used, omega 3 supplements, and diseases such as hypertension and diabetes can also cause bleeding. Outward or intra-tissue bleeding (hematoma) is a complication seen especially in the first 24 h, but it can be observed until the seventh day.

6.3.2 Infection

Infection, which manifests itself with complaints such as redness, purulent drainage, and tenderness in the operation area, is usually observed between the third and fifth postoperative days. When necessary, appropriate oral and local antibiotic treatments should be initiated by performing culture and antibiogram tests.

6.3.3 Wound Dehiscence

In the early period, the wound can be opened due to surgical technical defects. Wound dehiscence after the fifth day is due to infection, insufficient dressings, mechanical effects, impaired vascular circulation, or excessive tension of the tissue. If wound dehiscence develops after the second day after labiaplasty or perineoplasty operations, this should be left to secondary healing and revision should be performed if necessary after complete recovery (usually takes 2–3 months).

6.3.4 Excessive Wound Healing

Wound healing occurs with the common regulation of the three phases mentioned above. Excessive wound healing is characterized by continuous localized inflammation due to a defect in one of these three phases. Therefore, fibroblasts work exaggeratedly and ECM is produced and accumulated more than normal. Excessive wound healing manifests itself as a keloid or hypertrophic scar.

1. *Hypertrophic Scar*

   A result of excessive collagen production, it is scar tissue that is limited to the wound and generally does not exceed the skin level. Hypertrophic scars predominantly have Type III collagen. There are symptoms of edema, itching, and redness at the scar site due to a mild inflammatory process. Hypertrophic scars can regress over time and become completely normal (flat and pale).

2. *Keloid*

    The epidermis has thickened, protruding above the level of the skin and beyond the wound margins. There are excessive collagen and glycoprotein depositions in the incision line. The collagen here is known as hyalinized collagen or keloid collagen and consists mainly of disorganized Type I and Type III collagen. In the deep dermal layer, elastin content is higher than normal.

Keloids can cause itching and hyperesthesia symptoms. It is an aesthetic concern rather than a health problem. Their occurrence is due to the strong inflammatory pathological process. Keloid scars do not regress and will reappear if they are excised. While some parts of the body such as the shoulder and sternum are quite prone to keloid formation, the genital area is very fortunate in this regard.

It has been observed that the risk of scar formation is associated with a genetic predisposition. Also, it is more likely to occur in Blacks and those with darker skin. It has been reported to be more common in hypertensive people; this may be related to endothelial dysfunction.

Scar formation risk is more in the hood area and labia majora compared to labia minora (Fig. 6.1). To minimize the risk of scar formation, it is important to comply with general plastic surgery techniques, choose appropriate suture materials, protect the circulation as much as possible, avoid the use of aggressive electrocautery or laser, and prevent infection. Also, it has been claimed that long-term opening of the tissue in prolonged surgeries may increase the risk of scar formation.

Silicone gel layers or ointments, hypoallergenic microporous tape, or simultaneous steroid injection applications can be applied to people at risk of scar formation. It is thought that silicone gel layers, which have the most scientific evidence, may be effective by mechanisms such as improving hydration and occlusion at the wound site, increasing the temperature, and changing the mechanical tension of the scar.

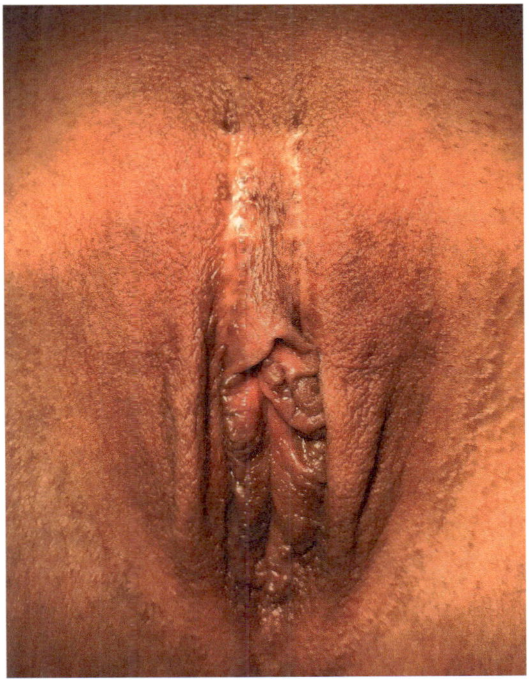

Fig. 6.1 Scar formation after clitoral hoodoplasty operation

Appendix

With the purchase of this book, you can use our "SN Flashcards" app to access questions free of charge in order to test your learning and check your understanding of the contents of the book.

To use the app, please follow the instructions below:

1. Go to https://flashcards.springernature.com/login
2. Create a user account by entering your e-mail address and assigning a password.
3. Use the following link to access your SN Flashcards set: ▶ https://sn.pub/tvlq7Q

If the link is missing or does not work, please send an e-mail with the subject "SN Flashcards" and the book title to customerservice@springernature.com.

References

1. Barbul A. Wound healing. Schwartz's principles of surgery. 8th ed. New York: McGraw Hill; 2005. p. 223.
2. Sherris DA, Kern EB. The wound. In: Basic surgical skills. Rochester: Mayo Foundation for Medical Education and Research; 1999. p. 8–12.
3. Wang PH, Huang BS, Horng HC, Yeh CC, Chen YJ. Wound healing. J Chin Med Assoc. 2018;81(2):94–101.
4. Bucknor A, Chen AD, Egeler S, Bletsis P, Johnson AR, Myette K, Lin SJ, Hamori CA. Labiaplasty: indications and predictors of postoperative sequelae in 451 consecutive cases. Aesthet Surg J. 2018;38(6):644–53.
5. Guo JJ, Yang H, Qian H, Huang L, Guo Z, Tang T. The effects of different nutritional measurements on delayed wound healing after hip fracture in the elderly. J Surg Res. 2010;159(1):503–8.

7 Preoperative Evaluation and Patient Selection

It is part of the cure to wish to be cured.

Seneca

Evaluations before the art of Aesthetic Genital Surgery (AGS) are very important. The surgeon performing the aesthetic operation should act like a psychologist during the consultations and as an artist while performing the surgical art, remembering that each patient is different from the others. It is extremely important to approach the external genital organs as a whole and to plan operations in line with the wishes and needs of the patient. Only in this way will the patient be fully satisfied.

Conversely, the surgeon should not recommend any genital aesthetic surgery to a patient who applies for a different reason such as a routine gynecological examination, smear test, etc. and does not express an aesthetic or functional problem related to her genital area. Otherwise, this attitude will not only be unethical but also harm the patient's body perception and self-esteem.

7.1 Preoperative Evaluation Stages

7.1.1 Detailed Anamnesis

The most important question to ask patients during the first visit is *"What is the primary complaint?"* Accordingly, the anamnesis is detailed. For example, *"What is the leading discomfort in your current situation?"* may be a good starting question. Later, other complaints should be heard (Table 7.1).

Afterwards, a detailed medical and obstetric history is taken. Obstetric history is important for vaginal tightening. Additional questions to be asked include whether she has any chronic diseases, past operations, regular medication, addictions, and allergies. Also, note the menstrual cycle and the date of the last menstrual period. It should also be inquired whether there is a complaint of urinary incontinence. All previous genital and non-genital aesthetic operations should be noted in the anamnesis.

Patients who apply for a revision surgery should be questioned about why they were uncomfortable with the previous operation, which problem or problems they had, and with what they were not satisfied.

In order not to be involved in a past operation questions such as *"With whom did you have surgery before?"* should be avoided. Such detailed questions, negative criticisms about the operation performed at the external center, or even just knowing who performed the operation may cause the patient to carry information between both

S. Eserdağ, *Aesthetic and Functional Female Genital Surgery*,
https://doi.org/10.1007/978-3-031-16019-6_7

Table 7.1 A sample of anamnesis form that can be used before labiaplasty operations

1. Are you not satisfied with the labia minora (hairless inner lips) or the skin around the clitoris? (Length, darkening, or asymmetry)
Yes/No Specify:
2. Do you feel pain, irritation, or discomfort while dressing, moving, or having sexual intercourse?
Yes/No
3. Are you ashamed of your genital area? Does it affect your social life? Can you wear tights, jeans, bikinis comfortably?
Yes/No
4. Do you feel pain in your genital organs due to stretching during intercourse? Or for any reason related to your genital organs, is your concentration impaired during intercourse?
Yes/No
5. Do you have hygienic problems due to excessive skin folds? Is it difficult to clean your genital area?
Yes/No
6. When urinating, does the urine stream spread in different directions instead of going straight down?
Yes/No
7. Do you have difficulty inserting tampons due to extra skin folds?
Yes/No
8. Have you ever had genital plastic surgery before?
Yes/No
If you have had surgery, why are you unhappy with the result? Specify:

physicians, to express words in distorted and exaggerated ways, and relate unpleasant events. Most legal problems arise as a result of negative statements made by another physician. Instead of saying, *"your operation was bad"* to the unhappy and seeking to remedy a patient who comes due to a revision, the modest approach of *"may be closer to what you desire if actually done this way"* would be more appropriate.

Some expressions used while taking anamnesis are important in terms of both understanding the expectations of the patient and evaluating her psychology. Unrealistic expectations need to be clarified (Table 7.2).

The patient who seeks a suitable physician for AGS must also be approved by the physician for the operation. Patients' expectations should be listened to during their first examination, and patients with unrealistic expectations or who are overly insecure, disrespectful, or obsessive should be politely rejected at the first meeting, if possible.

Table 7.2 Examples of some patients' unrealistic expectations

"I want my vagina to be tight, because that's why my husband is cheating on me!"
"I want my vagina to be narrow like I was at 18."
"Since last year I have completely lost my sexual desire towards my partner, so I want to have a vaginal tightening operation."
"I want my labia to be very small, even TO HAVE NO …"
"I want my inner lips to look NORMAL …"
"I want to be PERFECT, just like in this photo."
"I have never had an orgasm so far, so I urgently want a G-Shot© procedure…"

Body Dysmorphic Disorder (BDD) should be considered in patients with excessive body perception obsessions. Although the patient has undergone many plastic surgeries before, her body perception is still negative; making exaggerated and obsessive sentences such as *"I hate my vagina, my breasts, and my crooked nose"* may be an indicator of BDD or a low overall body image perception. Psychiatric consultation should also be requested when there is doubt about the patient's words and behavior.

7.1.2 Gynecological Examination

Gynecological examination should be done after taking a detailed anamnesis. Gynecological examination is in the form of examining both internal and external genital organs in lithotomy position.

In the examination of patients whose operation is planned, it is important to determine whether there are sexually transmitted infections (HPV, molluscum, herpes, etc.), vaginal infections (candida, bacterial vaginosis, trichomoniasis), skin inflammations (lichen simplex, eczema, dermatitis, etc.), varicosities and hemangiomas, and vulvar atrophy and dystrophies.

The presence of varicose veins in the legs or vulva of the patient scheduled for colporrhaphy indicates that the patient has a problem with collagen connective tissue. It should be kept in mind that varicose enlargement may also occur in the intravaginal vessels in these patients and carries a higher risk of bleeding (Fig. 7.1).

The patient should be strained during the examination to determine whether there are signs of rectocele, cystocele, uterine prolapse, and incontinence, and the operation should be designed accordingly. When necessary, perineal and vaginal ultrasonography should be performed in terms of POP findings.

It is more enlightening to give detailed information to the patient with a mirror placed in the patient's hand during the examination. Many patients examine their genital area closely for the first time in their lives; some may act timidly, ashamed, in an effort to get up from the examination table as soon as possible. Measurements related to the parts of the vulva are also made on the examination table and recorded in the patient file.

Patients who make a request after genital examination may also be shown pre- and postoperative photographs of patients whose consent was previously obtained. General information about the variations of the female genital anatomy should also be provided to all patients.

All patients should be given honest, unexaggerated, and clear information during consultations. Especially in labiaplasty operations, 100% symmetry should never be promised because sometimes, no matter how much attention is paid, complete symmetry cannot be achieved. It is never ethical to use exaggerated words such as

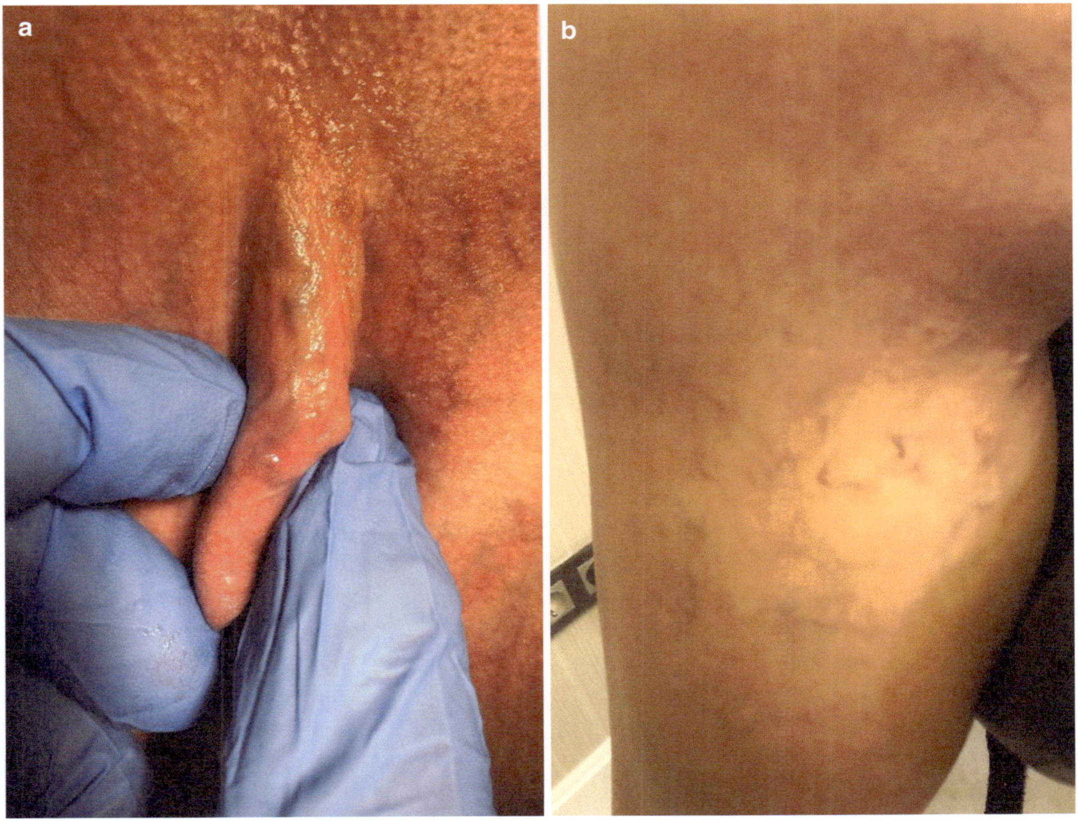

Fig. 7.1 Prominent varicose veins on the external genitalia of a patient (**a**) with diffuse varicose veins on the legs (**b**)

"it will be as if you have never given birth, you will be like an 18-year-old" for vaginal tightening operations!

The physician should know his/her own limits well without financial worries. The physician should clearly explain what he/she can do, what he/she cannot do, and always leave the final decision to the patient. In addition, patients who are considering surgery for reasons such as low body perception, psychological problems, and marital problems, but who do not have any anatomical problems during the examination should be given clear information about their situation, and these patients should be convinced that the operation is not necessary. Most of the patients who are convinced that their anatomy is normal give up the operation at this stage.

7.1.3 Planning the Surgery and the Following Process

The planned surgical method can be explained to the patient by a drawing. Patients are informed about the duration of the operation, the method of anesthesia, and the duration of stay in the office or hospital after the operation. Information is given about what will be encountered after the surgery, what to do and what not to do, how to change the dressing, when to take a bath, physical activities, business life, school, sports, horse or bicycle riding, and when to start or resume sexual activity. Information should also be given about alternative surgical and non-surgical methods by the surgeon, and costs and payment methods by the front office.

Afterward, a hospital or office appointment is made for surgery. Although there is no need for preoperative examinations in the office environment in healthy and young patients, in hospital operations, serological tests, coagulation profile, hemogram, fasting blood glucose, and liver function tests are routinely checked.

7.2 Photographs and Archiving

As in all aesthetic applications, it is extremely important to take before and after photos in genital aesthetics patients. It is important to inform patients about the purpose of taking photos (such as archiving, use in an article, use in a book, use on internet sites, sharing with patients who are considering surgery) before the photo shoot, and that photography and its purposes are included in the consent papers for patients to sign. All before and after photographs must also be archived. These photographs can protect the physician from difficult situations and conflicts that may later be claimed by the patient. However, it should always be kept in mind that good communication is a savior from many bilateral problems and legal processes that may arise in the future. Therefore, in the postoperative period, the patient's questions should not be left unanswered, listen patiently to the physician or assistant, and the necessary solutions should be produced.

7.2.1 Important Issues to Consider When Taking Photos

Before and after photographs should be taken in the same frame, at the same angle, with the same light source and light intensity. More daylight should be used and healing filters should be avoided. Shots should be made on the lithotomy table from the front, right and left laterals, oblique, top, and also standing and sitting position. Featured areas can be zoomed in on. Nowadays, many physicians use smart mobile phones for this purpose. Data can be archived periodically by transferring from a camera or mobile phone to a computer. Thus, the folders created for each patient can be combined with the photos taken during the follow-up/post-surgical periods. Care should be taken to hide patient information in terms of patient privacy, and facial images should not be included in the photographs.

It will also be beneficial for physicians who intend to work mainly on genital aesthetics to receive basic photography training. A good thing about the training on AGS is that it improves your visual skills. It is also important to create video recordings in special cases.

7.3 Body Dysmorphic Disorder (BDD)

The messages given by social media channels such as television, internet, magazines, Instagram, WhatsApp, Facebook, and Snapchat, where visuality is at the forefront, about the human body, are to highlight the image of a weak, thin-waisted, and well-defined sexy woman. The increase in pornography and nudity, easier access to cosmetic procedures, and social normalization of cosmetic procedures cause people to be more interested in their bodies and therefore need to make more changes to their bodies. This effect is particularly strong in adolescents.

BDD is a disorder associated with obsessive-compulsive disorder (OCD), characterized by excessive mental exertion of an imaginary defect that is small or absent in appearance. It is defined as dealing with an assumed defect in the person's appearance and engaging in compulsive behaviors to hide this defect. Mental engagement is most often associated with skin, hair, and nose. If there is a defect, the anxiety experienced in the face of this defect is much more intense than in people without BDD. BDD is frequently associated with reduced quality of life, personality disorders, and psychiatric problems. The disease usually begins at a young age and is more common in unemployed and isolated women. This shows the difficulties of these patients in establishing and maintaining relationships.

People with BDD cannot stop themselves from spending hours in front of the mirror examining the areas they see as flawed.

BDD is classified into "Obsessive-Compulsive and Related Disorders" in DSM-V (Table 7.3). Although its etiology is not known clearly, it has been determined that sociocultural, biological, and genetic factors play roles.

BDD diagnostic criteria are listed below.

Disability can also be seen in these patients as a result of depression, suicide attempts, frequent hospitalizations, and exposure to many unnecessary surgical procedures.

Quotes from one of my BDD patients:

"I have had numerous plastic surgeries so far, but I am still not happy with my body. I do not like my nose, the shape of my head, my legs and my genitals at all, I find them flawed. I constantly fall into negative thoughts about a different area, my tension increases more and more, then I find a doctor that I have thoroughly investigated and undergo surgery. This relaxes me temporarily, but later on I focus on a different part of my body, constantly thinking

Table 7.3 Diagnostic criteria of BDD according to DSM-V [1]

(A)	Preoccupation with one or more perceived defects or flaws in physical appearance that are not observable or appear slight to others
(B)	At some point during the course of the disorder, the individual has performed repetitive behaviors (e.g., mirror checking, excessive grooming, skin picking, reassurance seeking) or mental acts (e.g., comparing his or her appearance with that of others) in response to the appearance concerns
(C)	The preoccupation causes clinically significant distress or impairment in social, occupational, or other areas of functioning
(D)	The appearance preoccupation is not better explained by concerns with body fat or weight in an individual whose symptoms meet diagnostic criteria for an eating disorder
Disability can also be seen in these patients as a result of depression, suicide attempts, frequent hospitalizations, and exposure to many unnecessary surgical procedures	

about how ugly my area is, can't get it out of my mind, and finally go under the knife again to fix it. This vicious circle I can't get out of affects me so deeply that; I even thought about suicide countless times." The last thought of my patient I referred to psychiatry was that the occipital part of her head was too flat, and she had a video meeting with a foreign physician she had found on the internet to insert a silicone prosthesis into his scalp.

The prevalence of BDD is 5–13% in studies conducted without using structured tests; in studies conducted with structured clinical consultation, the prevalence was determined to be 0.7–3%. These rates are higher in patients who apply to dermatology, ear–nose–throat, or plastic surgery clinics for cosmetic treatments [2].

Obsessive-compulsive disorder, major depressive disorder, substance use disorders, and social anxiety disorders are frequently seen in BDD patients. In addition, paranoid and timid personality disorders may accompany the personality structures of these patients [3].

Most patients with BDD are not satisfied with their postoperative results. There is no change in the patient's anxiety and thoughts. In fact, their anxiety levels may increase. Therefore, cosmetic surgery procedures are contraindicated for this group of patients.

Appendix

With the purchase of this book, you can use our "SN Flashcards" app to access questions free of charge in order to test your learning and check your understanding of the contents of the book.

To use the app, please follow the instructions below:

1. Go to https://flashcards.springernature.com/login
2. Create a user account by entering your e-mail address and assigning a password.
3. Use the following link to access your SN Flashcards set: ▶ https://sn.pub/tvlq7Q

If the link is missing or does not work, please send an e-mail with the subject "SN Flashcards" and the book title to customerservice@springernature.com.

References

1. Substance Abuse and Mental Health Services Administration. DSM-5 Changes: implications for child serious emotional disturbance [Internet]. Rockville: Substance Abuse and Mental Health Services Administration (US); 2016. Table 23, DSM-IV to DSM-5 Body Dysmorphic Disorder Comparison. https://www.ncbi.nlm.nih.gov/books/NBK519712/table/ch3.t19/.
2. Altıntaş E. Body dysmorphic disorder in patients presenting for cosmetic treatment. Arşiv Kaynak Tarama Dergisi. 2015;24(3):324–38.
3. Veale D, Boocock A, Gournay K, Dryden W, Shah F, Willson R, Walburn J, Body dysmorphic disorder. A survey of fifty cases. Br J Psychiatry. 1996;169(2):196–201.

8 Instrumentation, Set-Up, and Anesthesia

He who works with his hands is a laborer.
He who works with his hands and his head is a craftsman.
He who works with his hands and his head and his heart is an artist.

Goethe

As in every surgical operation, the equipment used is important in Aesthetic Genital Surgery (AGS) to achieve the best results.

8.1 Tools and Devices Used

The tools and consumables used in AGS have some different features than those in classical gynecological operations.

The devices and tools needed are listed separately in Tables 8.1 and 8.2 and Figs. 8.1, 8.2, 8.3, and 8.4.

Table 8.1 Devices most frequently needed for aesthetic surgery procedures in office conditions and hospitals

– Gynecological operating table
– Mayo stand
– Halogen light
– Overhead lamp (optional)
– Smoke absorber (if cutting will be done with laser or RF)
– Bipolar and monopolar electrocautery
– Vaginal laser or genital RF device (optional)
– Ellman RF device (if a cut will be made with RF)
– Stool (with backrest)
– Air blast heater (if needed)

S. Eserdağ, *Aesthetic and Functional Female Genital Surgery*,
https://doi.org/10.1007/978-3-031-16019-6_8

Table 8.2 Instruments needed for surgical operations (*Eserdag*, set-up)

– Skin marker (Marker pen)
– Sterile surgical drapes
– Scissors: Metzenbaum scissors, iris scissors, curved and straight scissors
– Needle drivers: Crile Wood and DeBakey needle drivers, 15 cm for labiaplasty and 18 cm for vaginal tightening
– Forceps: DeBakey vascular clamp, Adson toothed and toothless forceps
– Clamps: Allis clamps for vaginal tightening, perineoplasty and hymenoplasty operations, Thoms-Allis tissue forceps (wide mouth), Collin hemostatic tissue forceps (triangular mouth), as well as straight or curved Rankin-Crile hemostatic forceps
– Vaginal retractors: Doyen vaginal speculum, Martin retractor, lone star retractor
– For fat aspiration: Lipoaspiration cannula, 20 cc or 60 cc gavage syringe, 10 and 5 cc Luer lock injectors, 3-way stop cock or filters, lipofilling cannula
– Scalpels (different numbers as shown below)

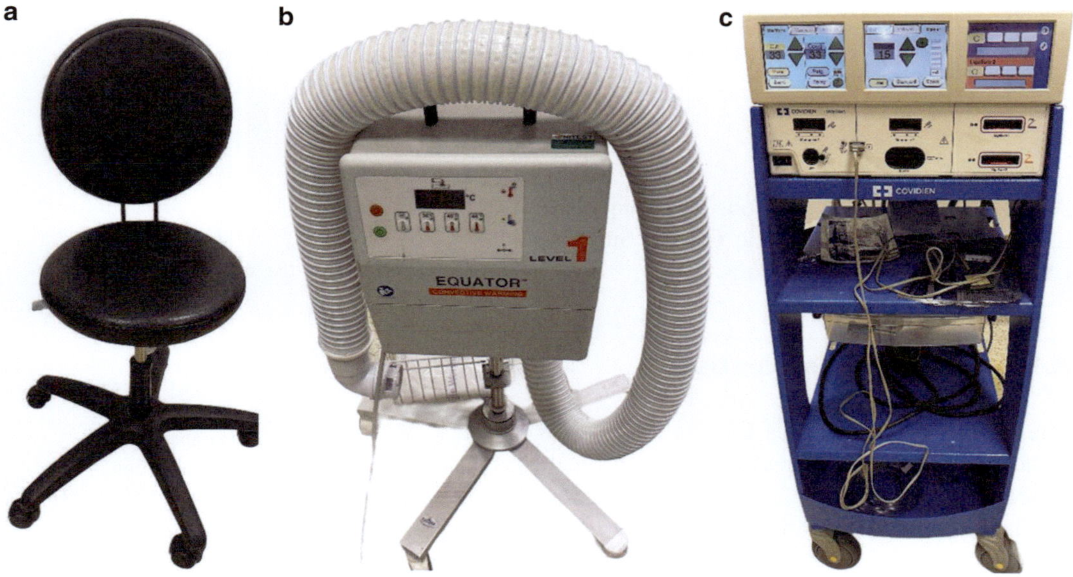

Fig. 8.1 Auxiliary equipment. (**a**) Ergonomic stool with backrest, (**b**) air blast patient warmer, (**c**) bipolar and monopolar electrocautery

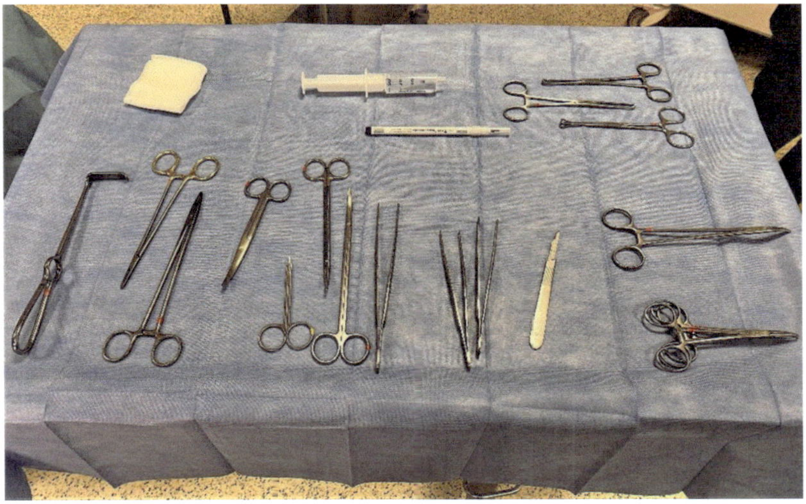

Fig. 8.2 Instrument desk

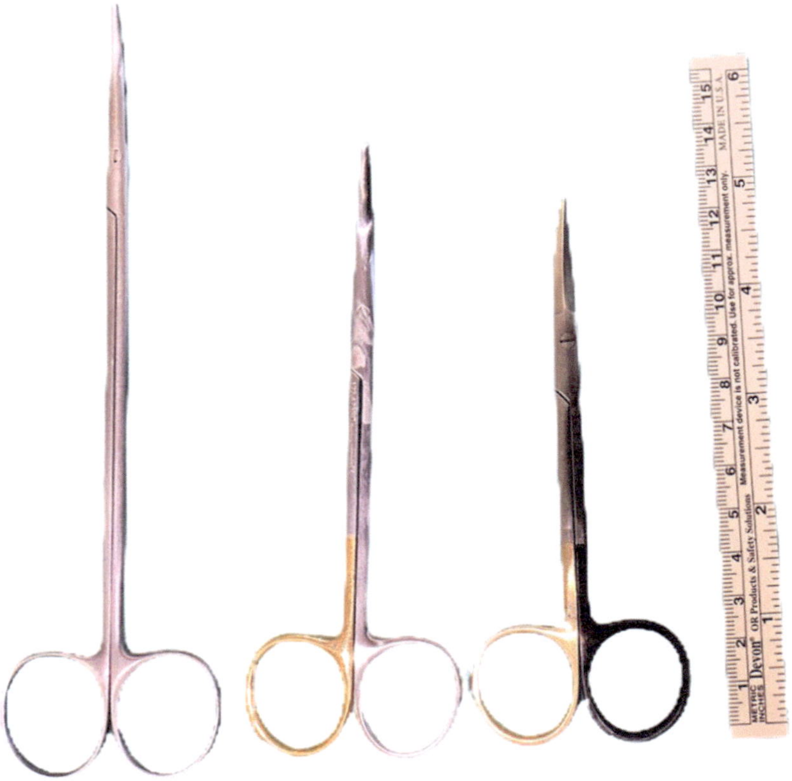

Fig. 8.3 Tissue scissors in different sizes

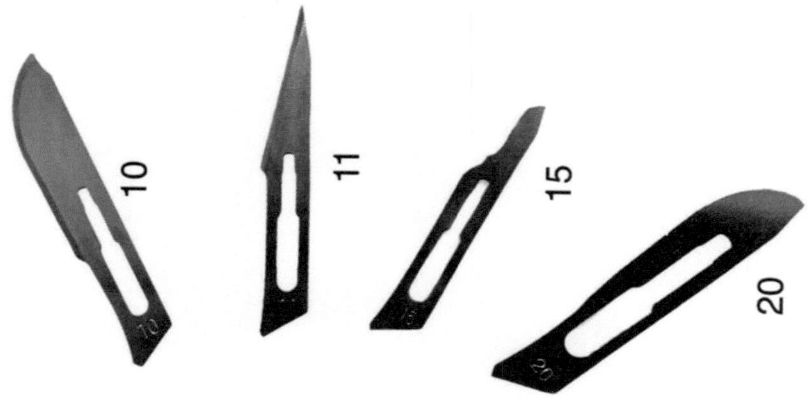

Fig. 8.4 Scalpels in different numbers used in cosmetic genital surgery

8.2 Suture Materials and Needles

8.2.1 Polyfilament (Braided) Sutures

Polyfilament rapid sutures are synthetic and fastest absorbable surgical suture materials with a predictable absorption time consisting of 90% glycolide and 10% L-lactide. These sutures are only intended for use when the need for wound support does not last more than 7–10 days. Because the suture is synthetic, the risk of an adverse tissue reaction is minimized. They lose their 50% of strength in 5 days. Complete absorption of these sutures through hydrolysis will occur within 42 days.

Vicryl™ (Ethicon) is a coated, braided, multifilament suture consisting of a copolymer made from 90% glycolide and 10% L-lactide. This suture has similar handling properties to polyglycolic acid but has more tensile strength. After tissue placement, polyglactin retains 75% of its tensile strength at 2 weeks and 50% at 3 weeks. It is essentially completely resorbed after 56–70 days. Vicryl™ is widely used in cutaneous surgery. Other brands of polyglycolic acid sutures include Pegesorb™, Pegelak™, Surgicryl™, Polysorb™, and Dexon™, all of which are manufactured by different companies.

8.2.2 Barbed Sutures

Knotless tissue devices like V-Loc™ 90 (Covidien) or Stratafix™ (Ethicon) provide strong, secure closure appropriate for high-tension areas such as fascia or vaginal mucosa, provide smooth tissue passage and a secure hold that helps control tension and achieve excellent tissue approximation.

8.2.3 Monofilament (Non-braided) Sutures

Monocryl™ (Ethicon) is another synthetic, absorbable suture composed of poliglecaprone 25, which is a copolymer of glycolide and epsilon-caprolactone. It comes both dyed (violet) and undyed (clear) and is an absorbable monofilament suture. It is slippery, making it easier to pass than a braided suture and generally used for soft-tissue approximation and ligation. Monocryl has a low tissue reactivity, maintains high tensile strength, and has a half-life of 7–14 days. At 1 week its in vivo tensile strength is at 50–60% undyed (60–70% dyed), 20–30% undyed (30–40% dyed) at 2 weeks, and essentially completely hydrolyzed by 91–119 days.

In labiaplasty surgeries, the subcutaneous tissue is usually closed in one or two layers with rapid absorbable 4/0 sutures. Open vessels should not be left due to the risk of hematoma before closure. In skin closure, 5/0 rapid absorbable sutures are generally used. It is the same in clitoral hoodectomy operations, with 4/0 or 5/0 rapid absorbable sutures used for subcutaneous closure and 5/0 for skin closure. Since the clitoral border is a very rich area in terms of nerves, cautery or laser incision in operations on this area is not recommended. It will be more appropriate to use scalpel or Metzenbaum scissors for cutting.

In vaginal tightening, after the mucosa is cut and removed, the rectovaginal fascia is usually closed with 2/0 delayed absorbable sutures. The same sutures can be used to approximate the levator muscles. Subsequently, the mucosa is covered with continuous sutures. The situation is the same in the perineum; the subcutaneous tissue of the perineal body can be closed with 2/0 and the skin with 4/0 delayed absorbable sutures because the perineum is exposed to much tension.

8.2.4 Needles

For soft subcutaneous tissue 3/8 circle taperpoint (round), for skin closure 1/2 circle conventional cutting needles can be preferred as shown in Figs. 8.5 and 8.6.

In AGS surgeries, it is important to be sensitive to the tissue, not to pull the thread in too many continuous sutures, and to work with as thin threads as possible.

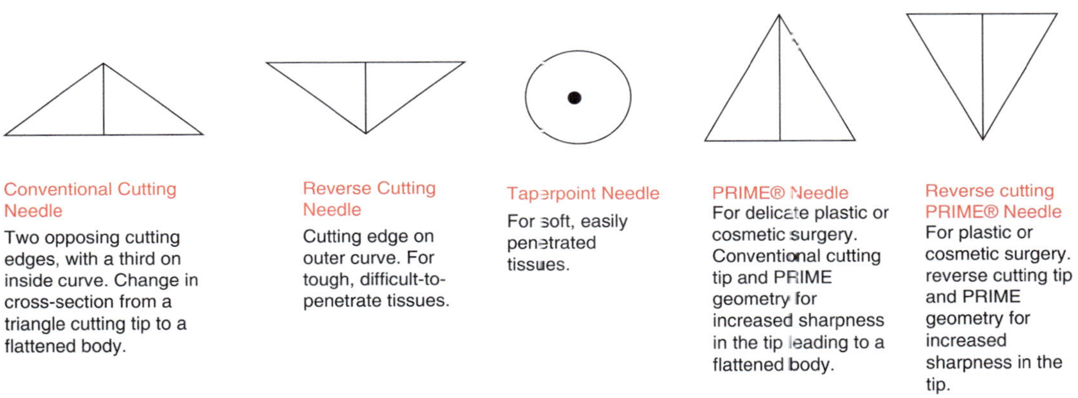

Fig. 8.5 Some types of needles (extracted from Ethicon product catalog)

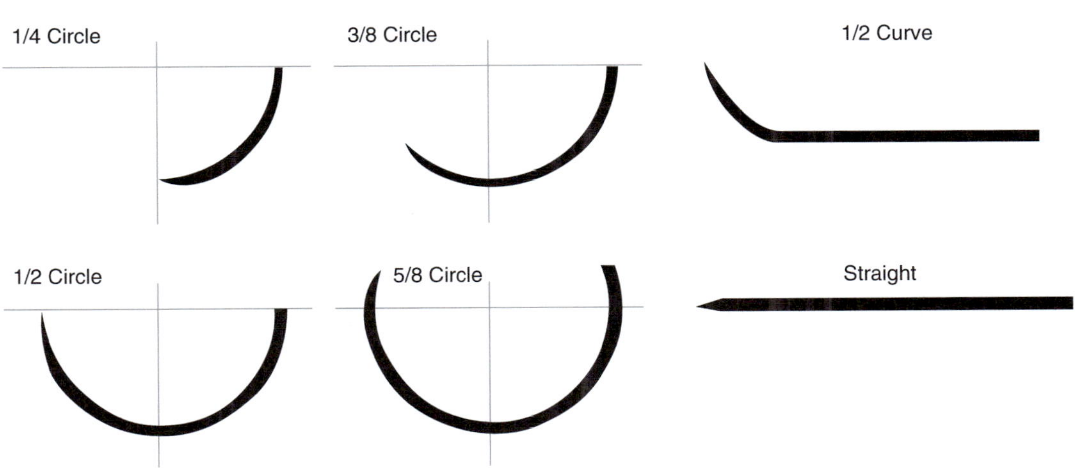

Fig. 8.6 Some shapes of needles (extracted from Ethicon product catalog)

8.3 Marking

Marking with a surgical skin marker pen, which plastic surgeons are quite familiar with, and obstetricians–gynecologists who will apply the art of AGS should know, is extremely important in determining the area to be operated on. Since surgical margins may be lost due to some swelling of the tissue after local anesthesia, the marking should be done before the local anesthetic injection, if it is done. Especially in labial surgeries, it is important that the labia are not wet while marking and that the inner labia are kept in a natural state without stretching during marking. After drawing with a single labia pen, the *"mirror image"* can also be taken by bringing it face to face with the other labia. A mirror image is important in determining the surgical margins, especially in asymmetry cases. In asymmetry cases, the short side is marked first, then both big labia are brought closer to each other and a mirror image is created on the opposite side (Fig. 8.7).

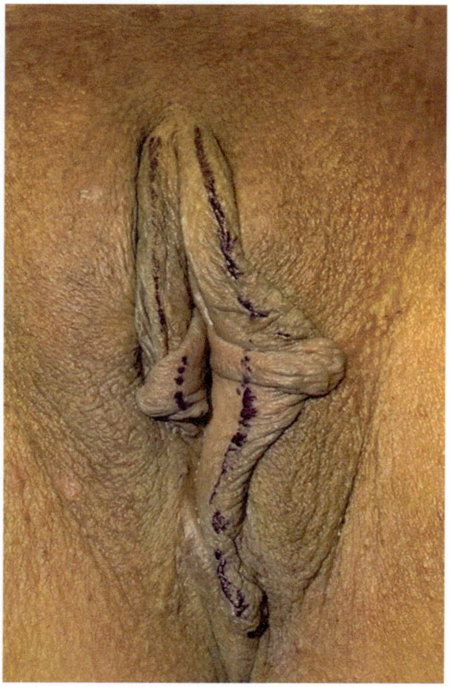

Fig. 8.7 Marking in a labial asymmetry case. First, the tissue to be removed from the short side is marked

Marking in labiaplasty is important for cutting the tissue properly. For this purpose, as a simplier method for the beginners, fine (30G) needles can be inserted into the marking area and guide the cutting process (Fig. 8.8).

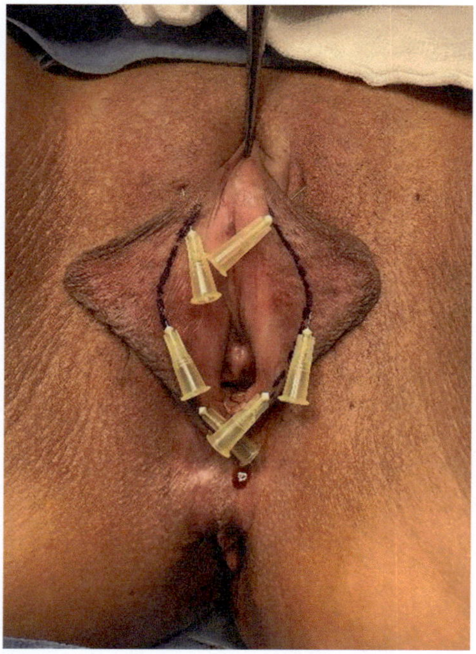

Fig. 8.8 Marking with fine needles. After marking with a pen in labiaplasty, fine needles can be used to determine the anterior and posterior areas before cutting so that cutting can be done more securely

In labia majoraplasty surgeries, performing the marking process after metric measurement is also a correct approach.

Marking should be done for the purpose of the procedure (Fig. 8.9).

Markings are made according to the incision or technique of the procedure. Metric measurements are taken when necessary. Sometimes customized marking is needed for specific or revision operations (Fig. 8.10).

Marking is important in all AGS operations. This process is important in determining the width of the operation to be performed. Labia minora *should not be stretched while marking* in labiaplasty. Otherwise, more tissue removal than normal may result.

The *"think 3 and cut 1"* general rule, which is important in all surgical procedures, is also valid here, because after the cutting is done, there can be no return. Scissors, scalpel, laser, and Ellman RF can be used for cutting in labiaplasty. Cutting

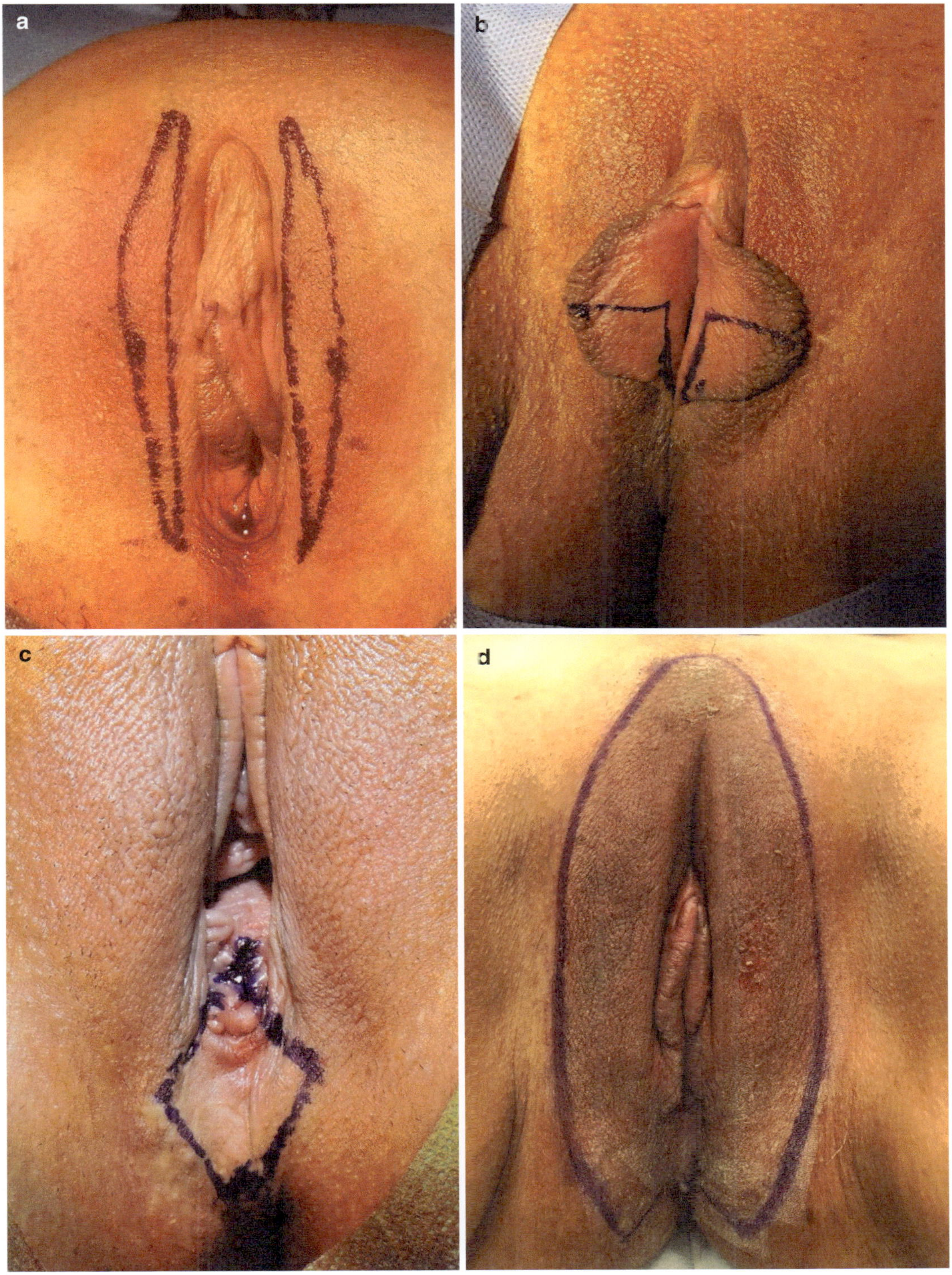

Fig. 8.9 Different drawings for marking. (**a**) Labia majoraplasty, (**b**) labia minoraplasty with wedge resection, (**c**) perineoplasty, (**d**) bleaching

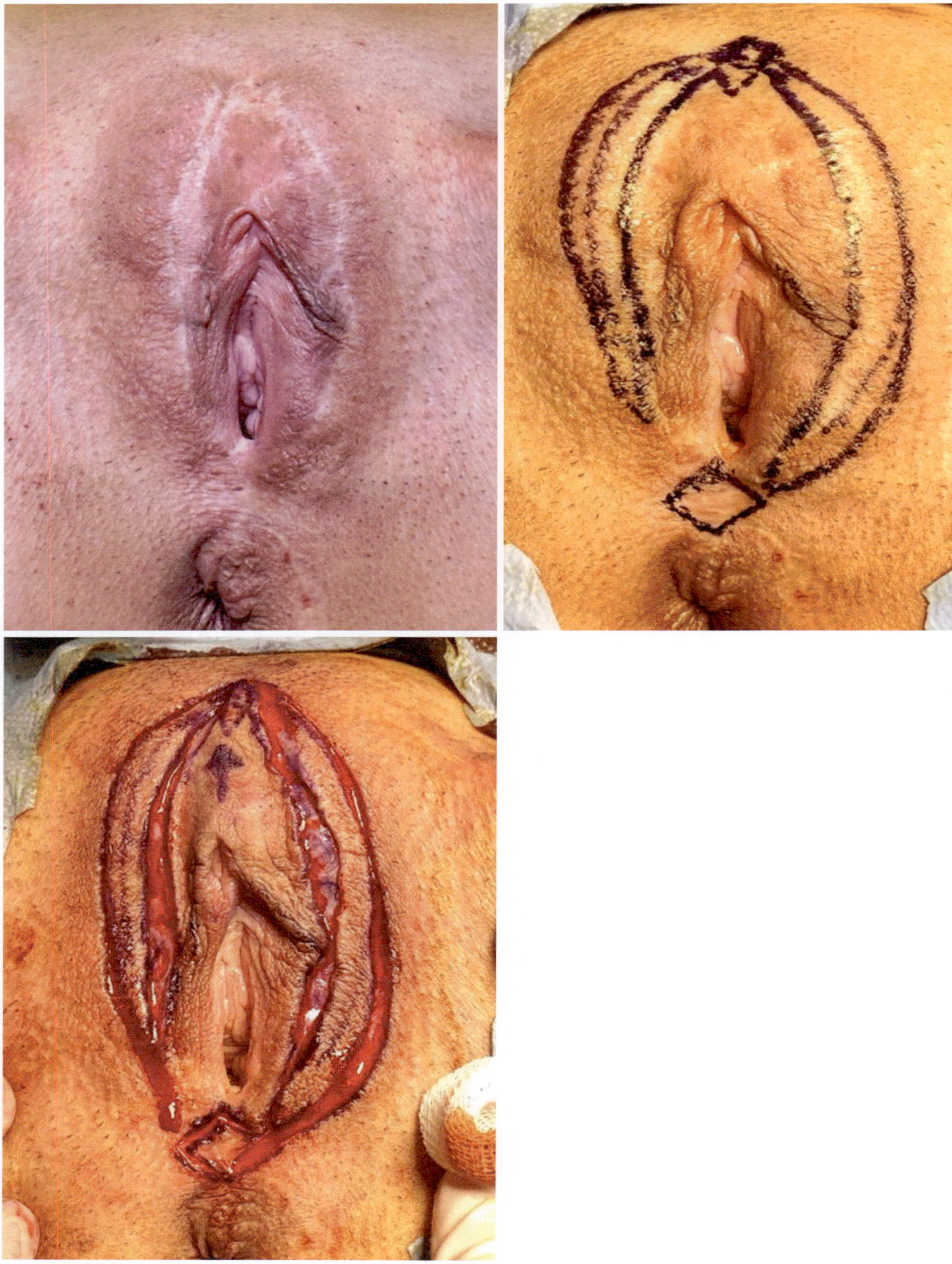

Fig. 8.10 Customized marking. Revision surgery for a patient who underwent majoraplasty, minoraplasty, and hoodoplasty. Marking lines are drawn by involving scar lines. Note the diamond-shaped markings for the anterior and the posterior commissures

the labia with monopolar cautery is not recommended because it will traumatize the adjacent tissue and delay wound healing.

As with any surgery, an experienced surgical nurse, well-trained staff, an operating room with ergonomic design, and the quality of the materials used are important to achieve the best result.

8.4 AGS Anesthesia

AGS anesthesia is an important issue. Operations can be performed in the hospital or, in appropriate cases, in an office, depending on the situation.

8.4.1 Surgery at Office Conditions

8.4.1.1 Local Anesthesia Applications

The most ideal cosmetic surgery:

- does not harm the patient,
- has highest patient satisfaction both functionally and aesthetically,
- is low cost,
- has the lowest risk ratio. For these reasons, patients who are considering labiaplasty, who are in good general health, and do not have severe hypertrophy of the labia, can be operated on under office conditions under local anesthesia.

The criteria for the ideal local anesthetic drug to be used in the office are to prevent pain without local irritation, to have a low allergic potential, to have a high therapeutic index, and to create a sensorial block instead of motor block [1].

All local anesthetics are drugs that stabilize the cell membrane; they reversibly slow down the rate of depolarization and repolarization in the membranes that can be excited such as pain receptors. Local anesthetics mainly act by blocking sodium entry into the cell via sodium-specific ion channels on the neuronal cell membrane. Thus, membrane depolarization is blocked and signal transmission is blocked. The potency of local anesthetics is largely the result of differences in lipid solubility, which enhances diffusion through nerve sheaths and neural membranes.

Advantages of local anesthetic applications:

- It is easy to see active vessels during the operation. Open-ended capillary arterioles that are overlooked due to hypotension in general anesthesia may cause postoperative bleeding.
- Does not include general anesthesia risks. It does not cause undesirable situations such as nausea, vomiting, and aspiration of stomach contents.
- It does not cause laryngeal irritation that may be caused by intubation.
- Patients can have a light meal even 1–2 h before surgery.
- Surgery can be scheduled in the afternoon.
- Patients can go home 2–4 h after surgery. They can drive car.

In addition, local anesthetic applications provide benefits such as predictable efficacy, high level of safety, minimal impact on physiology, and fast recovery time.

Disadvantages of local anesthetic applications:

- During the operation, the patient can distract the surgeon by talking.
- The patient may be agitated and panic. The patient may overreact, especially to local anesthetic injection.
- Situations such as syncope and temporary loss of consciousness may be experienced during injection due to vasovagal reflex.

Some ready-to-use local anesthetic preparations can be preferred according to surgeon's experience and duration of the operation as shown in Table 8.3.

Conversely, liposomal bupivacaine (Exparel™), a new local anesthetic derivative, is applied as a single dose to the operation area and is quite long acting. Its analgesic effect lasts for

Table 8.3 Some ready-to-use local anesthetic preparations and recommended doses

For infiltration anesthesia	Maximum single dose	Maximum total dose
2% lidocaine HCl +epinephrine (1:100,000)	7 mg/kg	500 mg/dose
2% lidocaine HCl + epinephrine (1:50,000)	7 mg/kg	500 mg/dose
4% Articaine HCl + epinephrine (1:200,000)	7 mg/kg	Determined by weight
4% Articaine HCl + epinephrine (1:100,000)	7 mg/kg	Determined by weight
0.25% Bupivacaine + epinephrine (1:200,000)	2.5–3 mg/kg	225 mg/dose
		400 mg/24 h
4% Prilocaine + epinephrine (1:200,000)	8.8 mg/kg	600 mg/dose
2% Prilocaine + levonordefrin (1:20,000)	6.6 mg/kg	400 mg/dose

approximately 96 h. It was approved by the FDA in 2011. In the USA, 266 mg (20 mL) dose is marketed for around $350.

Duration of Numbness

Local anesthetics vary in their duration of action due primarily to differences in their affinity for protein. The greater the affiliation to plasma proteins, the longer the anesthetic effect.

Duration of numbness is also influenced by the time a local anesthetic remains close to neural fibers. Sequestration of highly lipid-soluble anesthetics locally may allow for continual release to the neuronal membranes, prolonging duration, but the constriction of neighboring vasculature is more significant. For this reason, vasopressors are added to many formulations to delay absorption and prolong anesthesia, which is particularly important because local anesthetics vary in their ability to produce vasodilation. For example, lidocaine without vasopressors shortens its duration by vasodilatation, whereas mepivacaine and bupivacaine do not. Plain lidocaine formulations may be used for small interventions, but their efficacy is weak [2].

Drug Reactions

Reactions to local anesthetic agents can be classified as allergic, toxic, and autonomic. People undergoing genital treatments often exhibit autonomic (sympathomimetic) responses, such as tachycardia, sweating, and syncope. However, an autonomic response is usually mild. Allergic reactions, although rare, can be encountered during the operations. Mild allergic reactions usually occur because of histamine release in response to a particular agent. Such reactions are usually slow in onset and include responses such as rashes, angioedema, nausea, and itching.

Table 8.4 Local anesthetic toxicity

Serum concentrations		Symptoms
3–6 μg/mL	Subjective toxicity	Lightheadedness, restlessness, drowsiness, tinnitus, impaired vision, digital paresthesia, and circumoral numbness
5–9 μg/mL	Objective toxicity	Nausea, vomiting, tremors, confusion, excitement, psychosis, and muscular fasciculations
>10 μg/mL		Cardiac excitation followed by cardiac depression—bradycardia, asystole, convulsions, and coma
>20 μg/mL		Respiratory arrest
>26 μg/mL		Cardiac arrest

Local Anesthetic Toxicity

Systemic toxicity of local anesthetics attributed to dose-dependent (Table 8.4). After the injection, the blood concentration rises, and the peripheral nervous and central nervous systems are depressed in a dose-dependent manner. The generally accepted threshold level for lidocaine toxicity is 5 μg/mL. Evidence of lidocaine toxicity may commence at concentrations >5 μg/mL, but convulsive seizures generally require concentrations >10 μg/mL.

However, the level at which symptoms manifest varies with each patient. Subjective toxic symptoms are usually seen at serum concentrations between 3 and 6 μg/mL. Objective toxicity occurs at serum concentrations between 5 and 9 μg/mL.

Local anesthetics should be respected as central nervous system depressants, and they potentiate any respiratory depression associated with sedatives and opioids. Furthermore, their effects are increased during hypercarbia (elevated CO_2 in serum). The doses should be reduced in patients with cardiac, renal, or hepatic problems.

Local Anesthetic Allergy

It is not usual to meet the allergic effects of local anesthetics. Allergic reactions are more likely attributable to preservatives (methylparaben, bacteriostatic agent) or antioxidants (metabisulfite) contained in the solution. True allergic reactions to local anesthetics are possible but extremely rare.

AGS surgeries are operations with a high probability of bleeding due to their anatomical features. Even if the operation will be performed under sedation or general anesthesia, local infiltration anesthesia can be recommended to increase postoperative comfort and reduce the risk of intra/postoperative excessive bleeding.

The epinephrine content in local anesthetic ampoules is very low. It is never recommended to add additional epinephrine into these preparations that are available on the market because sudden sympathomimetic side effects can be seen when epinephrine passes under the skin into the systemic circulation.

In the vaginal tightening operation, a local anesthetic injection is performed as a subcutaneous application. Infiltration of the back wall of the vagina with a local anesthetic containing epinephrine both decreases the amount of bleeding and facilitates dissection.

Applying a 5% lidocaine-prilocaine mixture cream or 2% lidocaine pomade to the operation area 30–45 min before the local anesthetic application and covering that area with stretch film until the operation starts will relieve the injection pain.

Local anesthesia in labiaplasty should be performed with a thin (30G and long dental steel) needle, 0.5 cm lateral to the base of the labia minora. Injections made into the labium cause the tissue to swell and balloon, thus losing the surgical margin. In order to avoid postoperative asymmetry problems, local anesthetic injection into the labium should be avoided.

All local anesthesia applications can be done by diluting half with an isotonic sodium solution. Thus, drug-related side effects and overdose will be avoided.

The patients who will be operated on under local anesthesia should wear headphones and listen to music during the operation in order to significantly reduce anxiety. Supporting the thighs and lower parts of the knees with soft sponges in the lithotomy position will prevent nerve compression and increase comfort during the operation.

8.4.1.2 Tumescent Anesthesia

Tumescent anesthesia is a form of local anesthesia used for several plastic surgery procedures, particularly liposuction, and other disciplines, like dermatological, endocrine, and vascular operations. It is a technique in which a dilute local anesthetic solution is injected into the subcutaneous tissue until it becomes firm and tense. The word "Tumescent" means Tumid—Firm and Swollen. It is relatively safe, generally tolerated very well by patients, and can be applied in office procedures [3].

Tumescent local anesthesia was first described by Dr. Jeffrey A. Klein, a dermatologist from California, in 1985. For local infiltration anesthesia, the conventional dosage of lidocaine is up to 4.5 mg/kg, and with adrenaline is up to 7 mg/kg; however, in liposuction using tumescent anesthesia, the recommended maximum dose of lidocaine with adrenaline is up to 55 mg/kg [4]. Lidocaine with epinephrine in doses between 35 and 55 mg/kg is routinely used in liposuction. The American Academy of Dermatology (AAD) guidelines recommend a maximum dose of 55 mg/kg lidocaine with epinephrine to be safe for tumescent anesthesia for liposuction in patients weighing 43.6–81.8 kg (Table 8.5).

Lidocaine, the standard choice for use in tumescent anesthesia, is safe. Prilocaine has a similar effect as lidocaine and can be used as well.

Table 8.5 Standard Klein solution (local anesthetic–epinephrine–saline mixture) for lipoaspiration

• 50-cc bottle of plain 1% lidocaine
• 1 cc vial of 1:1000 epinephrine
• 1-L bag of isotonic NaCl solution (warmed)
• 10 mEq (10 mL 8.4%) $NaHCO_3$ (optional)

However, one of the metabolites of prilocaine, *O*-toluidine, can cause methemoglobinemia. Methemoglobinemia becomes life-threatening when methemoglobin levels exceed 50–60%, and it is managed using intravenous methylene blue, which reduces the hemes to their normal state. Nevertheless, methemoglobinemia attributed to prilocaine is unlikely when recommended doses are applied.

It has been suggested that a combination of lidocaine and prilocaine solutions may reduce the risk of toxicity from either drug and might be favorable in cases where a large volume of tumescent local anesthesia is needed [5]. However, bupivacaine is not recommended for this use due to the greater risk of cardiotoxicity and limited experience with its use.

Standard Klein Solution (local anesthetic–epinephrine–saline mixture).

After having the mixture, 0.05% lidocaine and 1:1,000,000 epinephrine would be obtained. To minimize the side effects, the dose of epinephrine in local anesthesia should not exceed 0.07 mg/kg. Lidocaine by itself and with epinephrine is highly acidic and causes stinging during infiltration. Hence, about 10 mEq of sodium bicarbonate ($NaHCO_3$) is added to 1 L of the tumescent solution to alkalinize the solution. Increasing the percentage of local anesthetic in the non-ionized form promotes its transit into cells, speeds the onset of analgesia, and reduces stinging.

Tumescent anesthesia ensures:

- Suitable and prolonged anesthesia,
- Low side effects,
- Hemostasis,
- Reduced postop pain,
- Minimal downtime,
  Outpatient management.

8.4.1.3 Pudendal Block

The pudendal nerve is located posterior to the sacrospinous process, next to the ischial process. The numbing of the pudendal nerve by injecting a local anesthetic agent transvaginally or transperineally is called "pudendal block." Pudendal block is a good anesthesia technique that can be applied in the clinical setting and can be preferred in combined surgeries, especially when the area to be numbed is large. The affected areas from bilateral pudendal block are the lower parts of the vagina, perineum, and labia minora and majora.

How Is a Pudendal Block Performed? RCOG Recommendations

An "Iowa Trumpet" or similar instrument can be used for the procedure. This instrument is 15 cm in length, has a tubular guide, and prevents entry of more than 1 cm into the tissue. If these instruments are not available, the procedure can also be performed carefully with a 22G spinal needle.

A total of 20 cc of 1% lidocaine is drawn into two 10 cc injectors. If the block is to be applied on the left side first, the forefinger and middle finger of the left hand are inserted into the vagina. After palpating the ischial protrusion with the forefinger, the Iowa Trumpet is held with the right hand and guided between both fingers. The needle is inserted into the 1 cm *posterior and medial part of the ischial process*. Since there are many veins in this area, negative aspiration must be applied. If no blood comes into the injector, 7 cc of local anesthetic is injected into the tissue. Then the same process is done to the other ischial protrusion. If necessary, the remaining 6 cc of local anesthetic can be injected into the perineum as an infiltration [6].

Although uterosacral block or paracervical block applications are recommended for genital esthetic surgeries, these methods do not cause vulvar numbness at the expected level.

Office Premedication

Preoperative premedication may reduce anxiety associated with the operation. For this, 10 mg diazepam (oral) can be given 1 h before the operation. Diazepam acts by interacting with specific benzodiazepine receptors in the central nervous system, maximizing pre- and post-synaptic inhibition of GABA at various synapses. Its inhibition in 5-HT and noradrenergic neurons provides anxiolytic and sedative effects. Conversely, diazepam is an effective amnestic and anticonvulsant. It also increases the toxic threshold value of local anesthetic drugs. However, it may increase discomfort and impair cooperation in some patients, although rarely. It is subject to green prescription in our country.

An antihistamine drug, 25–50 mg of hydroxyzine HCl (oral), may also be given 1 h before the operation in order to alleviate anxiety before the operation. Total daily dose should not exceed 100 mg. Hydroxyzine may prolong the QT period in ECG. It is not recommended for elderly patients; if it is to be used, it should not exceed 50 mg. Side effects such as dry mouth, weakness, dizziness, nausea, and agitation can be seen.

8.4.2 Surgery at the Hospital

8.4.2.1 Sedation

In some cases, sedation anesthesia can be applied with intravenous 1% propofol and/or midazolam-derivative drugs. However, if sedation anesthesia is to be applied, it is important that the operation time is less than 1 h. Care should be taken in terms of complications such as anaphylaxis, respiratory depression, and hypotension during intravenous sedation. Midazolam also has an amnestic effect and is subject to limitations in some countries. Some patients can be operated on after mild intravenous sedation supported by an injection of local anesthesia. Laryngeal mask airway (LMA), which is a supraglottic airway device, can also be used. It is designed to sit in the patient's hypopharynx and cover the supraglottic structures, thereby allowing relative isolation of the trachea.

8.4.2.2 General and Regional Anesthesia Methods

AGS operations can be performed in hospital operating rooms with general, epidural, spinal, and combined anesthesia methods in line with the medical history of the patient and her own request. Epidural and spinal anesthesia may be preferred in patients who have any contraindication of general anesthesia. Hypotension during the general and regional anesthesia may facilitate surgery by diminishing the intraoperative bleeding.

Appendix

With the purchase of this book, you can use our "SN Flashcards" app to access questions free of charge in order to test your learning and check your understanding of the contents of the book.

To use the app, please follow the instructions below:

1. Go to https://flashcards.springernature.com/login
2. Create a user account by entering your e-mail address and assigning a password.
3. Use the following link to access your SN Flashcards set: ▶ https://sn.pub/tvlq7Q

If the link is missing or does not work, please send an e-mail with the subject "SN Flashcards" and the book title to customerservice@springernature.com.

References

1. Weiniger CF, Golovanevski L, Domb AJ, Ickowicz D. Extended release formulations for local anaesthetic agents. Anaesthesia. 2012;67(8):906–16.
2. Becker DE, Reed KL. Local anesthetics: review of pharmacological considerations. Anesth Prog. 2012;59(2):90–102.
3. Uttamani RR, Venkataram A, Venkataram J, Mysore V. Tumescent anesthesia for dermatosurgical procedures other than liposuction. J Cutan Aesthet Surg. 2020;13(4):275–82.
4. Coldiron B, Coleman WP III, Cox SE, Jacob C, Lawrence N, Kaminer M, Narins RS. ASDS guidelines of care for tumescent liposuction. Dermatol Surg. 2006;32:709–16.
5. Augustin M, Maier K, Sommer B, Sattler G, Herberger K. Double-blind, randomized, intraindividual comparison study of the efficacy of prilocaine and lidocaine in tumescent local anesthesia. Dermatology. 2010;221 248–52.
6. https://elearning.rcog.org.uk//easi-resource/preparing-instrumental-delivery/analgesia/performing-pudendal

Part II

Surgical Operations in the Art of Aesthetic Genital Surgery

Labiaplasty

9

Primum non nocerum ("first, do no harm").

Hippocrates

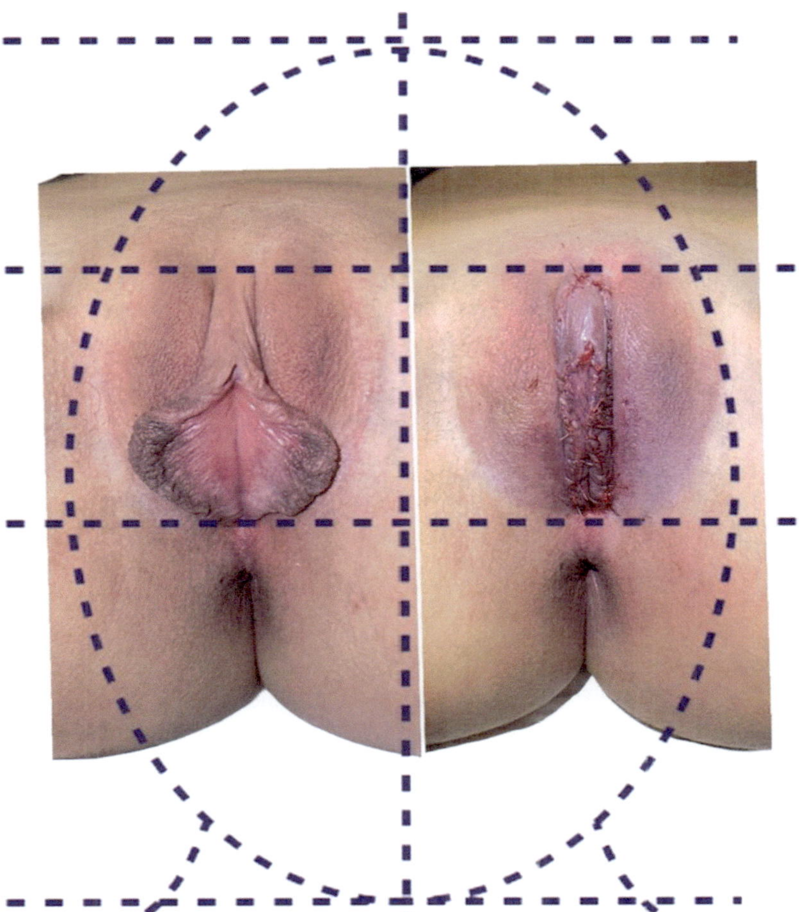

S. Eserdağ, *Aesthetic and Functional Female Genital Surgery*,
https://doi.org/10.1007/978-3-031-16019-6_9

Labiaplasty is an aesthetic surgery performed to reduce the size of the labia minora and to provide bilateral symmetry. It is also known as "labial reduction." In actuality, the term labiaplasty covers both internal and external genital labial aesthetics, but the term has mostly reserved for internal genital labia because these surgeries are much frequently performed. If we want to specify, the terms "labia minoraplasty" or "labia majoraplasty" should be used.

The labia minora are also known by names like "Nymphae" or "Labium Minus Pudendi." In France and some French-speaking regions of Canada, the term "Nymphoplastie" is more often used instead of the term labiaplasty.

9.1 Labiaplasty Indications

Labia minoraplasty is mostly performed for the purpose of eliminating hypertrophy, asymmetry, and aesthetic concerns that produce discontent, although there is no obvious structural problem. Deformities are often congenital and occur structurally (Table 9.1). However, excessive labial hyperpigmentations that develop over time, damages depending on vaginal deliveries, or Bartholin's gland cyst extirpations, deformities that may occur due to mechanical traumas such as traffic accidents, bicycle traumas, and falls may also be indications for labiaplasty. Although very rare, labiaplasty operations can be performed due to labial cysts, tumors, and varicose veins. Sometimes labiaplasty revision is performed in patients who have previously undergone labiaplasty operation but had undesirable results. Especially in recent years, in parallel with the increase in the number of operations performed, revision requests by patients have also increased.

Table 9.1 Labiaplasty indications for structural causes

Congenital defects
– Labial hypertrophy
– Asymmetry problems
– Congenital cysts and tumors
Acquired defects
– Excessive hyperpigmentation
– Development of labial cyst, tumor, and varicose veins
– Deformities due to vaginal deliveries, Bartholin's cyst extirpation, and mechanical blows by traffic accidents and straddle injuries, etc.
– Other iatrogenic problems

9.2 Labial Hypertrophy

Several classification systems have been proposed for labial hypertrophy. In the classification proposed by Franco and Franco in 1993, the length from the base of the labium to the tip is specified as below 2 cm (Type 1), 2–4 cm (Type 2), 4–6 cm (Type 3), and above 6 cm (Type 4) [1]. There are also those who consider 3 cm, 4 cm, or 5 cm and above as meeting labial hypertrophy criteria. In fact, when indicating labiaplasty, the physical complaints and emotional state of the patient should be considered rather than these measurements.

Labial hypertrophy is usually congenital and rarely acquired. Exposure to exogenous androgen hormones in childhood, sensitivity to topical estrogen, stretching the labia by pulling, dermatitis due to urinary incontinence, vulvar lymphedema (for example, Filaria sanguinis hominis infection involving lymph canal), and myelodysplastic diseases are acquired causes of labial hypertrophy. A high number of pregnancies can also cause hypertrophy [2].

Labial hypertrophy can cause psychological, cosmetic, hygienic, sexual, and functional problems. It can cause embarrassment and loss of self-esteem in some women. Excessively long and sagging labia cause pain due to stretch during sexual intercourse, chronic local irritation, hygiene problems during menstruation and after toileting, sweating and odor problems after exercise, irritation due to friction while wearing trousers, multidirectional urinary streaming, need for straining during urination, protrusion when wearing tight clothes, and may cause uncomfortable sensations while walking, cycling, and sitting [3]. Conversely, in our world where the use of social media and internet is widespread, the excesses of the internal labia can become larger in the mind and become an important focus problem that affects the whole life. Especially in Western society, it is the general expectation of patients that the labia minora do not protrude beyond the labia majora when standing and legs are closed. Having a straight cleft in the middle is accepted to be the ideal.

9.3 Labial Asymmetry

Labial asymmetry in women is quite common, just like in the breast and face. One side may be longer, thicker, more drooping, more in front, or a different color than the other. There may be asymmetrical appearances in the edges, frenulum, and hood structures. Also, if the base of one labium is located further forward or further back than the other, even if the metric lengths of both labia are the same, it may appear as if one is larger when viewed from the outside. These are the conditions that require the most surgical experience among labiaplasty surgeries.

The clitoral hood and frenulum regions on the labium side, which are hypertrophic in labial asymmetry, may also be hypertrophic (Fig. 9.1).

9.3.1 Labial Asymmetry Classification (Eserdag)

Labial asymmetry can be divided into four types according to the classification system as shown in Table 9.2.

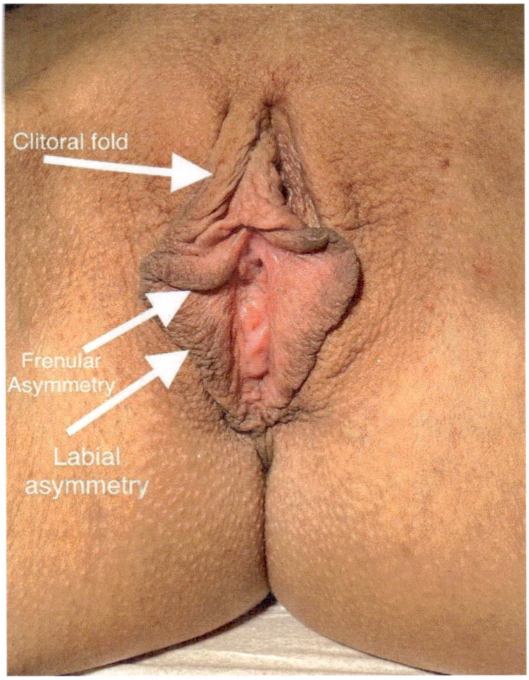

Fig. 9.1 Right labial asymmetry. In addition to the right labium, the right frenulum is hypertrophic, and there is even an extra fold of skin in the right clitoral hood. Therefore, the operation should be planned as bilateral equalization of all regions (labia, hood, and frenulum)

Sometimes a few type of asymmetries can be observed together.

According to our own observations, the visibly noticeable labial asymmetry rate is around 90% (Figs. 9.2, 9.3, 9.4, and 9.5) and needs different approaches.

In cases of asymmetry, pairing both labia with labiaplasty may be more difficult than labial hypertrophy alone.

Table 9.2 Labia Minora asymmetries (*Eserdag* classification) and management

Labial asymmetry classification (*Eserdag classification*)	Appearance	Surgical management
Type 1	Both labia are on the same plane, but one labium is more hypertrophic than the other. Hypertrophy can be in length or thickness. It is expressed based on the side of the larger labium. Right asymmetry if the right labium is larger, left asymmetry if the left labium is larger It is the most common and the easiest surgery to perform (Fig. 9.2a)	In a simple way, curvilinear resection can be performed by taking a mirror image after unilateral marking. Or, for those who want unilateral correction, equalization can be achieved by applying V-plasty to the hypertrophic labium
Type 2	Sizes can be the same or different. However, one labium is located more superior than the other. It is named according to the superiorly localized labium (Fig. 9.2b)	After unilateral marking, a mirror image is taken and curvilinear resection is applied
Type 3	Sizes can be the same or different. However, the bases of the labia connecting to the vulva are not in the same plane. One labium is more frontal than the other and is named according to the frontally localized labium. Operation is more difficult and requires advanced techniques compared to other types (Fig. 9.2c)	First, the skin fold that connects to the clitoral hood from the anterior labium is excised, then the labial edges are resected curvilinearly. In order for both labia to be seen equally when viewed from the outside the lower labium is left longer, and the upper labium is left shorter
Type 4 (unclassified)	The asymmetrical appearance may be different from the other three types. For example, some may have more serrated edges, darker color, or irregular structure	In this case, it is decided according to the condition of the tissue

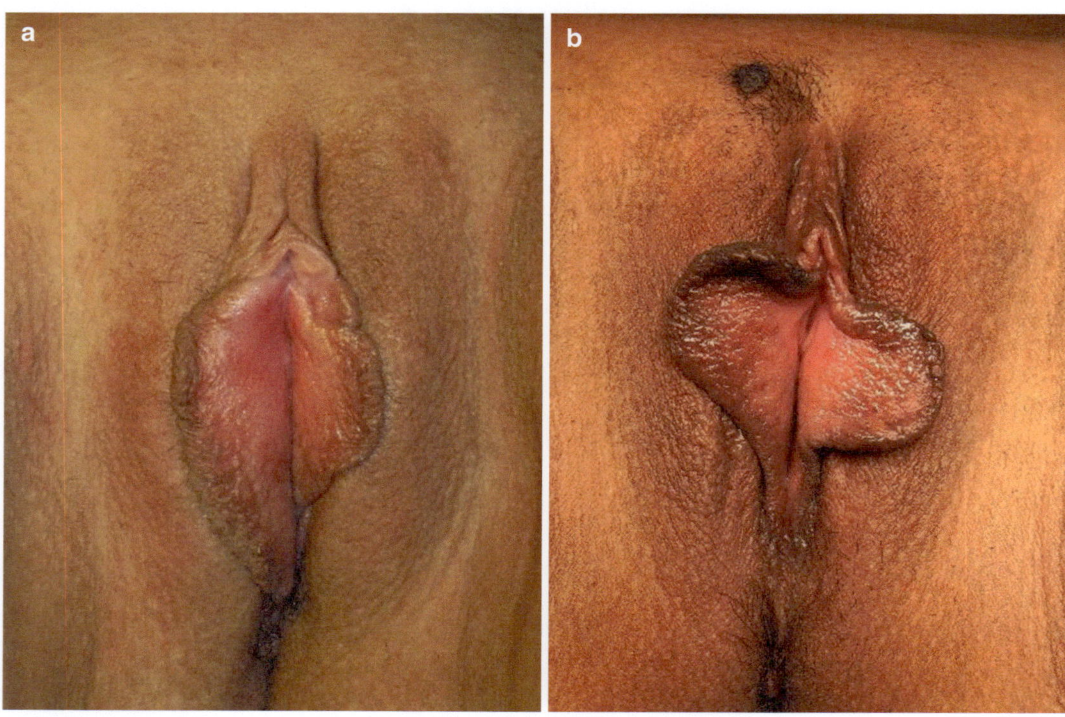

Fig. 9.2 Different labial asymmetry types. (**a**) Type 1 right asymmetry, (**b**) Type 2 right asymmetry, (**c**) Type 3 left asymmetry. (According to *Eserdag* Classification)

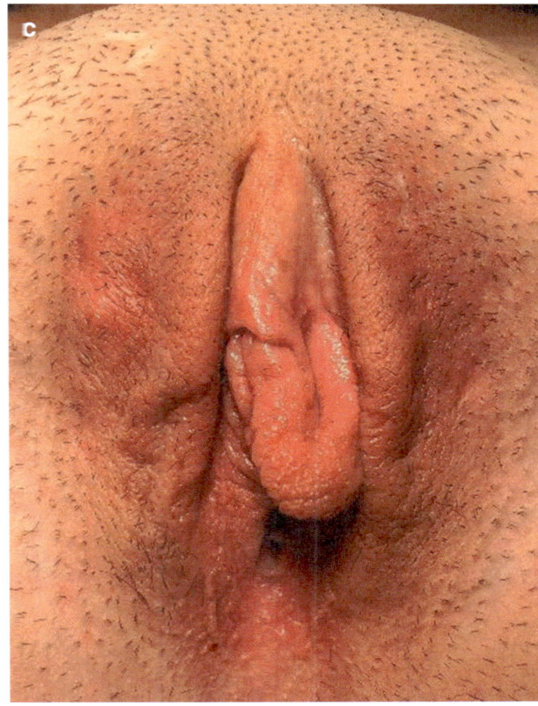

Fig. 9.2 (continued)

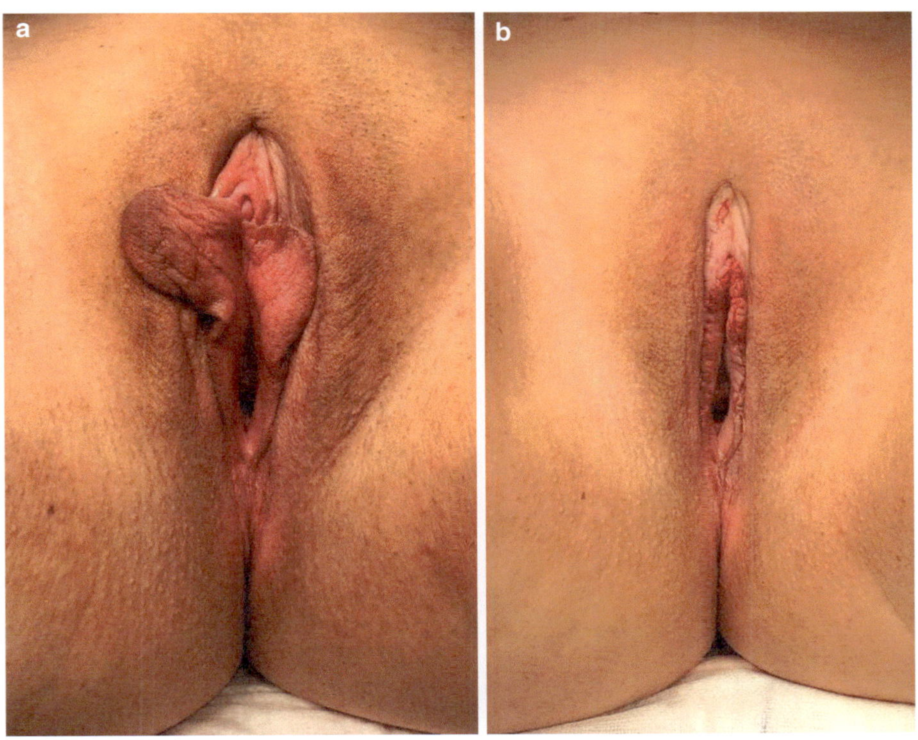

Fig. 9.3 Right labial asymmetry. (**a**). Equalization of the two regions by labiaplasty and clitoral hoodoplasty operations (**b**). Note that the clitoral border of the side with a larger labium is also more hypertrophic

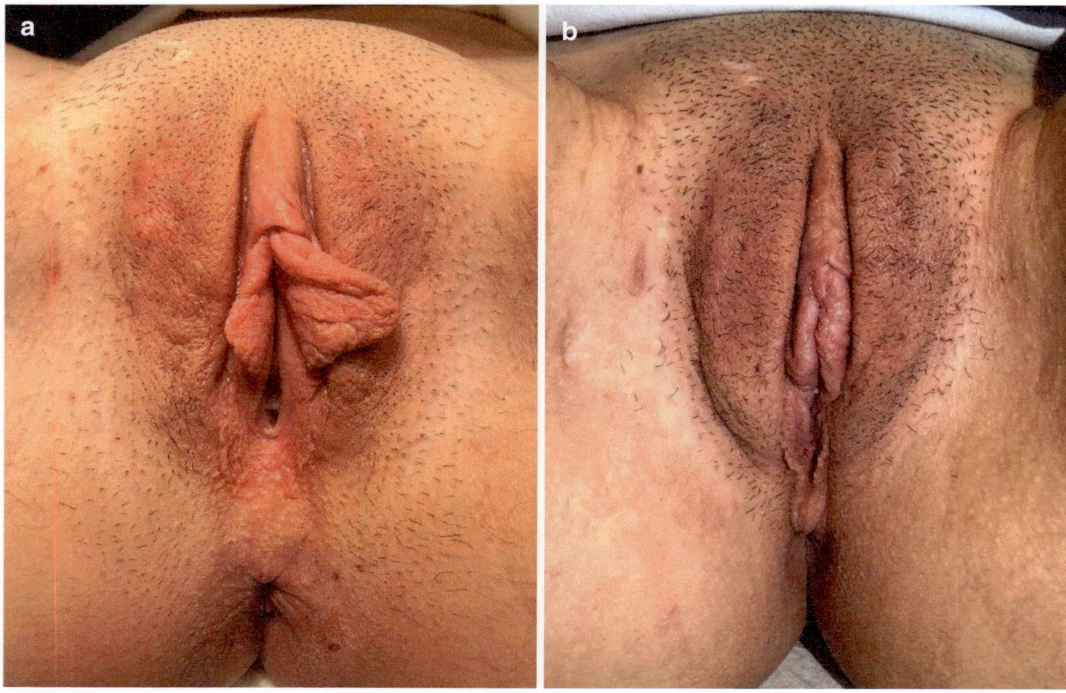

Fig. 9.4 Left labial asymmetry. Before (**a**) and 1.5 months after the surgery (**b**)

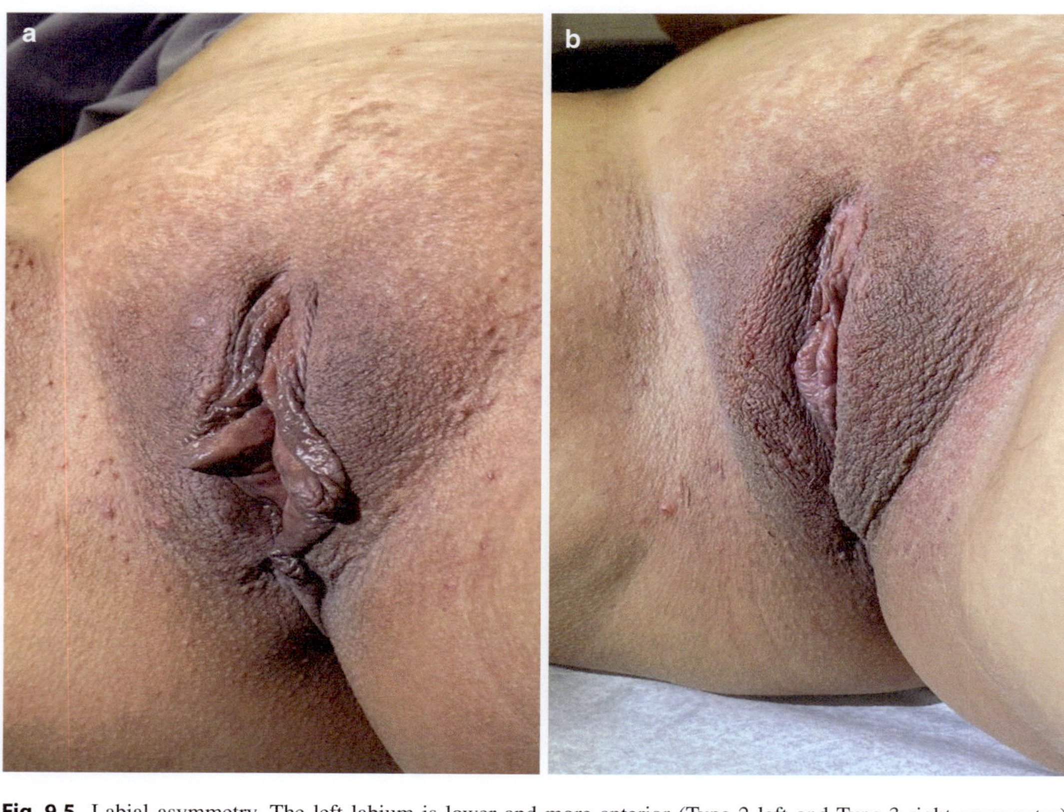

Fig. 9.5 Labial asymmetry. The left labium is lower and more anterior (Type 2 left and Type 3 right asymmetry). Appearances before (**a**, **c**) and 1 month after surgery (**b**, **d**)

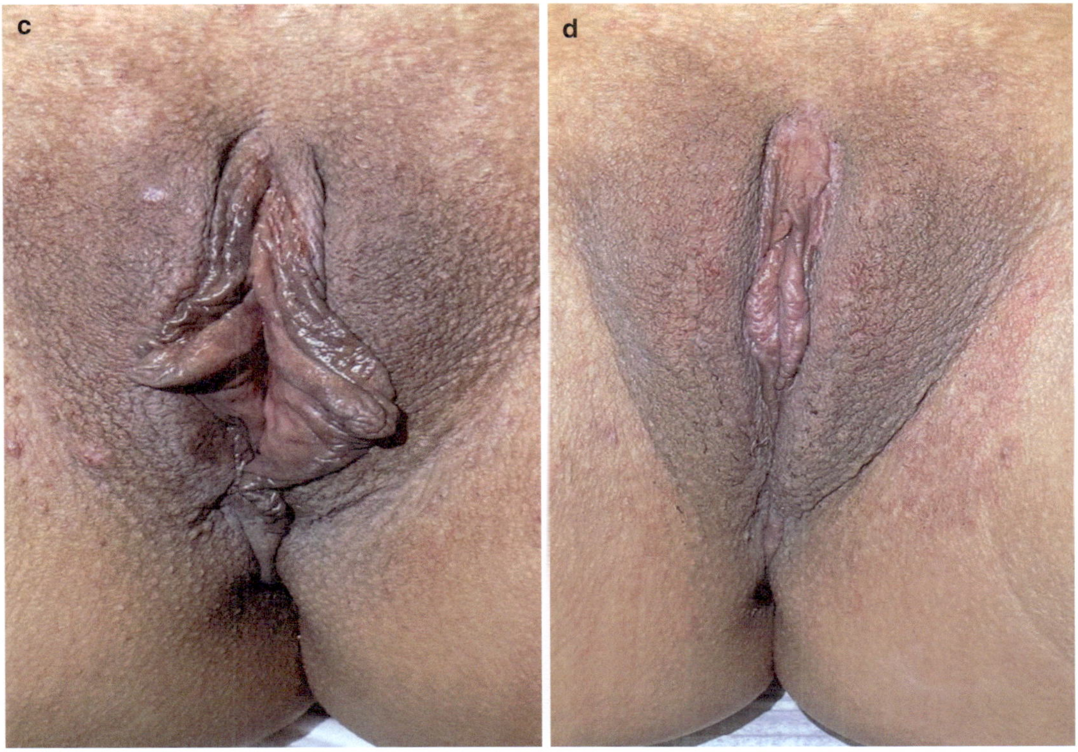

Fig. 9.5 (continued)

9.4 Other Psychological Causes

Some sexual traumas in childhood or adolescence can cause a desire for labiaplasty. The unconscious mechanism here may be the urge to *"be cleaned."* The surgeon planning the operation should try to understand the patient by asking different questions, to measure her expectations, and to discover whether her complaints are more psychological or functional by establishing empathy.

9.5 Operation Principles

When planning the labiaplasty operation, five important points should not be ignored:

1. Hypertrophic labia minora should be reduced.
2. Neurovascular structure should be preserved as much as possible.
3. Symmetry should be provided as much as possible.
4. Labial edges should be of optimal color and structure.
5. The vulva should be approached as a whole. If necessary, clitoral hoodoplasty, frenulaplasty, and perineoplasty procedures should be combined to labiaplasty.

It is a matter of debate whether the original (natural) edges on the lateral ends of the labia should be preserved. Some authors advocate that natural edges should be preserved so that nervous sensitivity does not decrease and the natural appearance is not lost. However, many patients are uncomfortable with the keratinized hyperpigmented appearance at the ends of the labia. It will be beneficial to consider the thoughts and demands of the patients while planning.

9.6 Historical Background

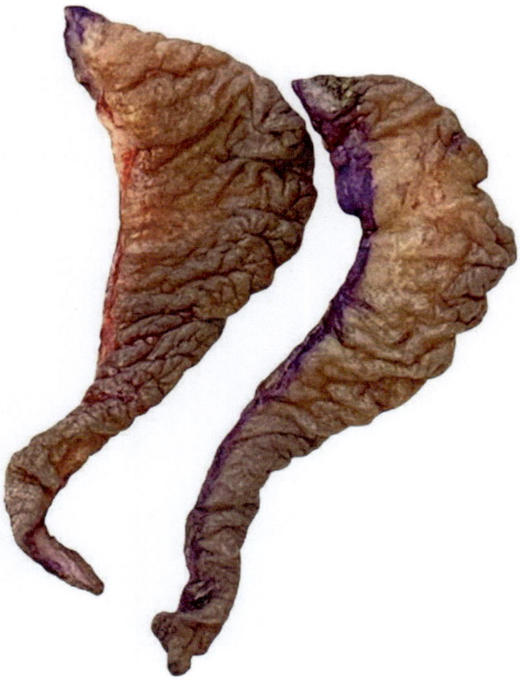

Labiaplasty is the most common aesthetic genital surgery in worldwide. Different techniques have been defined by different authors in the historical process (Table 9.3). However, no technique has a scientifically proven superiority over the others, and *there is no one-size-fits-all technique*. It is important for the physician performing the operation to have at least a few techniques mastered and to plan the operation in the most appropriate manner in accordance with the patient's tissue and wishes.

Preoperative evaluation and patient selection are described in Chap. 7.

Table 9.3 Labiaplasty techniques in the historical process [2]

Method	Author	Year	Number of patients	Indication	Advantages and disadvantages	Suture material
Elliptical incision	Hodgkinson	1983	3	– Difficulty in sexual intercourse – Shame	Easy	Prolene or chromic
Wedge incision	Alter	1998	4	– Shame	– Easy – Flexible planning	Vicryl
Posterior wedge excision	Rouzier	2000	163	– Aesthetic concern – Distress in sexual intercourse, exercise, and wearing pants	– Protection of free edges – Desired amount of tissue excision	Vicryl
	Munhoz	2006	21	– Shame – Poor hygiene – Difficulty in sexual intercourse		Absorbed sutures
	Alter	2008	407	– Shame – Pain during sexual intercourse – Lesions such as hemangioma	– Easy – Flexible planning	Monocryl
Zig Zag technique	Maas and Hage	2000	13		– Depigmentation	Absorbed sutures
De-epithelialization technique	Choi and Kim	2000	6	– Difficulty in sexual intercourse – Shame – Poor hygiene	– Preservation of natural color – Protection of labial edges – Preservation of vascular-nerve innervation	Catgut
Double wedge technique (star labiaplasty)	Matarasso	2011	8	– Shame	– During the surgery, incision can be made from different places	Chromic and Vicryl (sometimes dermabond)

9.7 Labiaplasty Techniques

Labiaplasty operations can be performed in different ways according to the condition of the patient's tissue, the patient's demands, and the surgeon's experience (Fig. 9.6).

These techniques are:

- *Curvilinear excision (Labial Trimming, Partial Resection)*
- *Wedge Resection (V-plasty)*
- *Extended Central Wedge Resection*
- *Bilateral De-epithelialization*
- *Zigzag Technique*
- *Modified Double Wedge Resection (Star labiaplasty)*
- *Laser Labiaplasty*

9.7.1 Curvilinear Excision

This is a slight elliptical removal of the edges of the labia. It is one of the most preferred techniques today. It is also known as "curvilinear amputation," "labial trimming," "edge trimming," and "partial resection." The first labiaplasty surgery in the literature was performed by Hodgkinson and Hait in 1984 with the curvilinear excision technique with the indication of social embarrassment and numbness during sexual intercourse.

In the partial resection technique, after the area to be operated on is cleaned with iodized solution and covered with sterile drapes, the area to be cut (in its own position) is marked with a skin marker without stretching. Afterward, a local anesthetic drug containing epinephrine is injected into the subcutaneous area about 0.5 cm laterally from the base of the labium. If the local anesthetic solution is diluted at a rate of 50–60%, the dose to be applied and the possibility of side effects related to this dose decrease. Local infiltration can be done with a 30G or fine dental needle.

Cutting can be done with scalpel, radiofrequency (RF), or Metzenbaum scissors. Cutting with laser or cautery is not recommended because of thermal energy damage to the adjacent tissue. Monopolar or less traumatic bipolar cautery for adjacent tissue can be used for post-incision hemostasis. Washing the tissue with 3% H_2O_2 (hydrogen peroxide) solution after the incision will be beneficial in terms of cleaning and disinfection of the surgical area.

In labiaplasty, when closing the subcutaneous tissue, round needle 4/0 and, when closing the skin, 5/0 rapid absorbable monofilament or polypropylene suture materials with sharp needles should be preferred. For the frenulum area, 6/0 rapid absorbable sutures can be used. Patients with thick subcutaneous tissue should be closed in two, sometimes even three layers without leaving a dead space. If there is an individual or regular incision line under the skin, it should be sutured continuously. The skin should generally be sutured continuously and without locking. It will be beneficial if the stitch intervals are tight. The suturing should be done without stretching the threads. After the skin is closed, extra security can be provided with one-by-one blocker sutures. Intradermal closure of the skin is not recommended due to the risk of dehiscence (Fig. 9.7).

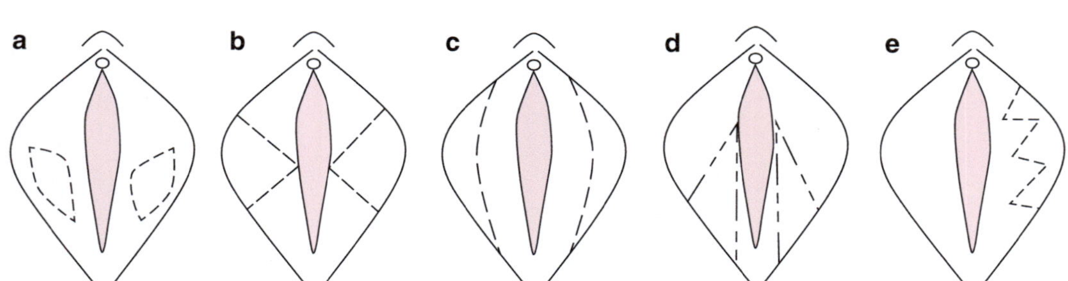

Fig. 9.6 Labiaplasty techniques with simplified narration. (**a**) De-epithelialization, (**b**) central wedge resection, (**c**) partial resection, (**d**) inferior wedge resection superior flap, (**e**) zigzag technique

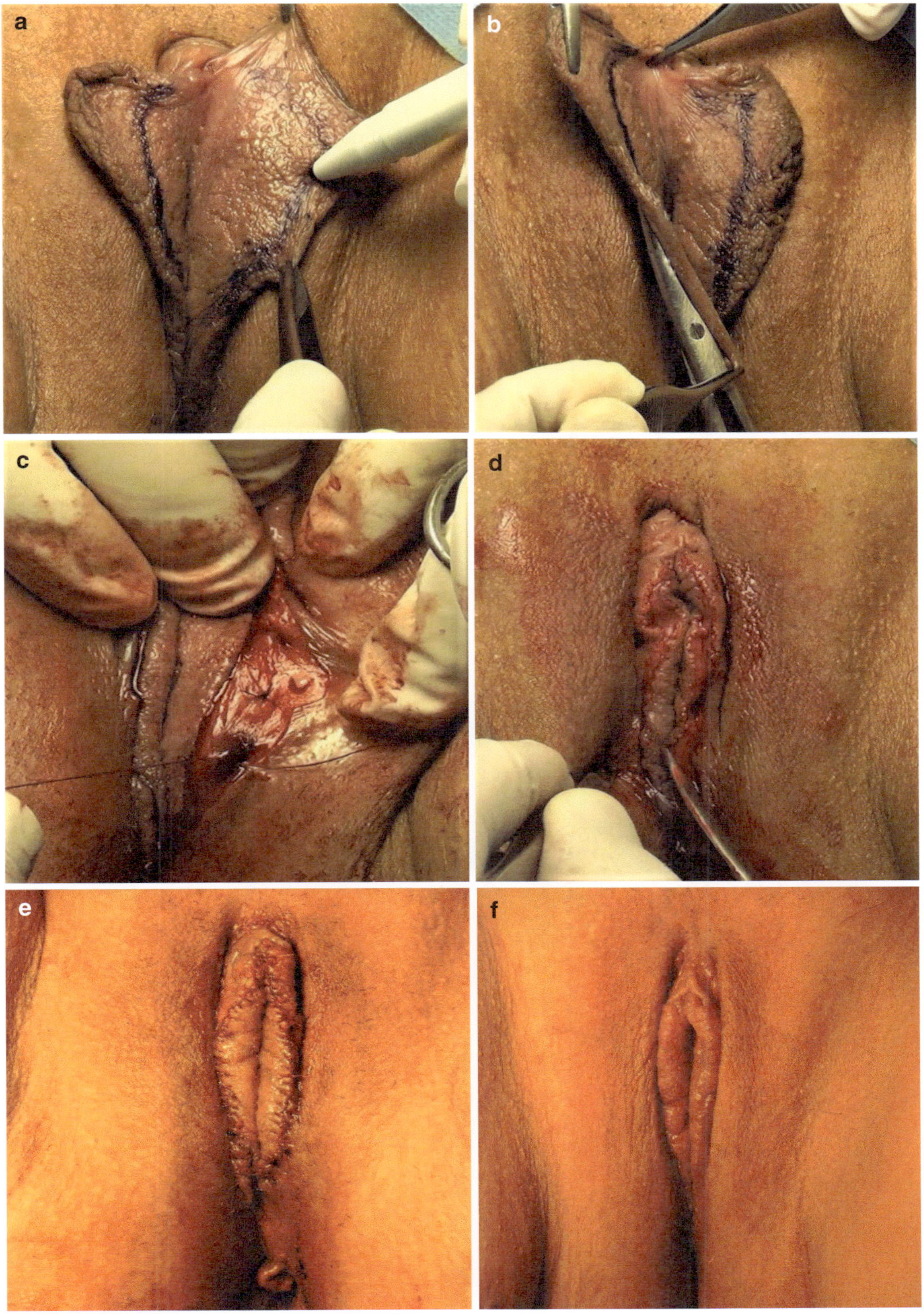

Fig. 9.7 A labiaplasty operation performed with curvilinear excision. Marking (**a**) and cutting the tissue with scissors (**b**). Subcutaneous closure with single sutures (**c**) and skin tissue closure with continuous sutures (**d**). Appearances just after the surgery (**e**) and 1 month later (**f**)

Step-by-step labiaplasty operation is outlined in Table 9.4.

In many studies, it has been suggested that the width of the labial tissue remaining after linear excision should not be less than one cm [4].

Table 9.4 The main stages of the labiaplasty operation

• Obtain pre-surgery images
• Mark the area
• Apply local anesthetic infiltration containing epinephrine to the area
• Cut out the marked area. *Do not stretch the tissue while cutting!*
• Re-trim with fine scissors the areas you see as excess after cutting
• Clean the incision area with H_2O_2
• Provide hemostasis by cauterizing open-ended vessels (bipolar cautery may be preferred)
• Approximate the subcutaneous tissues (4/0 or 5/0 suture materials)
• Close the skin (5/0 suture materials)
• Obtain post-surgery images
• Cover the surgical area by dressing with antibiotic ointments and take the patient to rest

Otherwise, urine may be distributed in different directions while toileting due to urethral orifice distortion. It is also beneficial not to extend the surgical excision to the posterior fourchette in order not to shrink the vaginal introitus. As a matter of fact, stiffness and tension due to perineal skin excision can cause sensitivity during sexual intercourse or perineal granuloma fissuratum.

In patients operated on under general or regional anesthesia, open vessels that do not bleed due to hypotension may be activated in the early postoperative period and cause bleeding. Therefore, all open vessels should be cauterized carefully and dead spaces should be closed. In addition, the hypotensive state can be made normotensive, and the subcutaneous can be closed after hemostasis is achieved.

In the curvilinear trimming technique, the structure and color of the original edges are not preserved (Fig. 9.8). Partial cutting is applied regardless of the localization of the vessels and nerves. Theoretically, although concerns are expressed that the sensitivity due to scar forma-

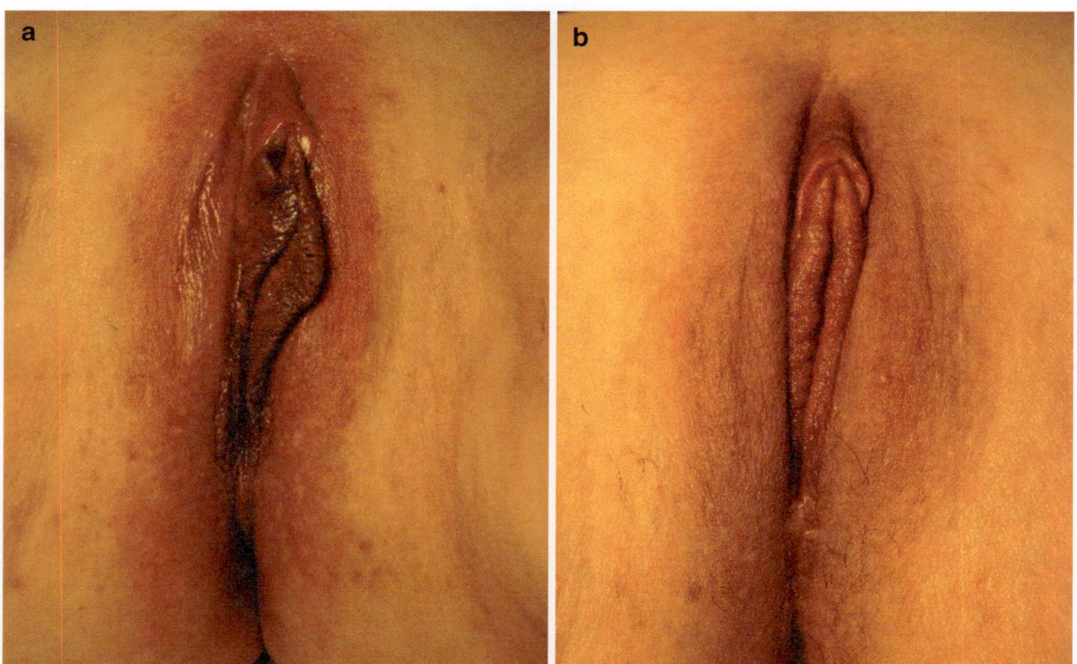

Fig. 9.8 Curvilinear labiaplasty. Hoodoplasty and skin perineoplasty were also performed, and the color of the original edges is not preserved. Before (**a**) and 1.5 months after surgery (**b**)

tion may be adversely affected after the incision made along the longitudinal line, such situations are rarely encountered in practice. It is an advantageous aspect of this technique that it allows excessive tissue removal especially in cases of severe hypertrophy.

One of the most common mistakes made in curvilinear labiaplasty operations is holding the labia longitudinally with curved or straight clamps before cutting. In this case, the remaining tissue will be damaged and the incision line will not be formed properly. Labia with excessive wrinkles should never be grasped with a Kocher Clamp before the incision.

In partial labiaplasty, two suggestions can be made for the new labial margins formed after the operation to not remain thick. The first is that the incision is made not perpendicular to the labial edges, but with a 45-degree inclination, and the other is that the subcutaneous tissue is thinned by trimming sufficiently after the incision. To sharpen the edge ends by inclining, it will be more appropriate to make the incision with an RF device or a scalpel. If the incision is made with scissors, it is more difficult to incline.

9.7.2 Wedge Resection (V-Plasty)

This is a technique that was first described by Gary Alter in 1998 with four cases [5]. Wherever there is a lot of excess tissue, the labia minora are reduced by resection in the form of a wedge (letter V). Wedge resection can be done from the upper, middle, or lower segment of the labium.

For the wedge resection (V-plasty) technique, the area to be operated on is first cleaned with iodized solution and covered with sterile drapes. The area to be removed is marked in a V shape with a skin marker. Later, the area is numbed with local anesthetics, as in curvilinear excision. After the tissue is excised, hemostasis is provided with bipolar cautery. Care should be taken not to impair circulation. Then the labia are closed in at least three layers. First, the subcutaneous tissue, then the inner and outer skin layers of the labia minora are sutured one by one or continuously with sutures that are absorbable in a short time such as 5/0 Monocryl. Critical areas can be supplemented with additional delayed absorbable sutures to prevent dehiscence (Fig. 9.9).

Tissue to be removed in a triangular shape in V-plasty should not be grasped with straight clamps before cutting. Otherwise, the remaining tissue will be damaged and the risk of dehiscence will increase.

With wedge resection, the original edges and colors of the labia can be preserved. However, because the two ends are brought closer to each other after resection, color contrast can also occur in the labial tissue. Some of the patients who undergo wedge resection may return to their surgeons in the future, demanding further reduction.

In the wedge resection technique, if the tissue is stretched too much, there are risks of dehiscence or windowing (fenestration) due to tissue avascularization. Therefore, it is essential to be meticulous during the operation. The following images show the stages of the surgery.

In cases where hypertrophy and darkening of the original edges are not evident, if there is a unilateral asymmetry problem, V-plasty can be performed unilaterally. Conversely, in some cases, V-plasty can be combined with a partial trimming technique in the same session (edge-wedge technique).

Unilateral V-plasty will be an appropriate choice, especially if the labial edges are regular and there is unilateral asymmetry (Fig. 9.10).

The postoperative healing process is faster and more comfortable in terms of pain in labiaplasty operations performed with V-plasty technique compared to partial resection.

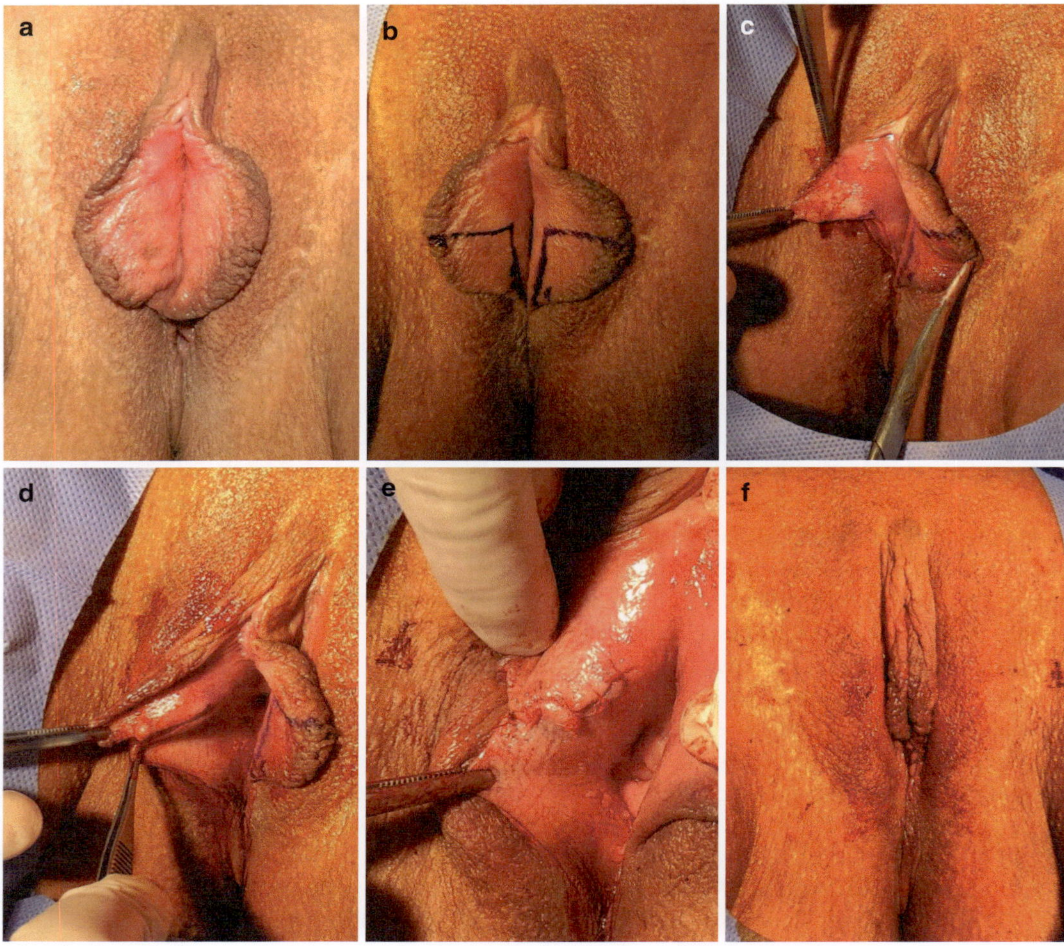

Fig. 9.9 Stage-by-stage lower segment V-plasty operation. Before the operation (**a**), marking (**b**), wedge resection (**c**), reapproximation of the submucosa by sutures after the hemostasis (**d**), closure of the internal labial mucosa and the external labial skin (**e**), just after (**f**)

9.7.3 Extended Central Wedge Resection

Gary Alter published a large series of 407 patients he operated on with the indication of aesthetic anxiety in 2008 [6]. In this technique, after removing the excess tissue with the classical wedge technique, clitoral hoodoplasty is added to the labiaplasty with the external wedge (hockey stick) made by extending the incision laterally and anteriorly (Fig. 9.11).

If wedge resections are done well, a rapid recovery is observed and postoperative comfort in terms of pain is also very high. However, if the correct technique is not applied, complications such as suture opening, scar formation due to tissue necrosis, and labial fenestration (windowing) can be seen. These situations are generally associated with the surgical technique. There are two important considerations to be done in order not to disturb the blood circulation of the tissue and to prevent suture opening (dehiscence). The first

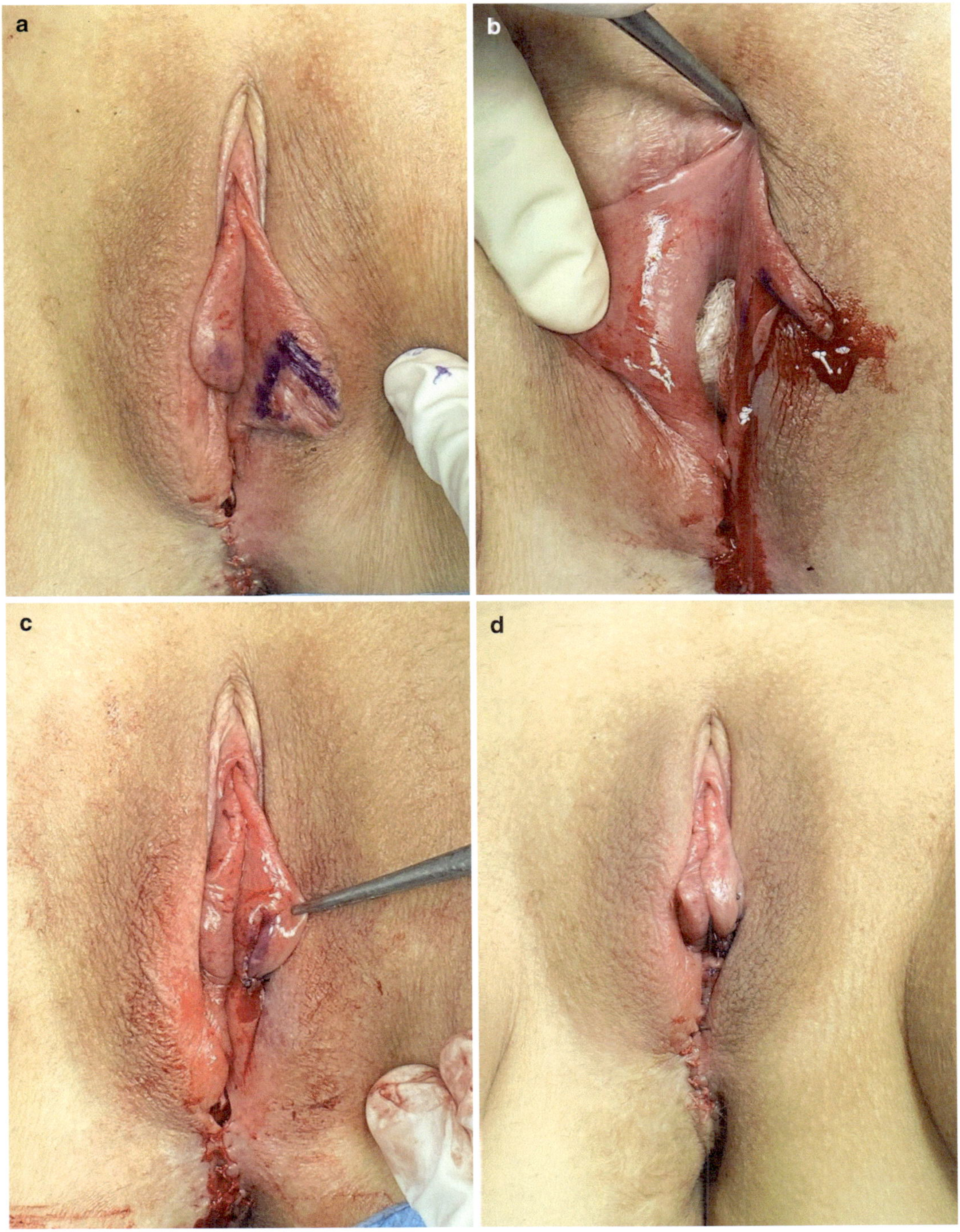

Fig. 9.10 Unilateral V-plasty. Marking of the left labium (**a**), excision of the excess tissue (**b**), repair of the incision in three layers (**c**), just after (**d**)

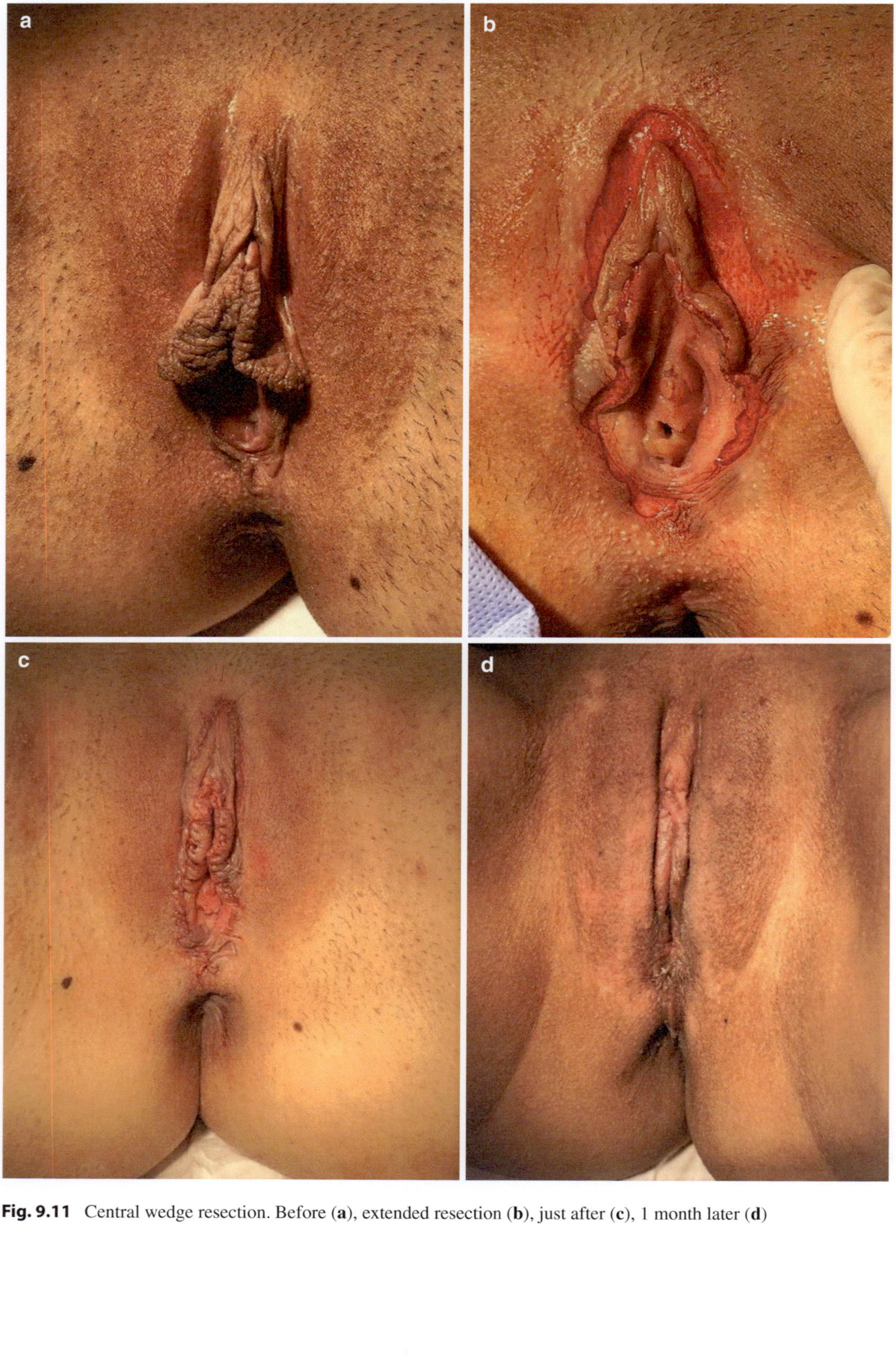

Fig. 9.11 Central wedge resection. Before (**a**), extended resection (**b**), just after (**c**), 1 month later (**d**)

is to provide good subcutaneous hemostasis. As a matter of fact, if hemostasis is not well achieved, sutures can open due to subcutaneous hematoma. The second is that no tension (pressure) is imposed on the reassembled tissues after V excision. If tension is placed on the reassembled labial parts, the risks of postoperative dehiscence and labial fenestration increase due to avascularization. Another important issue is that the surgical margins to be removed in the V shape are not held with Kocher clamps to prevent injury.

Wedge resection may be a suitable alternative in cases where the natural edges of the labia minora are smooth, not too thick or dark colored, or in cases of asymmetry requiring intervention in only one labium. Conversely, in order to determine the poorly vascularized area in V-plasty, a cold light source is used behind the labium in a dim environment with the transillumination technique, and after the vessel traces are determined, cutting can be performed. Thus, labial circulation will be less affected [7].

9.7.4 Bilateral De-epithelialization

This technique was first proposed in 2000 by Choi and Kim. A kind of epithelial peeling (de-epithelialization) is performed by cutting the areas with the most tissue excess both inside and outside the labia [8]. It is also called "delamination."

In this technique, unlike others, all original labial edges are preserved. Since the incision is not made completely, all vessels and nerves of the labia are protected. The disadvantage is the risk of scar formation. Also, only the vertical length of the labium is shortened. Therefore, it is not a suitable method for large labia. Conversely, tumescence and swelling may occur at the base and the appearance of hypertrophic tissue edges can cause psychological problems in the patient.

De-epithelialization can be a good alternative for patients whose labial width is not large, whose labial thickness is thin, and who are satisfied with their original edges and want them to be protected.

9.7.5 Zigzag Technique

This is a method defined by Maas and Hage with 13 patients. The edges are completely removed with a continuous zigzag incision applied to the labial edges. The aim is to make labial edges round. However, there is a loss of pigmentation along the labial edge. Maas and Hage also stated that the excision should not be extended to the clitoral hood and fourchette, and a minimum of 1 cm of tissue is left at the same time.

9.7.6 Modified Double Wedge Resection (Star Labiaplasty)

Star labiaplasty is a technique that was first described by Matarasso in 2011. It is also known as the double wedge technique. In this modified wedge technique, a star-shaped incision is made in the labium and excess tissue is removed.

9.7.7 Laser Labiaplasty

"Laser labiaplasty" is called when the cutting is done by laser light (Fig. 9.12). CO_2, potassium titanyl phosphate (KTP), Erbium:YAG, and Nd:YAG lasers are most frequently used in AGS. When CO_2 lasers are used, cutting is per-

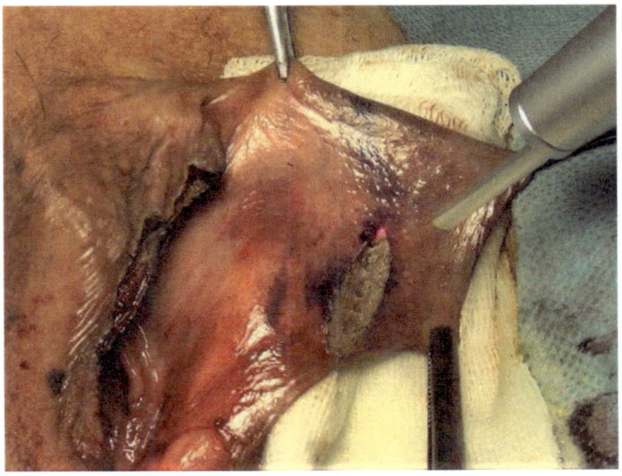

Fig. 9.12 Laser labiaplasty is performed by placing wet gauze behind the labium and excising the labia with laser's cutting probe

formed with 15–20 Watt energy. Patients find laser operations more acceptable (regardless of where on the body); the term *"laser labiaplasty"* is also attractive to patients. Laser labiaplasty surgeries are preferred to reduce bleeding. However, according to my observations, thermal damage in the adjacent tissues negatively affects the postoperative healing process in laser labiaplasty procedures. Moreover, manipulation of the laser coagulation and cutting apparatus is difficult. Different regions can be coagulated inadvertently.

In laser labiaplasty, the laser functions as continuous beat cutting and remote and intermittent beat coagulation. Nevertheless, cautery may be required where laser coagulation is not sufficient.

9.8 Labiaplasty According to Patient Expectations: *"Queens, Princesses, and Venuses" (Eserdag)*

We divide our patients who are considering labiaplasty into three groups according to their personality structures and surgery expectations: Queens, Princesses, and Venuses. This approach, somewhat witty, will guide the surgeon in terms of planning the operation to be performed and meeting the expectations fully. The surgeon performing the aesthetic operation should have an approach that suits the expectations of each patient, just like a tailor, because *"one size doesn't fit all."*

9.8.1 Queens

The queens, whose ages are generally over 40, prefer to remain as minimally invasive in their operations as possible and avoid taking too much risk with radical procedures. Their aim is to feel comfortable in functional aspects rather than aesthetics. Simple labial reductions due to their *"natural"* structure will meet the expectations of the queens (Fig. 9.13). After the operation, there is no problem if the inner lips extend slightly beyond the outer lips. Most of the time, they do not need a clitoral hoodoplasty operation or they avoid the operations on this area. This group says, *"I do not want to touch the clitoral area at all, surgery on that area scares me a lot, a slight recovery from my inner lips will be enough for me."* V-plasty operations may be a suitable option for them. In this way, labial reductions will be provided and the natural edges of the lips will be preserved. A superficial trimming (edge trimming) can also be done.

Queens mostly consider non-surgical procedures in the forefront among other genital aesthetic applications.

9.8.2 Princesses

The main purpose of princesses, who are generally in the age group of 30 and above, is to feel comfortable both aesthetically and functionally. However, the amount of inner lips remaining after surgery is neither as much as in queens nor as small as in Venuses. For princesses, it is sufficient to keep the inner genital lips at the same level with the outer lips (Fig. 9.14). A light partial trimming will meet their needs most of the time. In this way, the inner lips will be reduced and the keratinized, dark, and wrinkled edges will be eliminated. Although they do not know exactly what they want, they have a moderately cautious approach such as *"Doctor, I want to leave my surgery to you, but I do not want my lips to be removed in an exaggerated way."*

Princesses, whose thoughts are not very clear and who are in limbo while making many decisions in their lives, may knock on their doctor's door again after the surgery and request a revision such as *"I actually wanted my inner lips to be shortened more and not to be seen from the outside."*

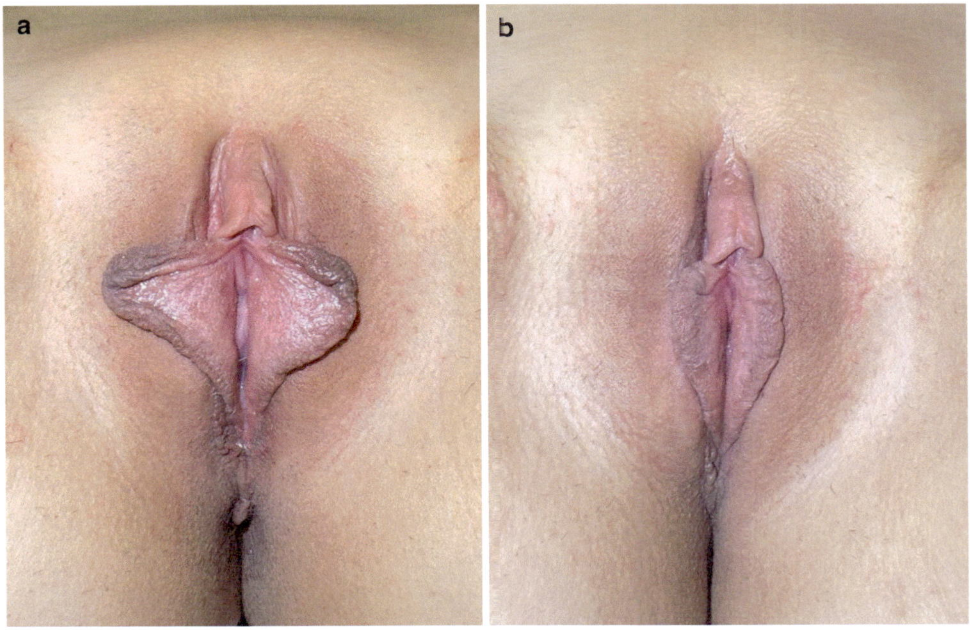

Fig. 9.13 Queen look labiaplasty. Before (**a**), 3 months after surgery (**b**). Labial edges were trimmed, but the clitoral hood was not reduced because the patient wanted a "natural look"

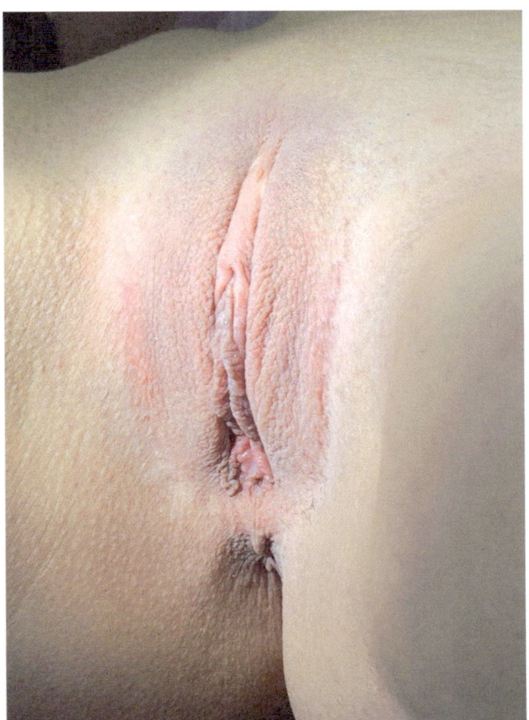

Fig. 9.14 Princess look labiaplasty. Appearance 1 year after labiaplasty surgery. The inner labia are level with the outer labia but do not protrude

9.8.3 Venuses

This is the most desired labial appearance in Western societies, and more than 90% of patients prefer the *Venus vagina* appearance including maximum labial reduction. The pornography industry in particular has idealized the rather short and pink appearance of labia. Although patients who desire a Venus vagina appearance are generally younger in age, they cover all age groups. In the Venus look, the inner lips are very short (often 0.5 cm or less) and are located inside the outer lips, invisible from the outside (Fig. 9.15). The clitoral hood is sometimes very slightly pronounced; sometimes it is inside the outer lips. Venuses, who take great care of their aesthetic appearance, are keen-minded about their labia to say, "*I've seen them for years, I don't want to see them anymore.*" The total excision of the labia is more of a "labiectomy" than a cosmetic operation and may lead to some negative consequences. For this reason, after the labia are resected, they should not be less than 0.5 cm.

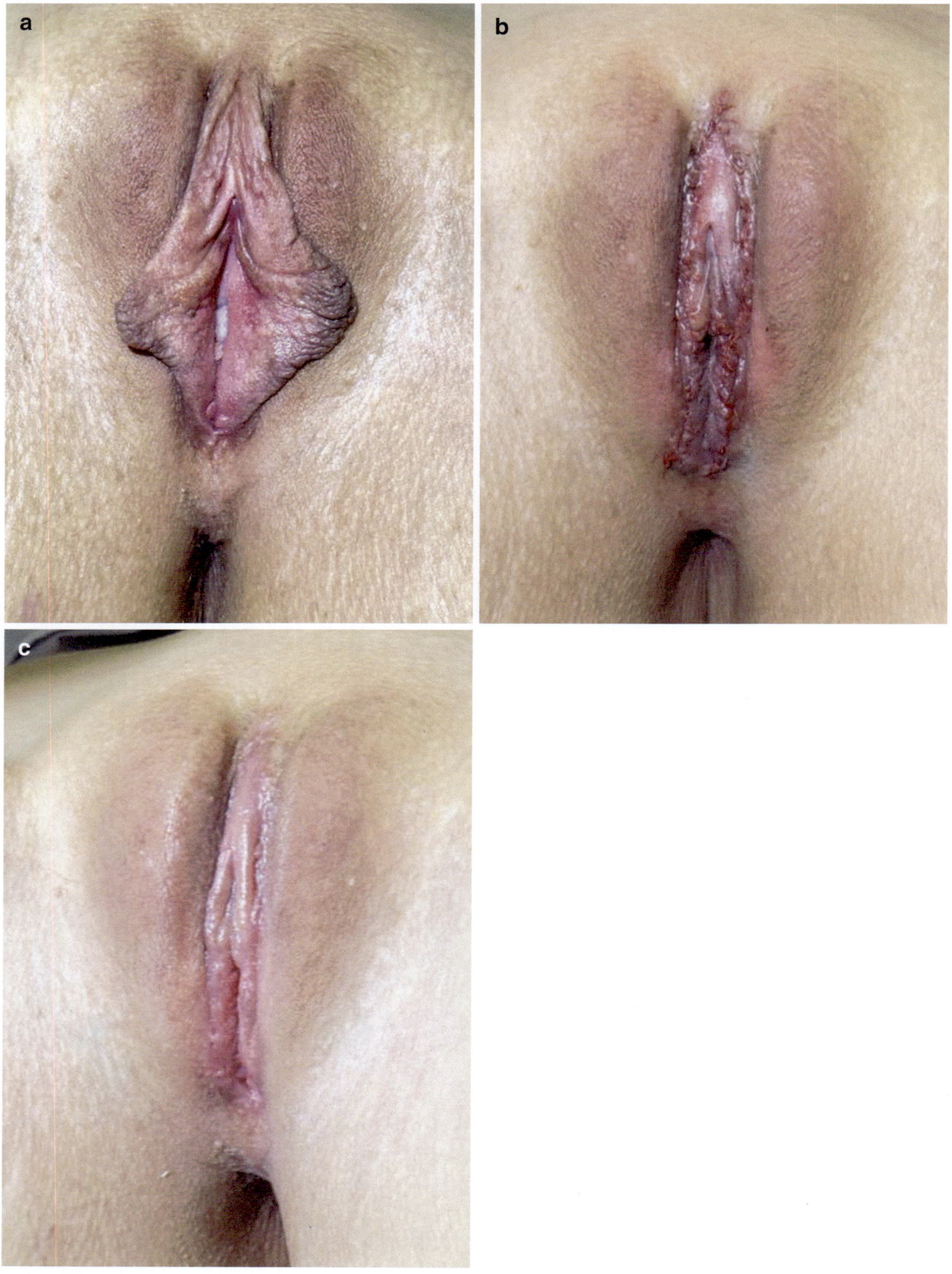

Fig. 9.15 Venus look labiaplasty. Before (**a**), just after (**b**), and 2 months later (**c**)

9.9 *Eserdag* 'Venus Vagina' Aesthetics Concept

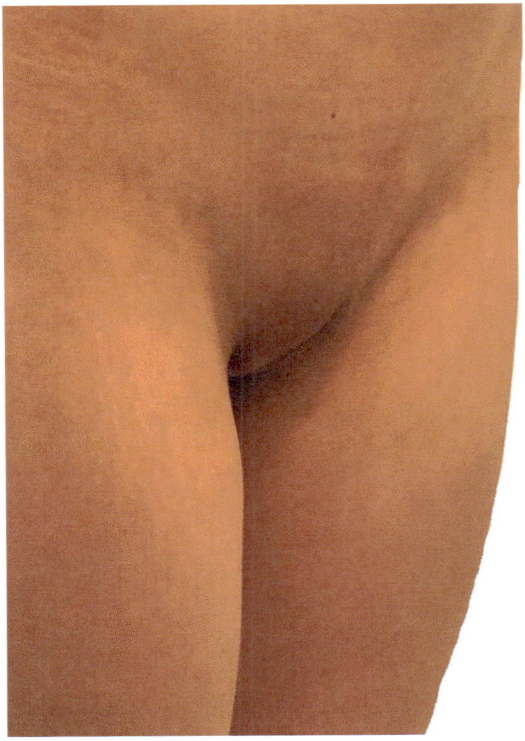

Venus is a Roman goddess, whose functions encompass love, beauty, desire, sex, fertility, prosperity, and victory. In the later classical tradition of the West, Venus became one of the most widely referenced deities of Greco-Roman mythology as the embodiment of love and sexuality. She is usually depicted nude in paintings."Venus vagina" is a term coined by us, describing the maximum shortening of the inner lips in labiaplasty. We have included some features into this technique.

The features of the "*Eserdag Venus Labiaplasty*" technique (Figs. 9.16 and 9.17) are as follows:

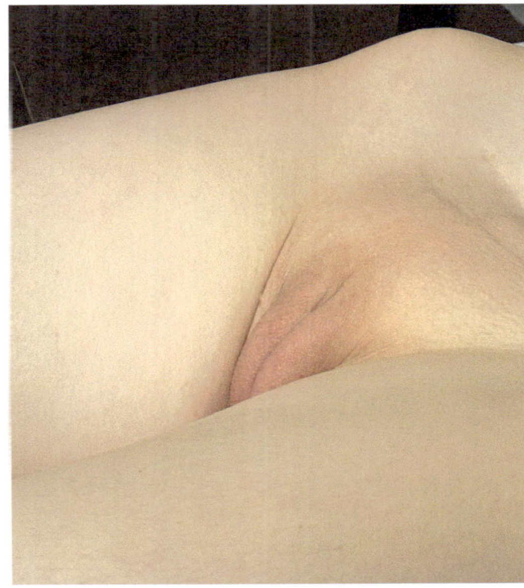

Fig. 9.16 "Eserdag Venus Labiaplasty" involving labiaplasty by trimming method, hoodoplasty by inverted-Y technique, and labia majora autologous fat transfer (postoperative second month)

- Shortening the labia minora as much as possible (maximum reduction)
- Clitoral hoodoplasty (maximum trimming of the clitoral hood with inverted Y-plasty technique)
- Augmentation of labia majora by autologous fat transfer or hyaluronic acid fillers (if the majora are too much thin or collapsed)

The purpose of Eserdag Venus labiaplasty is to prevent any tissue protruding outside while the person is standing or sitting position with closed legs, and to have only a thin, sexy line called "Venus Cleft" in the middle. The level of satisfaction with this appearance, which is frequently desired by patients, especially in recent years, is also very high.

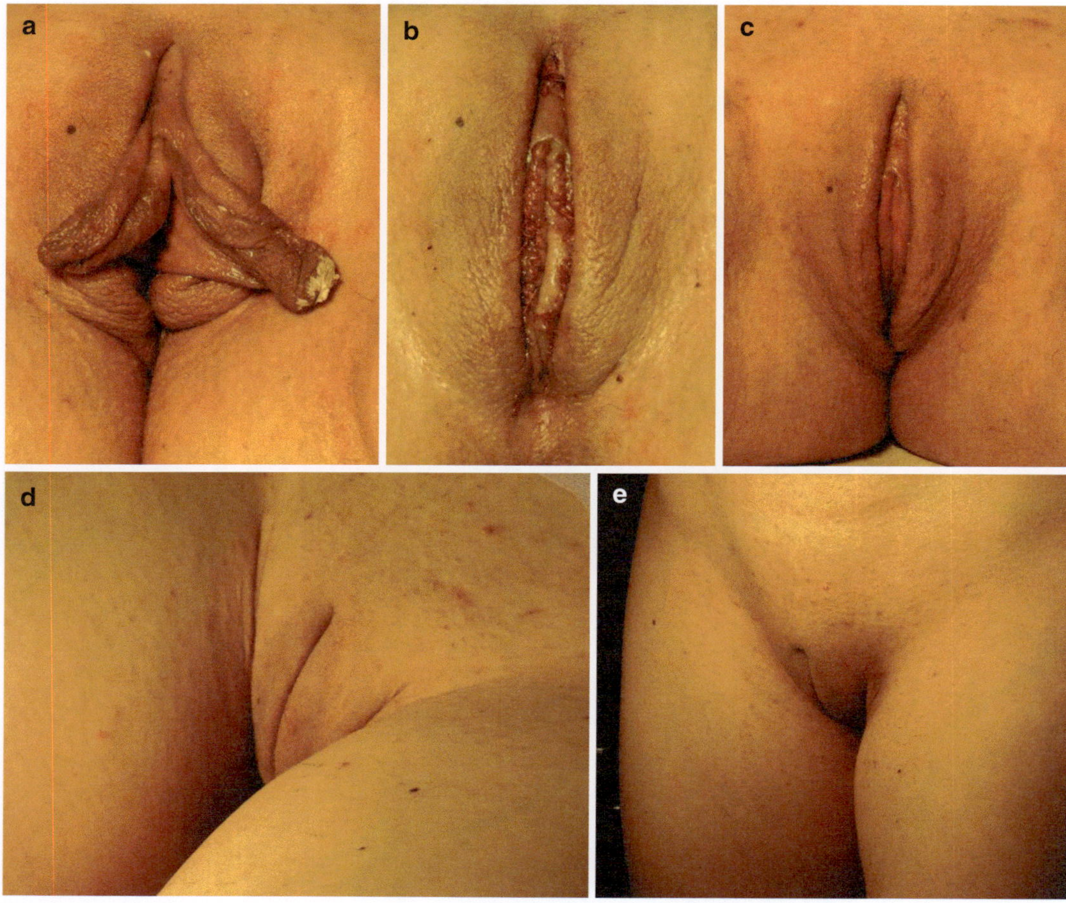

Fig. 9.17 The "Venus appearance" after labiaplasty. Before (**a**), just after (**b**), 1.5 months later in different positions (**c–e**)

One of the most important components in labiaplasty surgeries is the clitoral hoodoplasty operation, i.e., the trimming of the clitoral hood area, which is recommended to be done simultaneously (Fig. 9.18). In most patients, when only labiaplasty is performed, the dislocation of the clitoral area manifests itself more clearly, and this can be aesthetically uncomfortable. Clitoral hoodoplasty operations require more experience than labiaplasty surgeries.

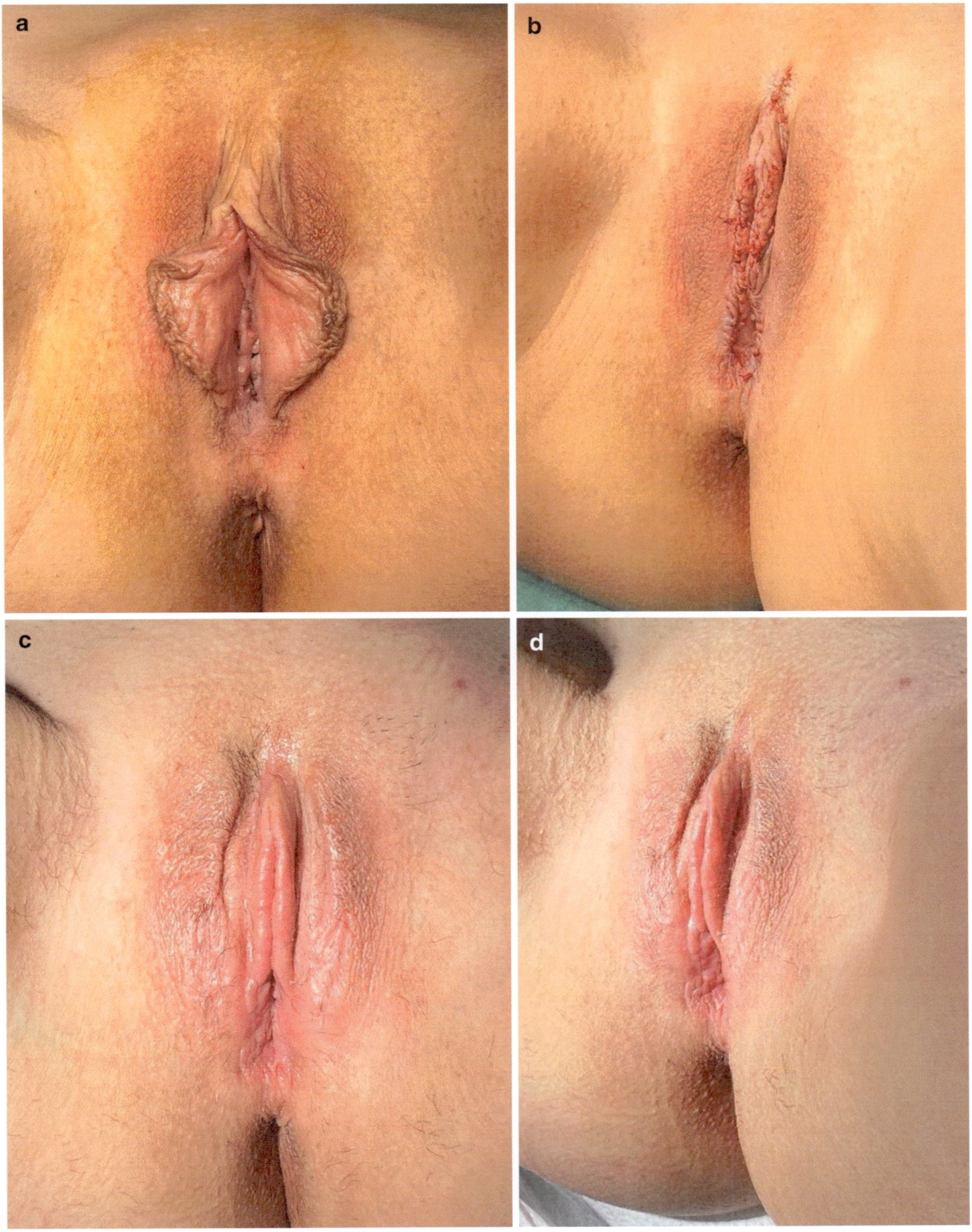

Fig. 9.18 A patient who underwent labiaplasty and inverted-Y clitoral hoodoplasty. Before (**a**), just after (**b**), 1.5 months later (**c**, **d**)

9.10 Office Labiaplasty

Labiaplasty operations can be performed in office conditions. The advantageous aspects are that the operation can be performed at noon, the patient does not have to go hungry, and the does not enter the hospital procedures and environment. However, for office labiaplasty, it is also important to have sufficient team and equipment support, to create hygienic conditions, and for the patient to have no chronic diseases such as asthma and heart disease. In addition, since the procedure will be performed under local anesthesia, the anxiety level of the patient is also important. In severely anxious patients, one should not insist on performing the operation under local anesthesia. The stages of preparation for the surgery in office labiaplasty and what can be done to increase the comfort of the surgery are listed below (Table 9.5).

9.11 Combined Procedures

A holistic approach is important in vulva aesthetics. For some, a simple labiaplasty is sufficient, while for others, procedures such as labiaplasty, clitoral hoodoplasty, frenulaplasty, and perineoplasty are required to be performed together. After general information is given to the patient during the examination, operations such as vaginoplasty, majoraplasty, or labia majora fat transfer can be performed simultaneously. Non-invasive procedures such as vaginal laser, vaginal RF, and hyaluronic acid filler applications can also be added to combined procedures. Some physicians state that recovery is accelerated with PRP injection to the surgical area immediately after the operation.

Combined methods are the crown jewel of the surgeon in terms of both patient satisfaction and

Table 9.5 Step-by-step preparation and some tips about in-office labiaplasty

• Listen to the patient before the operation, get her expectations, determine the technique to be applied, and inform the patient in detail
• Take verbal and written consent (must be taken by the physician)
• Apply topical anesthetic cream 45 min beforehand. However, topical creams sometimes can cause edema
• Give oral premedication. You can give mild anxiolytic or sedative oral medications half an hour before
• Insert IV catheter
• Take the patient to the gynecological table and take preoperative photos of the genital area in different positions
• Clean the vulva and vagina with disinfectant
• Drape the patient, then dry the genital area with gauze
• Mark the surgical site with the marker pen. Do this while the tissue is in a neutral position without stretching the labium while marking
• Infiltrate tumescent local anesthetic solution containing epinephrine with a fine-tipped needle and then wait for 10 min to reduce the risk of bleeding
Tumescent recommendation (Eserdag):
– 4 cc ampoule of lidocaine (20 mg/mL) + epinephrine (0.0125 mg/mL)
– 4 cc isotonic serum
– 2 cc tranexamic acid (100 mg/mL)
• Perform the operation in accordance with the condition and expectations of the patient's tissue
• *To increase comfort during surgery*
– Slow music will be relaxing
– By wearing an eye mask, the patient can be removed from the external environment
– The knees and thighs can be supported with silicone/sponge pillows
– To reduce the feeling of cold, the patient can be covered with a cover and socks can be worn on the feet
– The physician or assistant can help reduce the patient's anxiety by having the patient talk during the operation

aesthetic and functional results. The patient's wishes and the condition of the tissue during the examination are decisive when making a decision for combined surgery.

9.12 Botched Labiaplasty and Revision Surgeries

Although labiaplasty operations are considered minor surgery, they are operations that include many small details. Labiaplasty is a surgery not to be practiced without training. The fact that these operations are being performed more frequently in recent years by physicians who have not been adequately trained causes many medical and psychological problems for patients. In addition, they are the subject of many legal malpractice cases. Parallel to that, revision operations are also on the rise.

The most common mistakes made in labiaplasty surgeries are listed in Table 9.6.

Table 9.6 The most common reasons for requiring revision in labiaplasty

• Shortening the labia more or less than desired
• Irregular edges (Fig. 9.19)
• Wound dehiscence in V-Plasty operations (Fig. 9.20)
• Complete removal of the labia (labiectomy) (Figs. 9.21 and 9.22)
• Fenestration (windowing) due to avascularization, especially after wedge resection (Fig. 9.23)
• Exposition of the glans clitoridis (Fig. 9.24)
• Inability to achieve complete symmetry
• Formation of scar tissue at the incision site (Fig. 9.25)
• Dog ear appearances
• Formation of notches in the form of "saw teeth" on labial edges after the operation (scalloping) (Fig. 9.26)
• Formation of inclusion cysts due to skin islets buried under the skin (Fig. 9.27)
• Alteration in sensitivity (may develop as a result of not being gentle on the tissue, using thick sutures, cutting the clitoral neurovascular bundle, or nerve damage due to aggressive cauterization)
• Labiaplasty operation is performed without touching the clitoral hood area and therefore the appearance of "micropenis" occurs
• Dyspareunia due to overstretching of the perineum if perineum correction has also been made

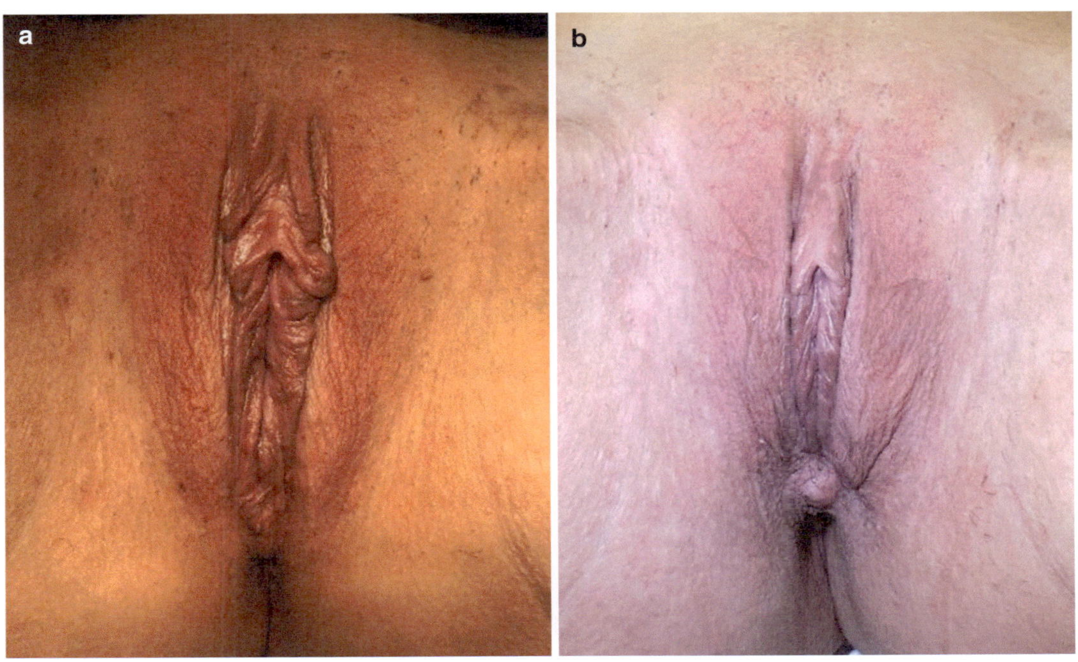

Fig. 9.19 Revision labiaplasty, clitoral hoodoplasty, vaginal tightening, and perineoplasty combined surgeries for a patient who had previously undergone labiaplasty operation but was not satisfied with the results, because of irregular edges. Before (**a**), 18 months after the surgery (**b**)

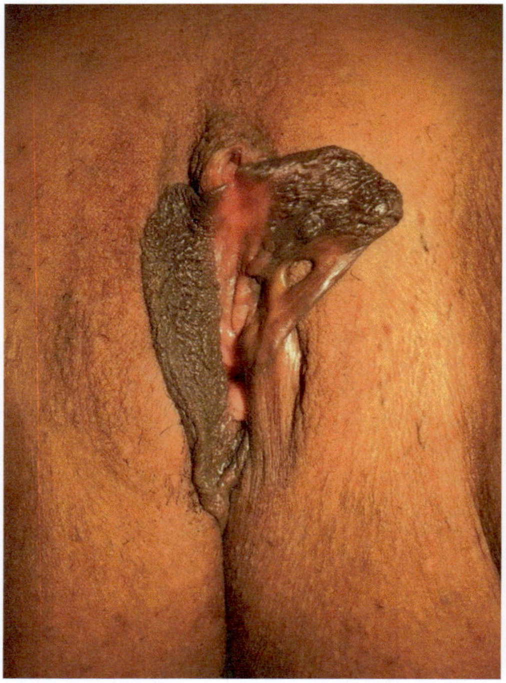

Fig. 9.20 Botched labiaplasty. Dehiscence in the left labium after V-plasty. This complication usually depends on the overstretching of the tissue and deterioration of the circulation

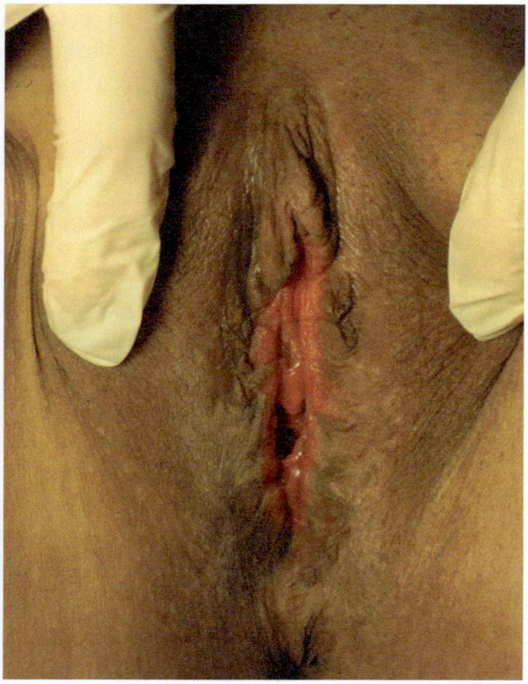

Fig. 9.21 Botched labiaplasty. Labia are completely removed, scar tissue has formed. The clitoral area was not treated. The patient was severely anxious and had vaginal dryness during sexual intercourse

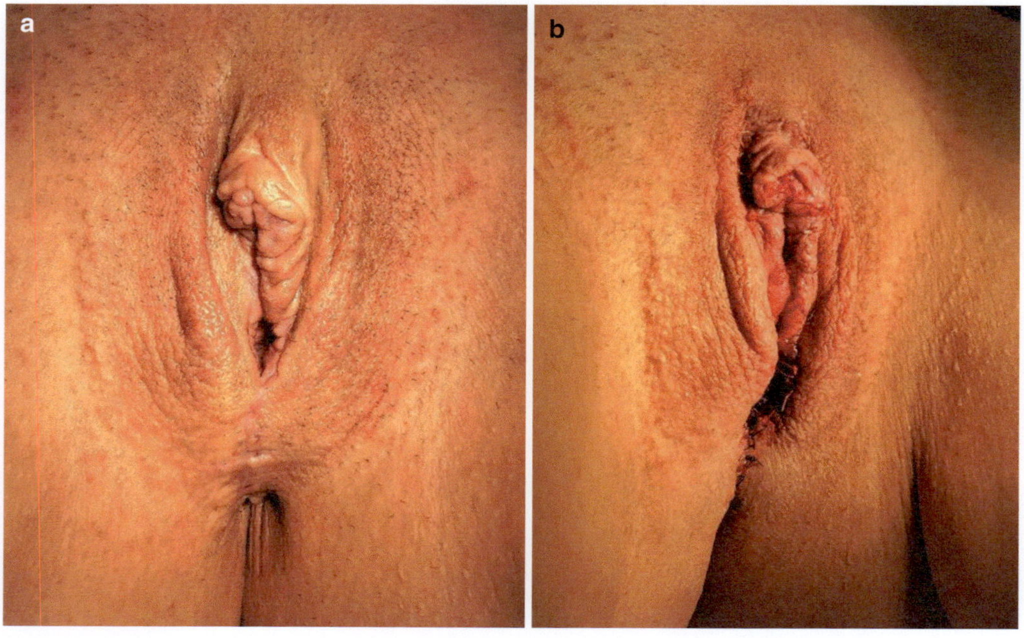

Fig. 9.22 Botched labiaplasty. Before the operation (**a**): the right labium is completely removed, the hood is untouched, coitus cannot occur because the perineum is raised excessively. After the revision (**b**): the right labium was reconstructed, the border was reduced, and the perineal entrance was enlarged

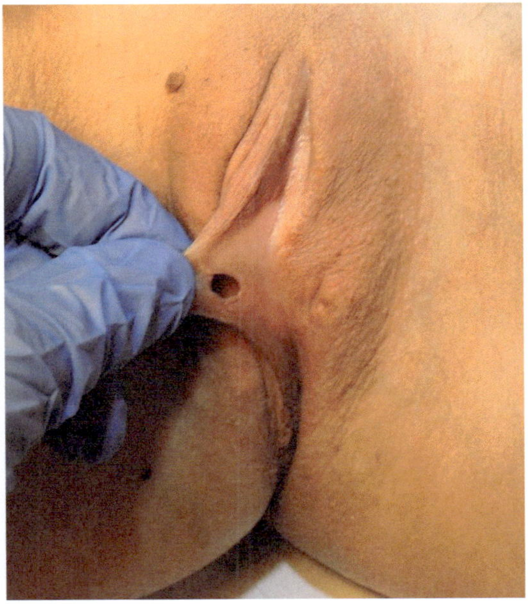

Fig. 9.23 Fenestration

As in the example I always give to my patients, "*labiaplasty operations are like building a house on an empty plot, whereas revision operations are like repairing a collapsed house.*" Therefore, a revision will never be as successful as an initial surgery. The aim is to bring the tissue to a better position in terms of aesthetics and functionality.

Sometimes, a revision may be required due to traffic accident, or removal of Bartholin's cyst, or deformations after vaginal surgery (Fig. 9.28).

Infrequently labial retransposition can be needed for a revision surgery (Fig. 9.29).

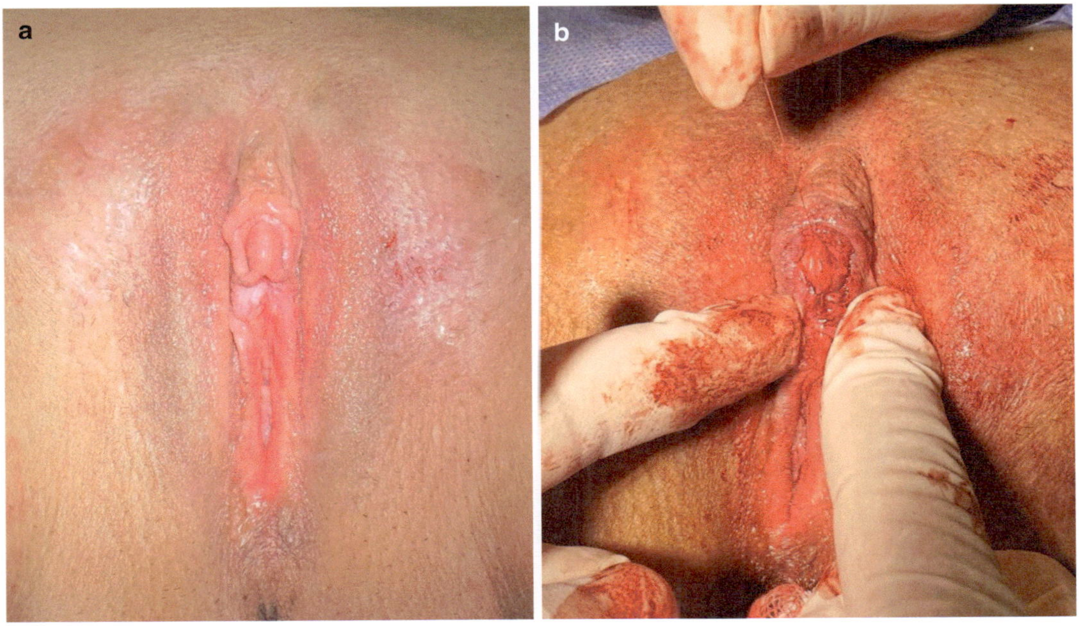

Fig. 9.24 Glans exposition due to excessive reduction of hood skin in labiaplasty (**a**). This situation causes chronic irritation and extreme discomfort. Therefore, the patient covers her genital area with a plaster. You can also see the traces of plaster allergy (**a**). The glans is placed inside the hood (**b**). The images below are just after surgery (**c**, **d**)

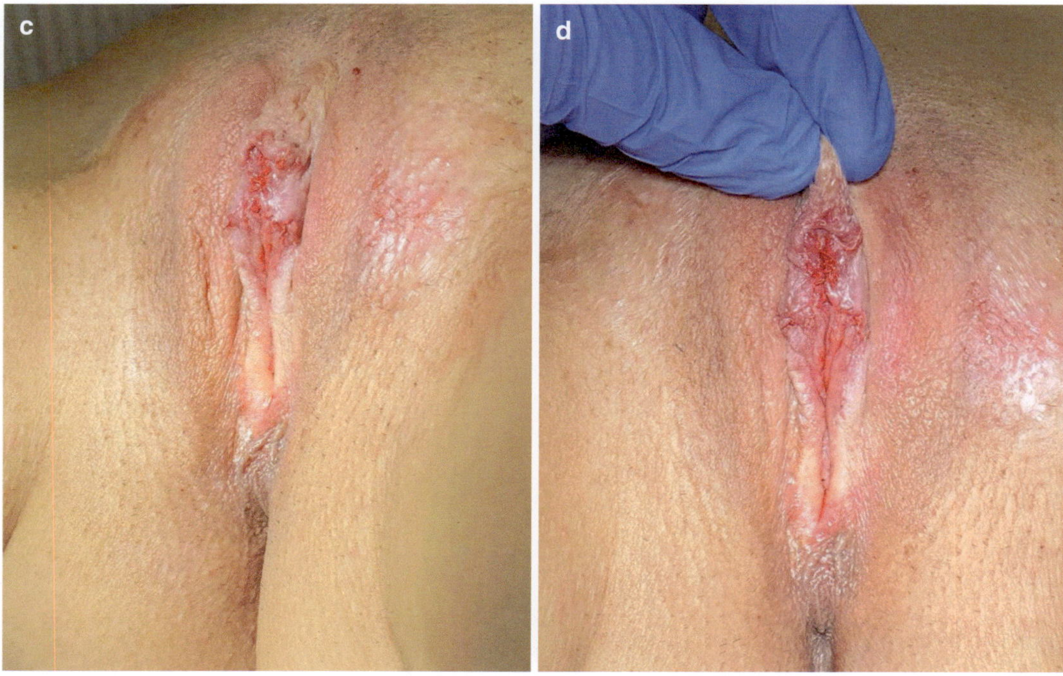

Fig. 9.24 (continued)

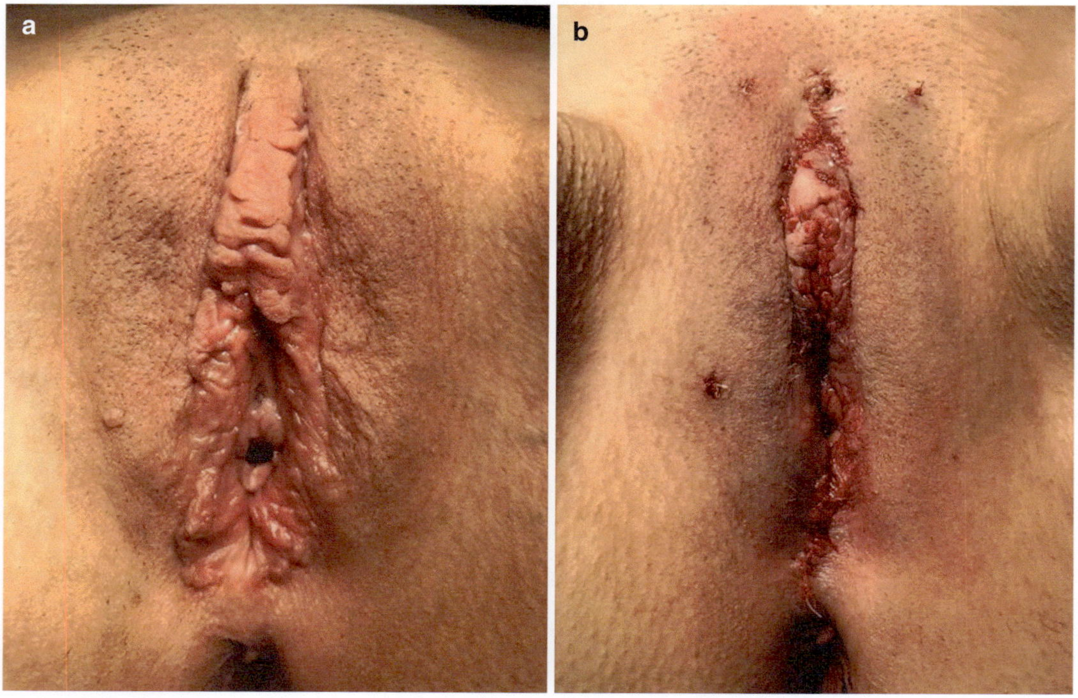

Fig. 9.25 Botched labiaplasty revision. Labial scar tissue removal, perineoplasty, and transfer of up to 15 cc of fat to each majora. Before (**a**), just after (**b**), and 2 years after the surgery (**c**)

Fig. 9.25 (continued)

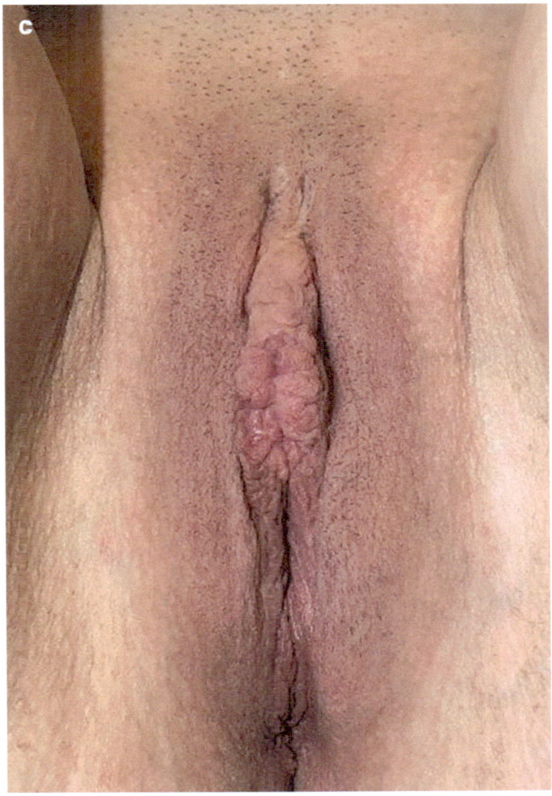

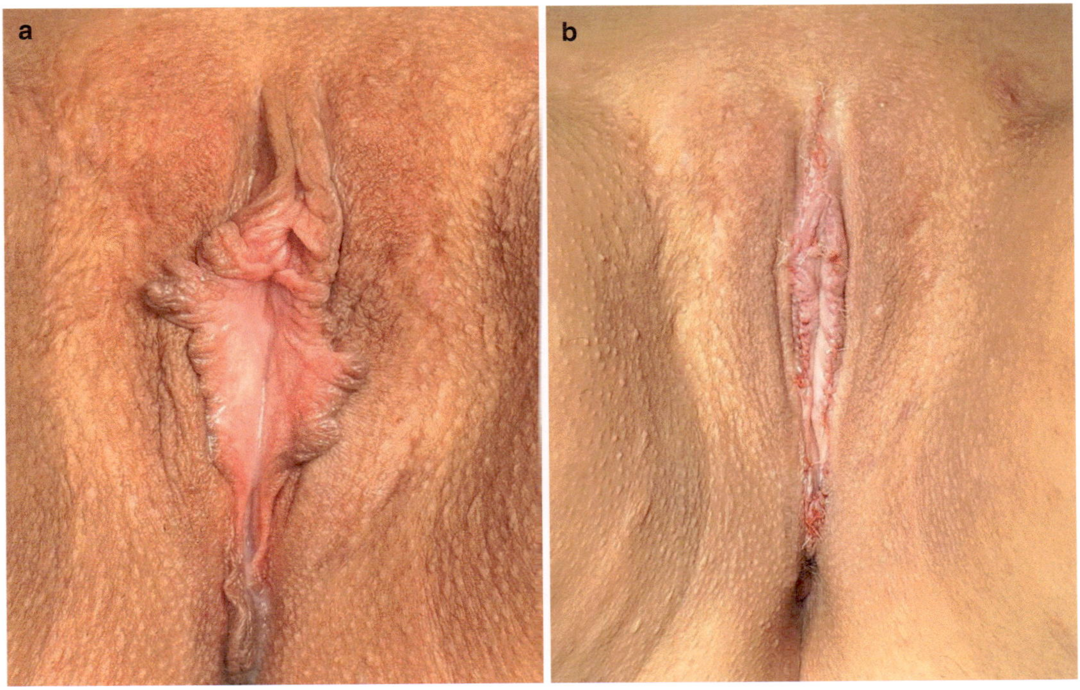

Fig. 9.26 Sawtooth appearance (scalloping) after labiaplasty. Preop (**a**) and just after (**b**) appearances. Labial revision, hoodoplasty, and removal of excess perineal skin were performed

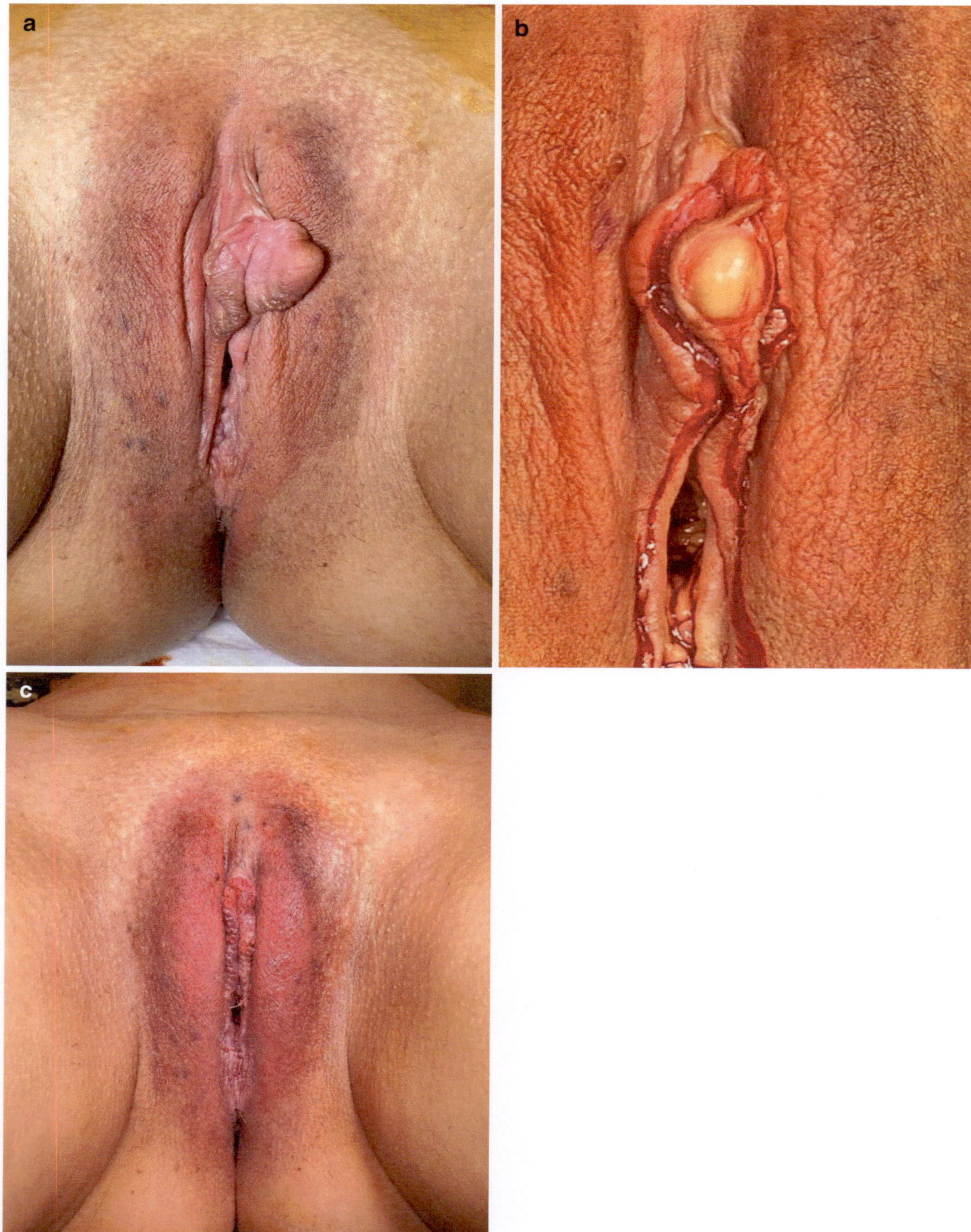

Fig. 9.27 The patient who had labiaplasty revision surgery (**a**). The inclusion cyst in the upper part of the left labium was removed (**b**), and also autologous fat tissue was transferred to the labia majora and perineum (**c**)

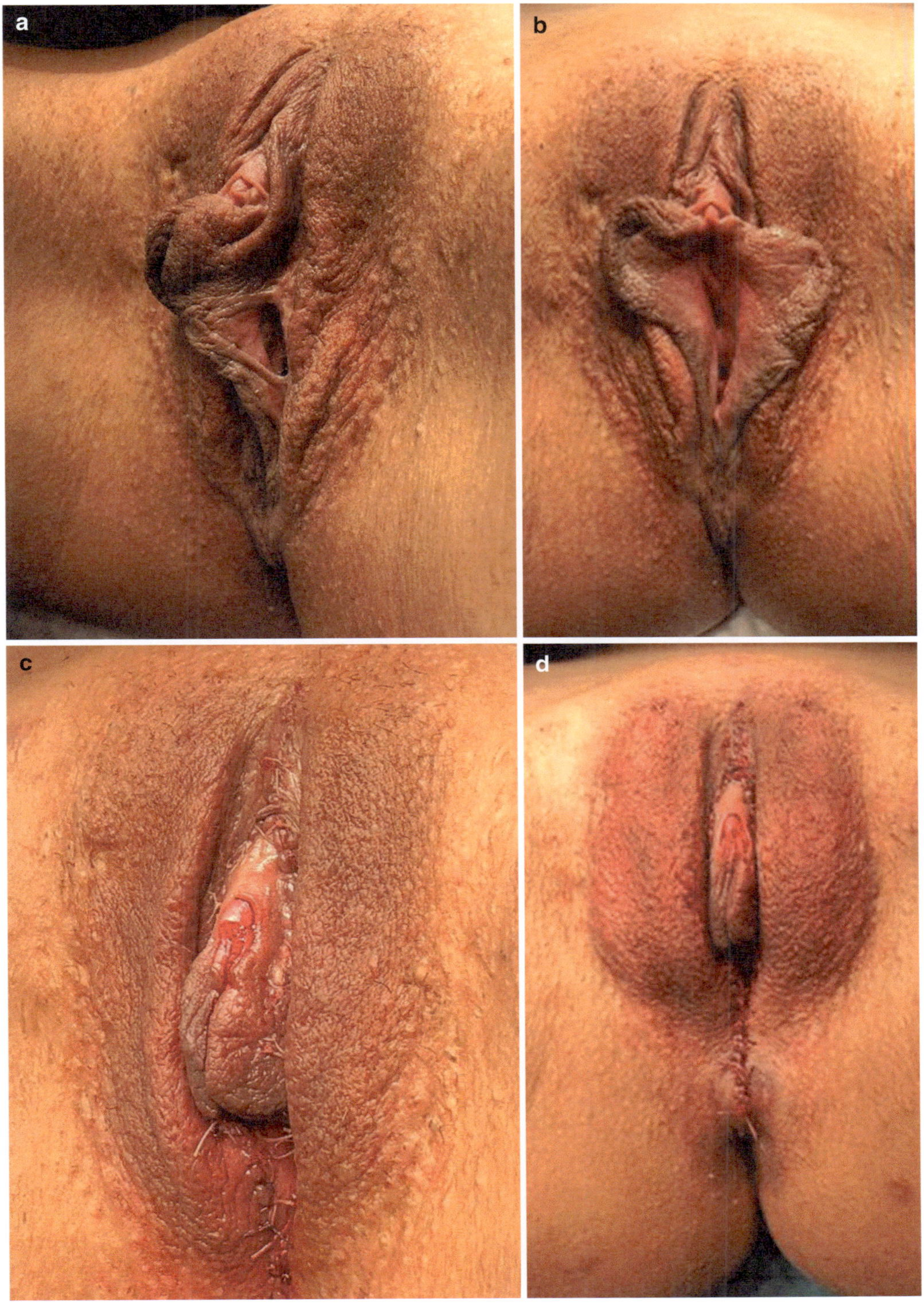

Fig. 9.28 Labial reconstruction. After Bartholin's cyst extirpation, fenestration depending on the tissue necrosis due to silver nitrate administration as well as complaint of vulvar laxity. Labium revision with V-plasty, hoodoplasty, perineoplasty, and majora fat transfer procedures were done. Lateral and frontal views of the before (**a**, **b**) and just after the surgery (**c**, **d**)

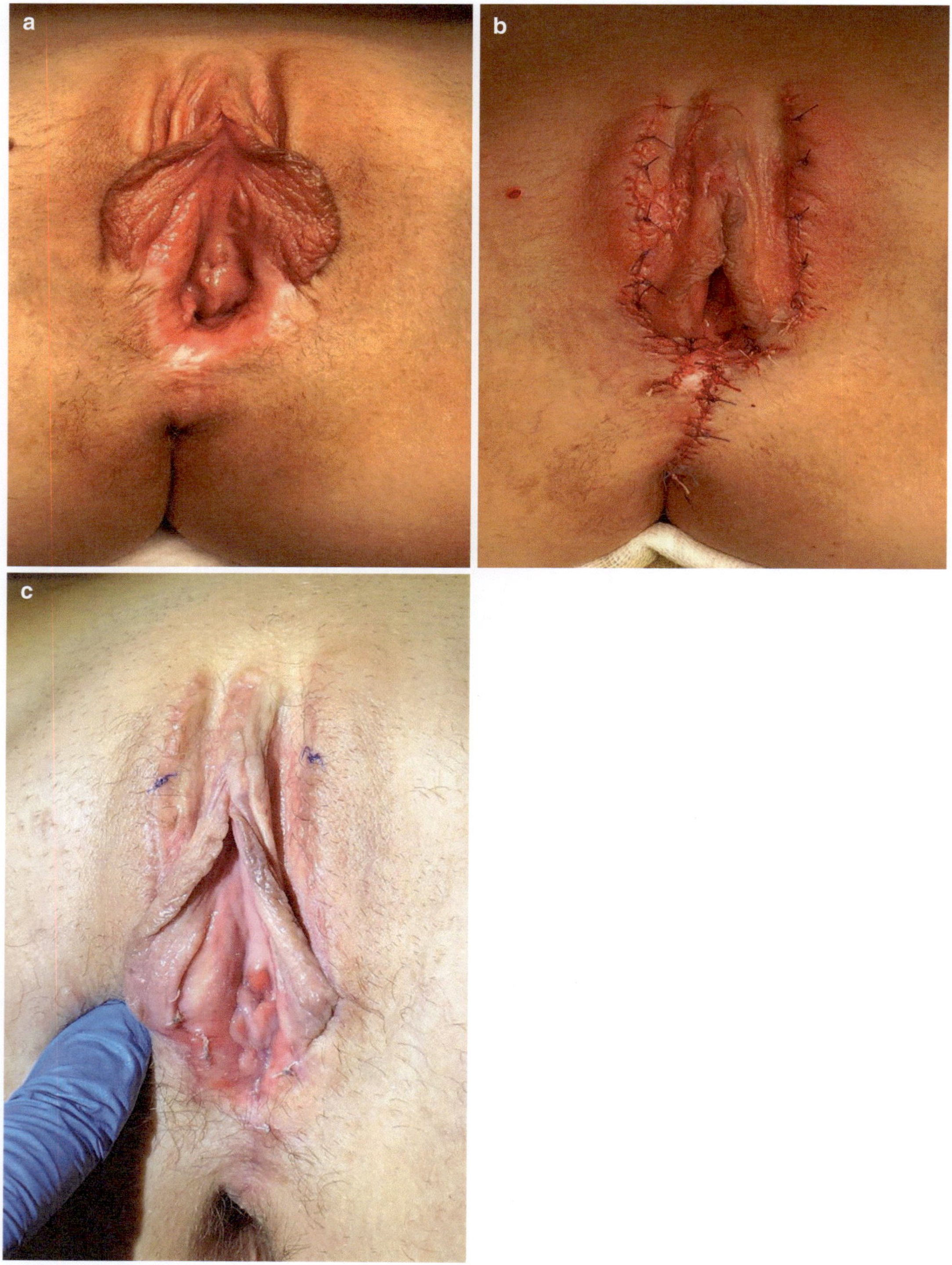

Fig. 9.29 Labial retransposition (*Eserdag*). Appearance of a patient who had previously undergone combined operations of vaginal tightening, labia minoraplasty, and majoraplasty (**a**). Perineal scar tissue caused dyspareunia, the labia were cut and moved upwards, and there was a scar on the incision line in the majora area. Labial retransposition was done (labials were cut from the base and moved down again), perineoplasty was performed, and majoraplasty scar was revised. Just after (**b**), and 1 month after the surgery (**c**)

9.13 Neolabiaplasty *(Eserdag)*

Some patients apply for revision purposes with one or both inner labia removed, i.e., labiectomized. It is not an easy procedure to recreate the completely removed inner labia. However, with a method that I named as "Neolabiaplasty," I was able to reconstruct the labia in about 10 patients with dissection and square (mattress) stitches (Fig. 9.30).

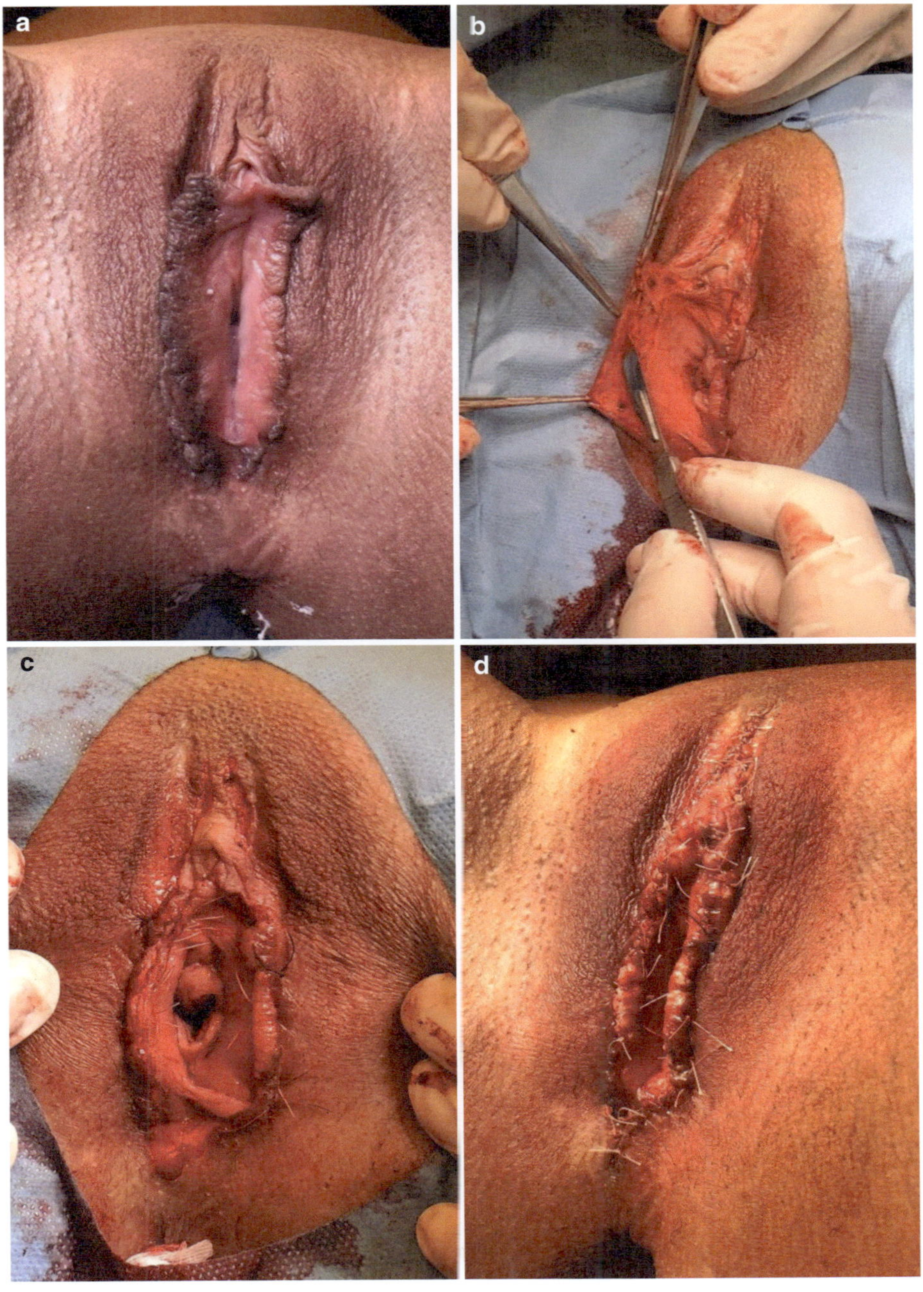

Fig. 9.30 Neolabiaplasty (*Eserdag*). Right labiaplasty, clitorohoodoplasty, and left neolabiaplasty (re-labial formation) operations in a patient whose left labium was completely excised and right labium was deformed. Before (**a**), dissection of left labium for having a skin fold (**b**), slight trimming of the right labium and having square (mattress) sutures on the left labium (**c**), just after the operation (**d**)

Below are the revision stages of a 32-year-old patient who had labiaplasty 3 months prior (Fig. 9.31).

Another approach in the revision surgeries of patients who have undergone labiectomy is the transfer of a flap extracted longitudinally from the clitoral hood area to the amputated labial area by rotating 180°.

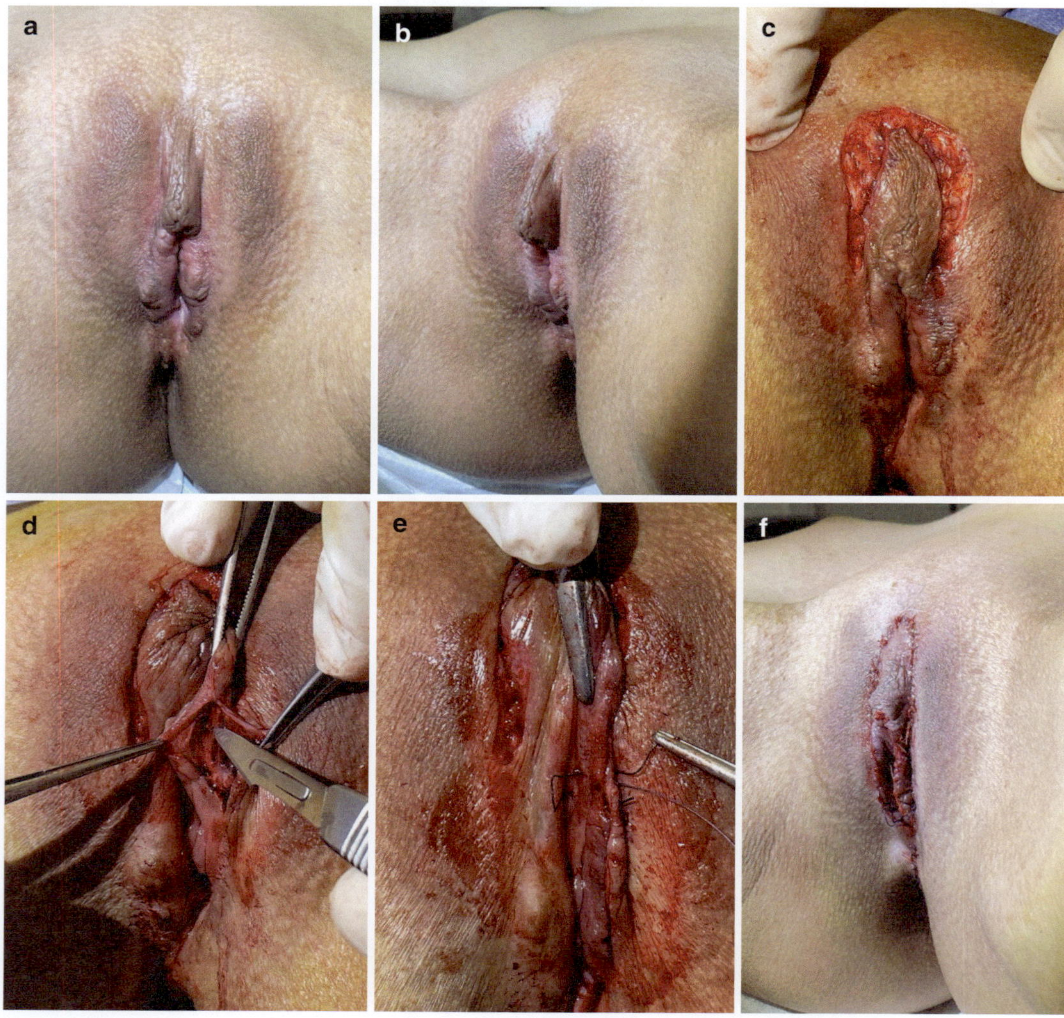

Fig. 9.31 Revision surgery. In the previous labiaplasty, the left labium was completely removed, very little tissue was left in the right labium, and the hood region protrudes in the form of micropenis since hoodoplasty was not performed (**a**, **b**). The hood area is pulled down by sutures in hoodoplasty with an extended inverted-U incision (**c**). After linear incisions are made on both residual labia, new skin folds are formed by bilateral dissection (**d**). Later, skin folds were made more prominent with mattress sutures (**e**). Postoperative lateral and frontal views (**f**, **g**), and from the patient's vision clitoral hood area before the surgery (**h**), and after the surgery (**i**). Clitoral protrusion was completely disappeared and neolabia was formed

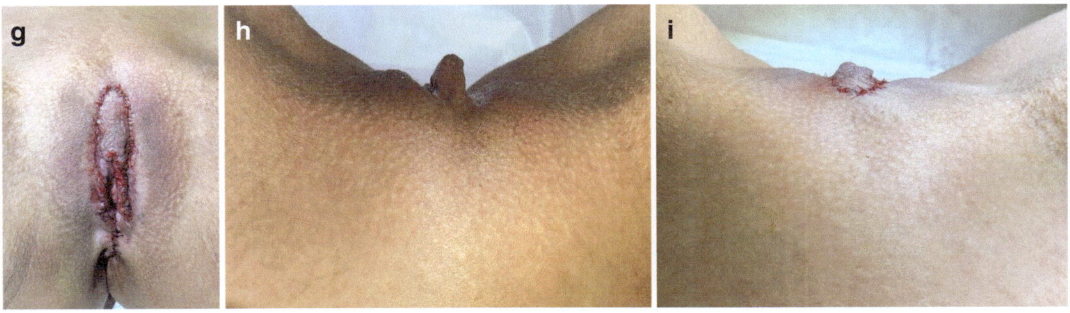

Fig. 9.31 (continued)

9.14 Common Complaints After the Operation

Some possible outcomes experienced by patients after labiaplasty can be uncomfortable and worrying. For this reason, it is important to inform the patients before the operation and to write the possible outcomes, side effects, and potential complications on the consent forms.

9.14.1 Vasovagal Reflex

In operations performed under local anesthesia, syncope attacks due to vasovagal reflex that develop during the intraoperative period, when first standing up, and sometimes even hours after the operation can be observed. Head trauma may occur because of syncope. Hypotension as a result of sudden bradycardia due to excessive anxiety and pain usually plays a role in syncope.

If the operation is to be performed with local anesthesia, the measures that can be taken include the patient's arrival with a lightly full stomach, eliminating anxiety before the operation as much as possible, and diluting the local anesthetics to be used.

Sudden loss of consciousness that develops during office labiaplasty is very disturbing for the surgeon. In this case, it is important to open the airway by interrupting the operation, to provide oxygen support, and, if there is severe bradycardia, atropine injection, sodium isotonic, and IV fluid support are important.

9.14.2 Bleeding

Bleeding in the postoperative period is usually light and leaky and limited to the first few days. Sudden bleeding, extended bleeding lasting longer than a week, and swelling in the operation area are conditions that should be considered. Anti-bleeding measures will be discussed later.

9.14.3 Pain

Pain is a common complaint, especially in the first 12–24 h. If the procedure is performed under local anesthesia, throbbing pain usually peaks 6–8 h after the absorption of the local anesthetic agent, and then it starts to decrease. During this period, the use of pain medications, ice application, providing elevation by placing a pillow under the legs, taking mild sleep-inducing drugs, and bed rest are among the measures that can be taken. In the USA, injectable local anesthetics containing liposomal bupivacaine (Exparel™) create a local anesthetic effect for 3–5 days postoperatively.

In the postoperative period, pain is more intense, especially in the clitoral area. The pain is expected to subside over time. The throbbing pain in the first days will continue in the form of burning, pricking, and stinging for a few weeks. Intense pain, bleeding, confusion, and rapidly developing stiffness or swelling in the operation area suggest the possibility of hematoma.

9.14.4 Itching

Itching, especially after 4–5 days, is very uncomfortable for most patients. Perhaps it is the biggest problem in the subacute period due to inflammation in the wound healing process and usually occurs at night. In these cases, antihistaminic creams or oral medications, such as hydroxyzine can be used. In severe cases, hydrocortisone containing creams can also be applied to the wound area. Usually, itching recovers after 2–3 weeks with the disappearance of the sutures. Itching is the most common cause of complaints by many labiaplasty patients. Sometimes, vaginal yeast infections that develop due to antibiotics can also cause itching.

9.14.5 Edema

Edema, which develops 24 h after the operation, lasts for a few days, and is generally observed in different amounts on both operated labia can be alarming for patients. Edema can be common, sometimes covering the labia majora. This situation, which develops due to the wound healing process, usually reduces rapidly from the first week. However, in rare cases, especially in atopic bodies, or extended surgeries prolonged edema can be observed.

Ice compression is recommended in the first 3 days to minimize edema and can be done every half hour. Thus, the risk of bleeding and edema decreases. Goulard's extract (subacetate of lead) can be prescribed as a magistral solution after extensive labiaplasty and hoodoplasty surgeries. Topical creams of chondroitin polysulfate or arnica montana can also be preferred. These creams will also provide faster healing of subcutaneous ecchymosis that develops after the operation.

9.15 Complications

Although labiaplasty is not difficult, it is an aesthetic intervention that contains many pitfalls, tips, and tricks. First of all, it is never a procedure that can be done by making quick decisions without fully understanding the patient's expectations or evaluating the tissue condition fully.

Especially in recent years, increasing patient demands and physicians' doing this operations without training has brought many victims with it. Forums like *"labiaplasty victims"* and negative posts on social media have reached a level that damages the reputation of doctors in recent years. Malpractice lawsuits that have increased as a result of botched labiaplasty are another aspect of the business.

9.15.1 Acute Term

Acute complications that can be seen intraoperatively/postoperatively in labiaplasty operations include bleeding, hematoma, and allergic reactions to drugs or anesthetic agents used. If the procedure is performed in the office and under local anesthesia, hypotension and temporary loss of consciousness due to vasovagal reflex can also be observed.

Common varicose veins seen in the labium and clitoral hood in some women tend to bleed. Genital varicose veins are more common, especially in those who have given birth multiple times (Fig. 9.32).

Bleeding risk increases especially in overweight patients, those with bleeding diathesis or

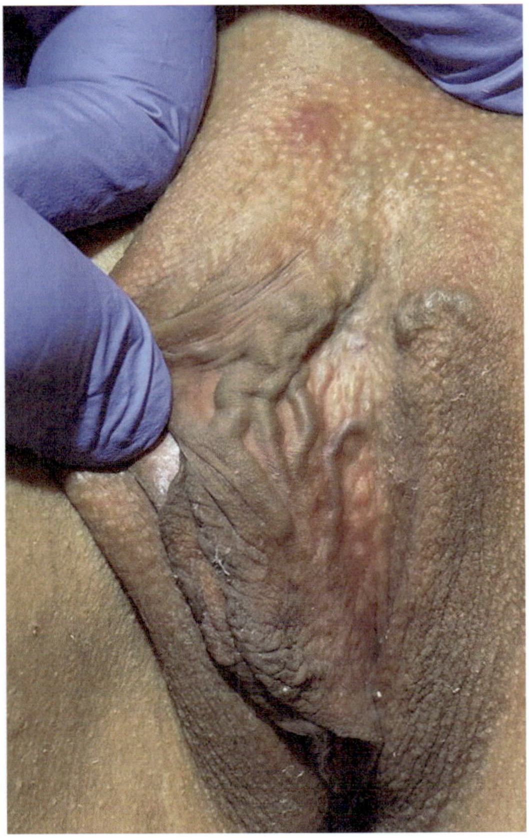

Fig. 9.32 Prominent varicose veins in labia and clitoral hood area

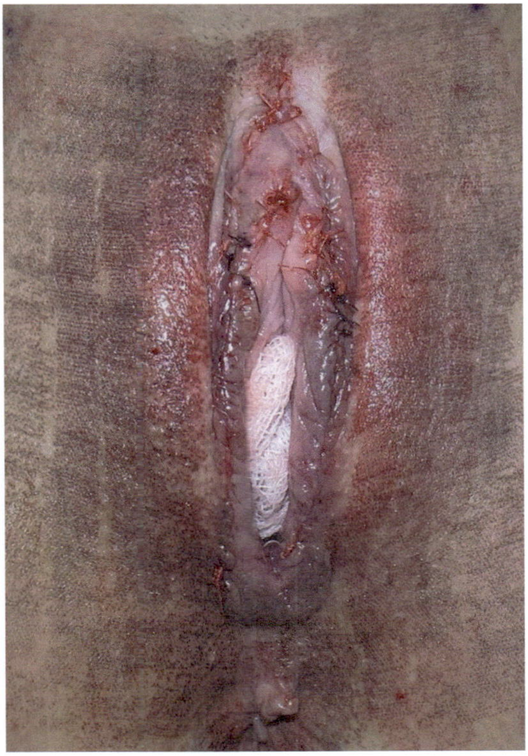

Fig. 9.33 Compression after labiaplasty. During the operation, compression can be performed with gauze placed in the introitus in patients with excessive bleeding

diffuse varicose veins. This risk is also higher in those with severe labial hypertrophy: Indeed, *"larger the organ, higher the vascularization and higher the risk of abnormal bleeding."*

In order to reduce the risks of bleeding that may occur in the intraoperative and postoperative periods, 10–15 mg/kg (500–1000 mg) IV tranexamic acid (TXA) can be administered prophylactically 20 min before surgery. It can be followed by infusion of 1 mg/kg/h postoperatively. TXA is a synthetic derivative of the amino acid lysine and binds the five lysine binding sites on plasminogen. This inhibits plasmin formation and displaces plasminogen from the fibrin surface. It may also directly inhibit plasmin and partially inhibit fibrinogenolysis at higher concentrations. TXA is also thought to exert an anti-inflammatory effect and may improve platelet function in certain circumstances. Preoperative intravenous TXA reduces perioperative blood loss and transfusion requirements in a variety of surgical disciplines without increasing the risk of thromboembolic events. Therefore, it should be considered for prophylactic use in surgery to reduce operative bleeding [9]. TXA should not be used in patients with a history of hypercoagulopathy, renal failure, embolism, thrombosis, and deep vein thrombosis.

Conversely, platelet-rich plasma (PRP) or platelet-rich fibrin (PRF) injections can also be performed in patients with excessive bleeding during the operation. These injections will both reduce the risks of bleeding and hematoma formation as well as accelerate the wound healing process.

In patients with more resistant bleeding during the intraoperative period, wet gauze placed in the introitus will reduce the risk of bleeding via a compression effect (Fig. 9.33).

9.15.2 Subacute Term

Complications such as excessive edema, wound infection, and dehiscence may occur during the subacute period (usually on the third-fifth days). Skin/subcutaneous bleeding can sometimes continue as leakage for 7–10 days after the operation. Wound infections generally develop due to subclinical anaerobic non-specific vaginitis. Vaginal infections may cause wound infections, and wound site infections may cause suture opening. Other reasons for wound dehiscence include non-compliance with surgical principles, subcutaneous bleeding, hematoma, and avascularization. Especially in wedge excisions, it is not uncommon for circulation problems due to the tight closure of the tissue or dehiscence that occurs as a result of incomplete closure of the wound edges while suturing.

9.15.3 Chronic Term

In the chronic period, complaints such as scar formation, abscess formation, asymmetry, sawtooth appearance of the edges (scalloping[1]) (Fig. 9.34), windowing (fenestration) due to necrosis of the tissue on the labium (Fig. 9.35), prolonged edema (Fig. 9.37), sensation changes, and dyspareunia may occur.

In some labiaplasty cases, more bleeding than expected may occur and more hemostasis sutures may need to be placed. In this case, Z-sutures should be avoided, especially when suturing the skin tissue. Instead of Z-sutures that cause a sawtooth appearance, the suture technique called "square suture," a kind of mattress suture, is more suitable for both hemostasis and aesthetics (Fig. 9.36).

Tissue stiffness and scar formation seen after labiaplasty may develop depending on the surgical technique used. Reasons such as too frequent suturing, use of thick suture material, locking in continuous repair, use of aggressive cautery, and suturing the wound edges without bringing it to the end both disrupt wound healing and cause scar formation. There may also be a problem of numbness in the tissue. Labiaplasty surgeries require patience, meticulousness, and sensitivity to tissue. Conversely, postoperative hematoma or infections increase the risk of scar formation by prolonging the inflammation phase of wound healing.

Perineum correction can also be performed during labiaplasty, and if hard scar tissue develops in this region, problems such as strain, pain, and tearing during intercourse will occur. In order to avoid development of scar tissue in the perineum, excessive tissue removal that may cause stretching of this area and frequent suturing with thick threads that will negatively affect vascularization should be avoided.

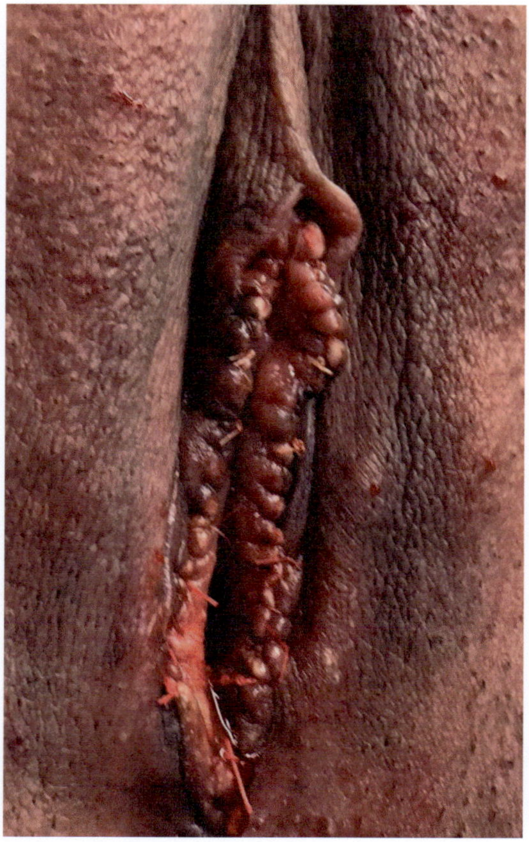

Fig. 9.34 Scalloping. Frequent and tightly laid suture materials lead to a sawtooth appearance in the future

[1]Scallop: This is the name given to some species of bivalves in English. It is the name given to this appearance because the shells of the scallop protrude just like saw teeth.

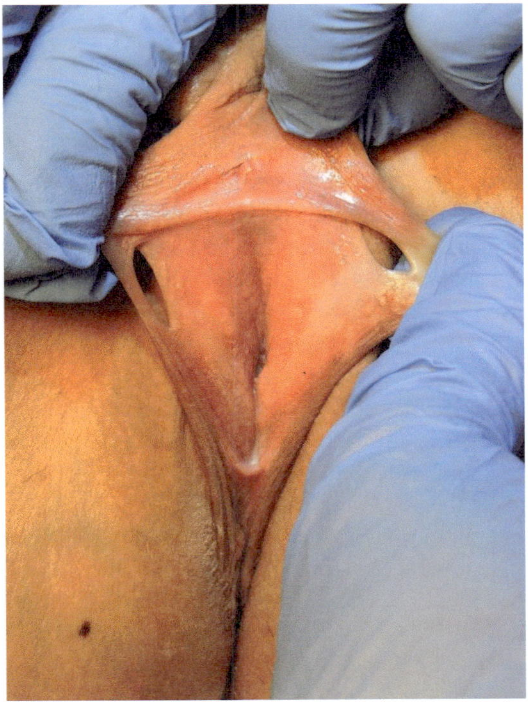

Fig. 9.35 Bilateral fenestration due to tissue necrosis after V-plasty

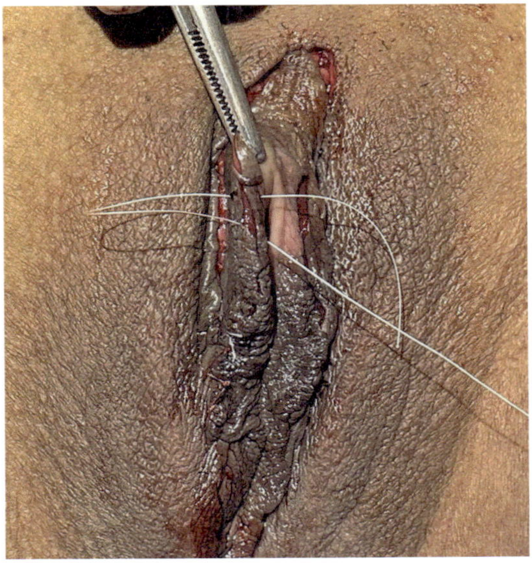

Fig. 9.36 Square sutures *(Eserdag)*. The square or mattress sutures used in a patient undergoing labiaplasty and hoodoplasty provide hemostasis and prevent the sawtooth appearance (scalloping) of the labial edge

When the V-plasty technique is applied, tense suturing of the superior pedicle to the lower segment, frequent sutures for hemostasis, or the use of aggressive cautery may lead to tissue necrosis due to avascularization and tissue dehiscence and labial windowing.

Long-term edema can also be seen as a result of impaired venous circulation. Tissue damage due to the use of electrocautery for hemostasis or incision is the most common cause of edema. Sutures that are placed too often and too tightly may disrupt the circulation and cause long-term edema. Postoperative edema mostly occurs in the clitoral hood area. Prolonged edema may also develop due to the trauma of the operation or allergy to the suture materials used; this situation will usually improve over time (Fig. 9.37).

Asymmetry after labiaplasty is one of the most common problems. Asymmetry can cause physiological problems such as urine flowing in

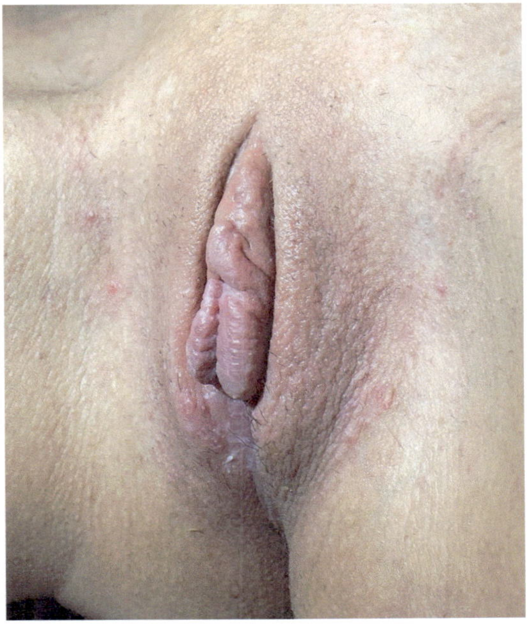

Fig. 9.37 Prolonged edema. Although it is the postoperative 40th day, significant edema in the labia and hood area continues. The reason for this edema that developed after minimally invasive labiaplasty operation is tissue allergy. Edema disappeared rapidly after the second month. It is important for this group of patients to avoid genital irritations such as wearing tight pants, using a pad, and cleaning the genital area with soap or shampoo

different directions, as well as negatively affecting patients psychologically. Especially in patients with symmetry obsession, psychological effects are quite high even in cases of mild asymmetry.

One of the most common mistakes is removing the labia completely, that is, a "labiectomy" procedure. Labiectomy is both a cause of poor aesthetic appearance and may cause problems such as vaginal dryness and dyspareunia. This situation is actually a genital mutilation, and it is not easy to reconstruct the labia.

An unpleasant appearance for patients is that labial reduction is not in the desired amount. In general, most patients desire the maximum possible tissue removal.

Another problem is that although the labia are shortened too much, the clitoral hood is not similarly adjusted. As a result of this situation, the clitoral hood takes on the appearance of a "child's penis," which is very disturbing for the patients.

In patients with thick labia, the short and thick appearance of the new edges (stumping) after the incision is made with scissors can be aesthetically disturbing. In these patients, the stump appearance can be prevented by trimming the subcutaneous tissue sufficiently. Another precaution is to make the incision not perpendicular to the labial edge, but with a 45-degree inclination. The new edges will be sharpened, especially with the inclined incisions that can be made with RF or scalpel.

If revision is required after labiaplasty operations, at least 3 months should pass before the secondary surgery. However, the aesthetic results obtained after revision surgeries will never be as good as if the first operation had been well performed. Therefore, all operations should be done with great care and meticulousness.

9.16 Vulvar Hematoma and Management

Hematoma is bleeding under the intact epidermis. It is divided into obstetric and non-obstetric. It is a serious complication that usually occurs during the acute phase of labiaplasty operations. Apart from labiaplasty, falls, bicycle accidents, traumatic coitus, especially in those who without prior sexual experience, sexual penetration without foreplay, foreign body insertion into the vagina, or masturbation may cause hematomas. Many hematomas are small or medium in size and self-limiting, but sometimes enlargement may impair hemodynamic stability.

In the post-labiaplasty period, if there is a unilateral, localized, fluctuating, purple-colored firm mass that is accompanied by pain and/or anxiety, hematoma should be first considered. The difference between vulvar edema that can occur in the postoperative period and hematoma is that vulvar edema is more common, soft, pale-colored, and painless on palpation. Edema can sometimes become broad.

9.16.1 Approaches in Hematoma

9.16.1.1 Passive Management

If the hematoma margins are clear and do not grow, try to drain it by pressing it manually. Vital signs are checked periodically, and the patient is followed up with coagulation and hemogram tests. If necessary, the size of the hematoma can be measured with ultrasound. During this period, try to reduce the patient's pain and anxiety by applying ice compression and analgesics.

In acute bleeding, 1000 mg of tranexamic acid can be given as an IV infusion over 10 min.

Treatment can be continued as 1000 mg IV administration 8 h after the initial infusion. Tranexamic acid is a competitive inhibitor of plasminogen and synthetase lysine analogue, with a half-life of approximately 120 min. By binding to plasminogen, it blocks the interaction of fibrin and plasmin and thus enables the formation of a fibrin plug. Oral tranexamic acid medications may also be prescribed for prolonged bleeding after discharge.

9.16.1.2 Active Management

If the hematoma is growing and the patient's complaints of pain increase, active treatment should be started. Because of the patient's severe pain and intense anxiety, the incision line is opened and subcutaneous clots are emptied, usually with sedation or general anesthesia. The hematoma area is very fragile. Hemostasis is provided with cautery and sutures, and the wound is closed without leaving any dead space. If there are persistent leaks of unknown origin, a Penrose drain is placed under the skin.

In the postoperative period, the patient is given IV fluid support. Analgesic and antibiotic drugs are also prescribed, and ice compression is recommended for a few days. Eau de Goulard (2% lead subacetate) solution to prevent vulvar edema and intense inflammation after the operation may be prescribed. This solution reduces edema in the wound healing process and increases comfort with its anti-inflammatory effects. Topical heparinoids containing mucopolysaccharide polysulfate (chondroitin polysulfate) (Hirudoid gel™) or Arnica Montana Flower healing herb (Arnica gel/cream™) can also be applied to reduce edema, eliminate ecchymosis, and accelerate healing.

Vulvar hematoma can rarely occur in the late postoperative period, even 5–7 days after the operation (Fig. 9.38). Prolonged bleeding in the form of leakage after surgery may be a sign of an approaching hematoma.

The preventative measures to reduce bleeding in labiaplasty are listed in Table 9.7.

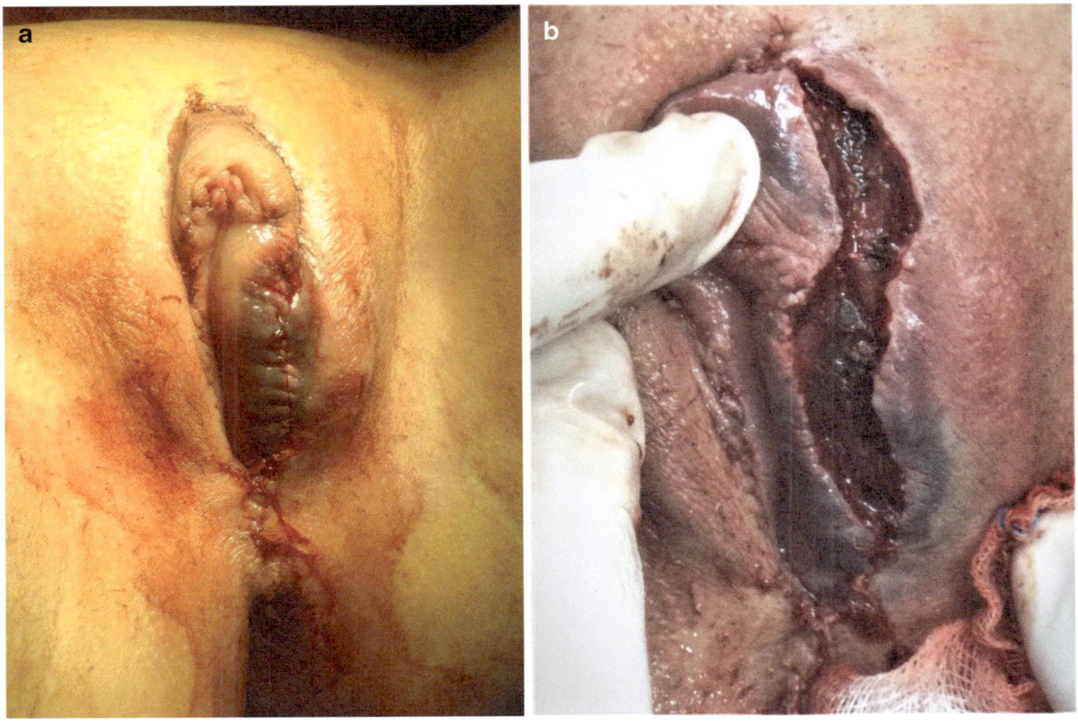

Fig. 9.38 Vulvar hematoma (**a**). Acute hemorrhage and hematoma on the left side, which started 8 h after a rather bleeding-free labiaplasty operation. Due to excessive bleeding, the incision areas were opened (**b**), and after ensuring hemostasis, the incision was closed (**c**)

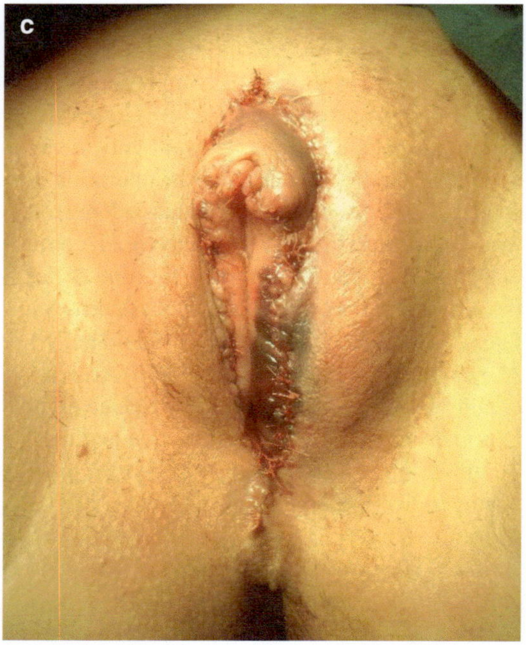

Fig. 9.38 (continued)

9.17 The Postoperative Term

Four to 6 h after the operation, the patient can be discharged to the home or to the hotel, after the medical dressing is changed. For the first day, folded gauze that is placed over the labia and tight underwear that apply slight compression will reduce the risk of bleeding. Patients should be advised to regularly use the prescribed NSAIDs such as ibuprofen and penicillin or cephalosporin-derivative antibiotics for 5 days. They should also be advised not to stand for long periods of time during the first 3 days. Standing excessively during this period may increase the risk of edema and bleeding. Patients can usually return to their work/school life within 3–5 days after surgery.

Intermittent ice applications for 3 days after the operation will be useful for pain, edema, and bleeding complaints. Ice application should not exceed 3 days, and the application should be

Table 9.7 The preventative measures to reduce bleeding in labiaplasty

• The patient should stop green tea, omega 3, aspirin, supplements containing gingko biloba, or coumadin-derivative drugs at least 1 week before the operation
• Question the amount of bleeding during menstruation, previous births, or surgeries in the anamnesis
• Obtain INR measurement, especially in patients with chronic diseases or a history of abnormal bleeding
• Inject local anesthetics containing epinephrine in the form of infiltration to the base of the labia before the procedure (even if the procedure will be performed under general anesthesia). 250 mg tranexamic acid can also be added in local anesthetic solution
• Wait for 15–20 min before the incision is made after the local anesthetic injection
• Use RF for cutting of excessively thick, vascularized, and hypertrophic labia
• Provide hemostasis by using bipolar cautery and square (mattress) sutures in excessive bleeding
• If there is excessive hypotension under general anesthesia, this may prevent open vessel ends from being activated. In this case, the anesthetic gases can be reduced, so that blood pressure is increased, after controlling of hemostasis, the skin can be closed
• Inject PRP locally in abnormal bleeding (PRP may also accelerate wound healing)
• Apply 500 mg IV tranexamic acid 20 min prior to the surgery (this can be performed as a routine application in patients without hypercoagulopathy)
• In cases with excessive bleeding, place a thin gauze pad in the introitus for compression

done intermittently. In addition, direct skin contact should be avoided by wrapping the ice in a sterile compress.

Compliance with hygiene rules and dressing with topical antiseptic or antibiotic creams for 7 days reduces the risk of infection. Three days after the operation, an outpatient shower can be done without rubbing the surgical area. It is not recommended to take a bath in a bathtub for the first 7 days.

Smoking after labiaplasty disrupts the oxygenation of the tissue and slows wound healing. This process is especially important in the first month. Patients should be advised against smoking.

There is a *rule of 3 days, 3 weeks, and 3 months* for labiaplasty and also for other aesthetic operations. In the first 3 days, the edema begins to resolve; after 3 weeks, complaints such as pain, burning, and stinging decrease; and after 3 months, complete well-being occurs, and the tissue is fully shaped. Even though, total healing of the wound takes 6 months. There may be a process for some patients to feel psychologically ready for the newly formed genital areas.

Patients should avoid heavy sports training, fitness, hair removal, yoga and pilates, cycling, horseback riding, and sexual intercourse for 1 month after labiaplasty. If perineoplasty is performed simultaneously, sexual avoidance increases to 1.5 months.

Patients should be advised that the final appearance after surgery is usually formed at the end of the second month, so the genitals should not be inspected with a mirror until this period. Moreover, both labia are healing asynchronously. That is, one side will swell more, one side will hurt more, and localized complaints will occur more in certain areas.

Giving all this information to the patients in advance reduces postoperative anxiety and prevents the patient from unnecessarily occupying the physician with questions. Normal and abnormal situations that may be encountered in the postoperative period and the things to do and avoid should be given in writing to genital aesthetic patients.

Patients can be routinely called for follow-ups on the second day, first week, and second month after the operation. However, this follow-up process may be interrupted in patients coming from outside the city. During the follow-up visits, it is important to obtain written and verbal permissions and postoperative photos of the patients to follow the healing process and to archive the work done.

9.18 Long-Term Results

Whether the genital lips reduced after labiaplasty will enlarge again is one of the questions frequently asked by patients. Although very rare, such a situation may occur. Chronic irritations, especially horseback riding, cycling, and constant scratching can cause regrowth of the reduced labium. Apart from that, it does not seem possible to form labia again in the cut area.

Re-keratinization may also develop over time in the margins of the labia minora reducted by partial resection (Fig. 9.39).

However, patients whose operations were performed with techniques such as V-plasty or delamination may return to their physicians for a labial re-reduction and getting rid of keratinized labial edges.

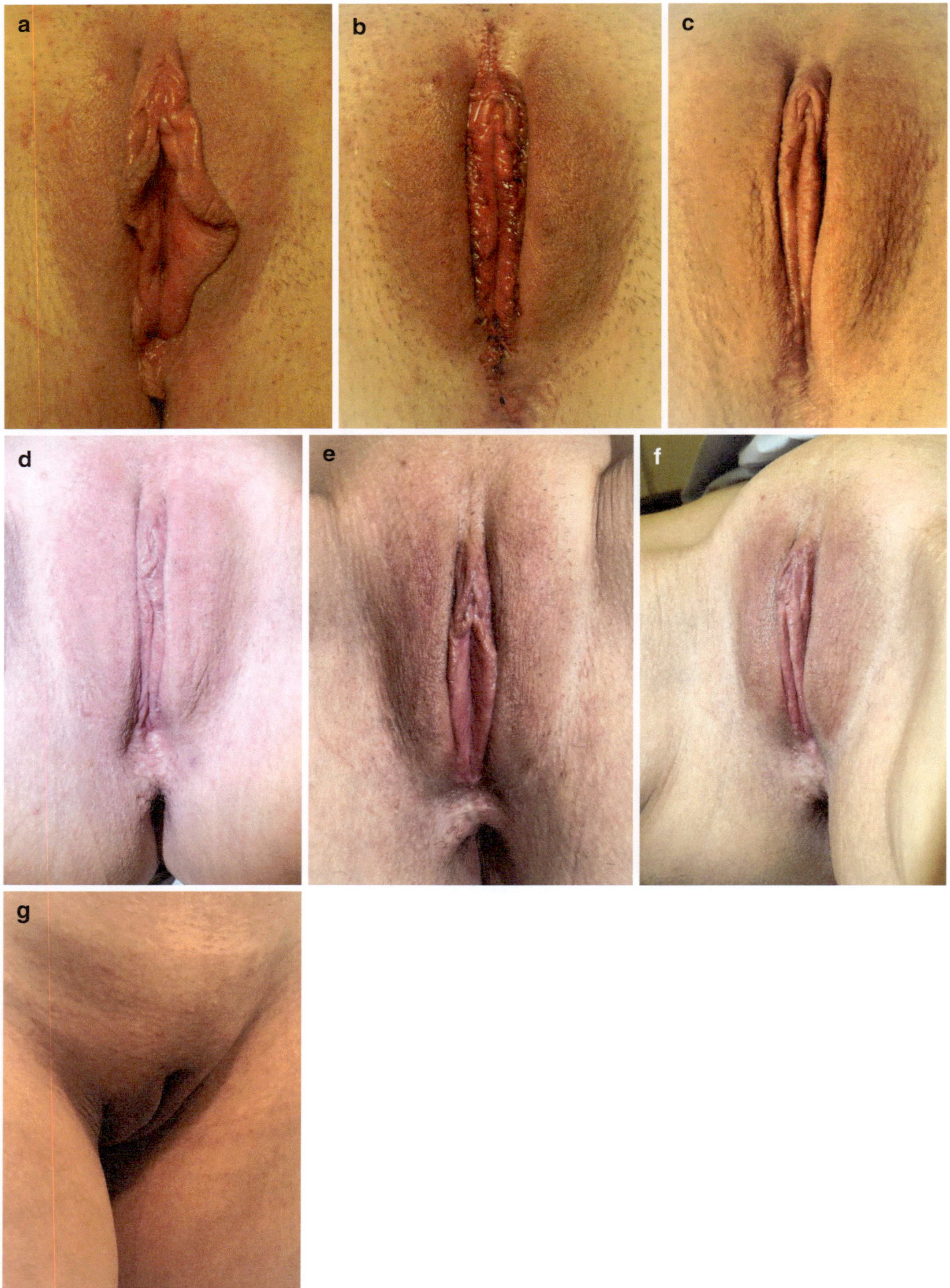

Fig. 9.39 Long-term results after labiaplasty and hoodoplasty [10]. Before (**a**), just after (**b**), postoperative sixth month (**c**), postoperative fourth year (**d**), and postoperative sixth year in different positions (**e–g**)

9.19 Postoperation Psychological Effects

Generally, patient satisfaction level is quite high in labiaplasty operations. While even simple labial reduction may be sufficient for some patients, the situation may differ for others, especially in those with excessive symmetry obsession and in patients with excessive expectations. Extreme dissatisfaction becomes a very uncomfortable dimension for the physician. Even for some patients, a new genital appearance after the operation may be more severe than expected. The adjustment period can be a long time. In this case, it is psychologically relieving to share pre- and postoperative photos with the patient.

Conversely, some women who have been abused in childhood and feel *"dirty"* may also seek different types of genital aesthetic operations for spiritual relaxation or *"emotional cleansing,"* even though these operations are not indicated. These patients must be referred to a psychologist or psychiatrist. Chronic persistent pain in the genital area with no physical cause can be seen after unethical aesthetic applications performed on patients who had been abused in childhood. This may be due to the reopening of the psychological wound (trauma) that was buried well in the past.

Appendix

With the purchase of this book, you can use our "SN Flashcards" app to access questions free of charge in order to test your learning and check your understanding of the contents of the book.

To use the app, please follow the instructions below:

1. Go to https://flashcards.springernature.com/login
2. Create a user account by entering your e-mail address and assigning a password.
3. Use the following link to access your SN Flashcards set: ▶ https://sn.pub/tvlq7Q

If the link is missing or does not work, please send an e-mail with the subject "SN Flashcards" and the book title to customerservice@springernature.com.

References

1. Franco T, Franco D. Hipertrofia de ninfas. J Bras Ginecol. 1993;103:163.
2. Tepper OM, Wulkan M, Matarasso A. Labiaplasty: anatomy, etiology, and a new surgical approach. Aesthet Surg J. 2011;31(5):511–8.
3. Radman HM. Hypertrophy of the labia minora. Obstet Gynecol. 1976;48(1 Suppl):78S–9S.
4. Motakef S, Rodriguez-Feliz J, Chung MT, Ingargiola MJ, Wong VW, Patel A. Vaginal labiaplasty: current practices and a simplified classification system for labial protrusion. Plast Reconstr Surg. 2015;135(3):774–88.
5. Alter GJ. A new technique for aesthetic labia minora reduction. Ann Plast Surg. 1998;40(3):287–90.
6. Alter GJ. Aesthetic labia minora and clitoral hood reduction using extended central wedge resection. Plast Reconstr Surg. 2008;122(6):1780–9.
7. Kaya AE, Dogan O, Yassa M, Basbug A, Çalışkan E. A novel technique for mapping the vascularity of labia minora prior to labiaplasty: cold light illumination. Geburtshilfe Frauenheilkd. 2018;78(8):775–84.
8. Choi HY, Kim KT. A new method for aesthetic reduction of labia minora (the deepithelialized reduction of labiaplasty). Plast Reconstr Surg. 2000;105(1):419–22; discussion 423–4.
9. Heyns M, Knight P, Steve AK, Yeung JK. A single preoperative dose of tranexamic acid reduces perioperative blood loss: a meta-analysis. Ann Surg. 2021;273(1):75–81.
10. Eserdağ S, Anğın AD. Surgical technique and outcomes of inverted-Y plasty procedure in clitoral hoodoplasty operations. J Minim Invasive Gynecol. 2021;28(9):1595–1602.

10 Clitoral Hoodoplasty and Frenulaplasty

Science is fortune in good times, a shelter and a good guide in bad times.

Aristo

The clitoral hood or "preputium" is the superior part of the labia minora. The tissue excess here disrupts sensitivity and sexual function and produces dissatisfaction in terms of aesthetic appearance [1].

Surgery to reduce the clitoral hood area aesthetically is called "clitoral hoodoplasty." It is also referred to by names such as "clitoral hoodectomy", "clitoral trimming", or "clitoral hood resection."

10.1 Why Is Hoodoplasty Required?

Since the clitoral hood is a part of the labia minora, clitoral hoodoplasty should be performed simultaneously with labial surgery because, in general, if labial hypertrophy is present, the excess tissue continues toward the clitoral hood area. Even unilateral labial hypertrophies usually have excess skin on the same side of the clitoral hood. Isolated hypertrophies are less common.

A physician who is not familiar with different clitoral hoodoplasty techniques should not perform labiaplasty operations. As a matter of fact, if a hoodoplasty procedure is not added to most labiaplasty operations, a much worse *"micropenis appearance"* appears compared to before.

10.2 Isolated Hoodoplasty

Sometimes hoodoplasty is needed to be applied alone:

- Most often in revision patients who had prior labiaplasty without hood reduction and therefore have aesthetic concerns,
- In isolated hood hypertrophy or clitoral dominance (Fig. 10.1),
- In cases of pseudoclitoromegaly,
- In cases of buried clitoral glans in diseases such as lichen sclerosis,
- In cases of clitoral hood tumors (rare) or abscess.

Hoodoplasty requires more surgical experience compared to labiaplasty because of its features and anatomical location.

Clitoral hoodoplasty is a completely safe and highly necessary operation. When applied with the right technique, it does not affect sexual plea-

S. Eserdağ, *Aesthetic and Functional Female Genital Surgery*,
https://doi.org/10.1007/978-3-031-16019-6_10

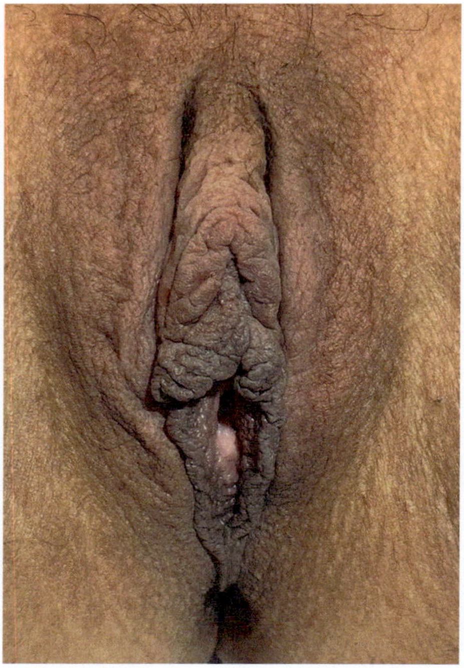

Fig. 10.1 Isolated hood hypertrophy. Hypertrophy of the hood area alone, with the patient's clitoris and labia being of normal size

sure. In fact, for many women, excess skin on the clitoris, wrinkles, and protruding appearance of the area negatively affect body perception and concentration in sexual intercourse. Having a thicker skin-subcutaneous tissue above the clitoris or the clitoris being embedded under this tissue may reduce sensation during sexual intercourse. The removal of excess skin on the clitoris both positively affects the body perception and increases the mechanical effect on the clitoral body during intercourse. However, evidence-based data are needed on this subject.

10.3 Classification and Management of Clitoral Hood Abnormalities

The classification and management of clitoral hood abnormalities were first made by Adam Ostrzenski in 2013 [2]. Ostrzenski divided the problems in the clitoral hood area into three main categories and suggested a separate interventional practice for each category as shown in Table 10.1.

Table 10.1 Classification and management of clitoral hood abnormalities according to Ostrzenski

	Explanation	Anatomy	Management
Type 1	Closed (occluded)	The clitoris is completely or partially buried under the clitoral hood	Hydrodissection with inverted V-plasty
Type 2	Hypertrophic-open	Clitoral hood skin long and thick	Modified Hydrodissection with inverted V-plasty
Type 3	Asymmetrical with subdermal hypertrophy	The thickness of the clitoral skin is not even	Subepithelial reduction

10.4 Hoodoplasty Techniques

Several surgical techniques have been proposed in the literature for hoodoplasty. We also added some techniques we have implemented. These include:

- *Bilateral longitudinal skin excisions (classical method)*
- *Inverted V-plasty (extended central wedge resection)* [3]
- *Hydrodissection with inverted V-plasty* [4]
- *Inverted Y-plasty (inverted Y-plasty, Eserdag)* [5]
- *Inverted-U extended hoodoplasty (inverted-U extended hoodoplasty, Eserdag)*
- *Hat trimming (Hat trimming, Eserdag)*
- *Subepithelial hoodoplasty (Ostrzenski)* [6]
- *Edge-wedge labiaplasty (edge-wedge technique)* [7]

10.4.1 Bilateral Longitudinal Skin Excisions (Classical Method)

This is a technique in which longitudinal incisions are made from both laterals of the clitoral hood, along the interlabial sulcus, and tissue is excised from this area. Thus, the clitoral hood will be made tighter, the wrinkles on it will be cleared, and the protrusion on this area will be slightly reduced (Figs. 10.2 and 10.3).

The advantage of this technique is that the incision scar is hidden in the interlabial sulcus. Also, since it is far from the glans, it does not cause postoperative sensitivity in this area. However, if the excess tissue in the clitoral hood is too large, this technique is not suitable. If too much tissue is removed along the interlabial sulcus, the hairs on the labia majora may

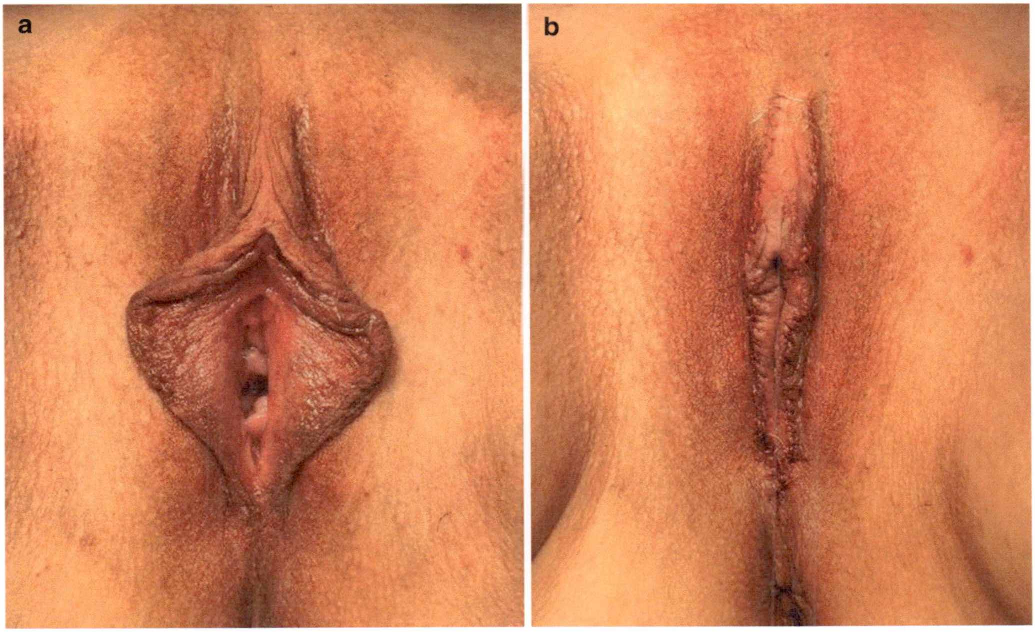

Fig. 10.2 Labial trimming and hoodoplasty by classical incision (**a–c**). Lines that do not converge on the hood

c

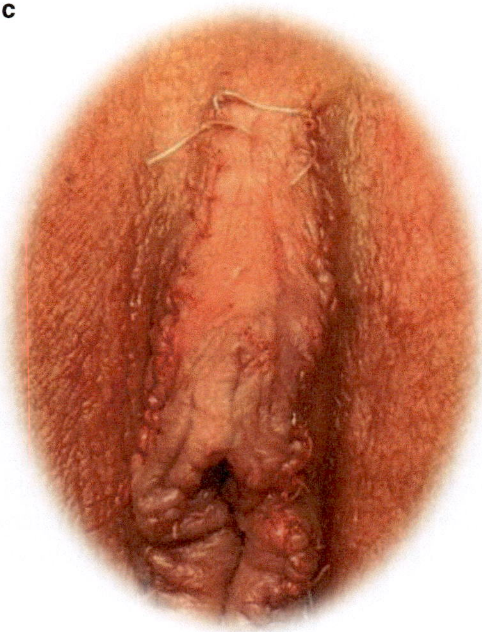

Fig. 10.2 (continued)

cause irritation by approaching the clitoral area. In this case, the only thing that can be recommended is laser epilation in the postoperative period.

10.4.2 Inverted V-Plasty and Extended Central Wedge Resection

In this technique, which was popularized by Gary Alter, clitoral hood resection is performed after the labia are reduced bilaterally by wedge resection. In hoodoplasty, the incisions starting from the interlabial sulcus of both labia are joined to the clitoral midline and excess tissues are removed along the incision line (Figs. 10.4 and 10.5). If the amount of tissue in the superior medial region of the clitoral hood is excessive, this technique may be insufficient.

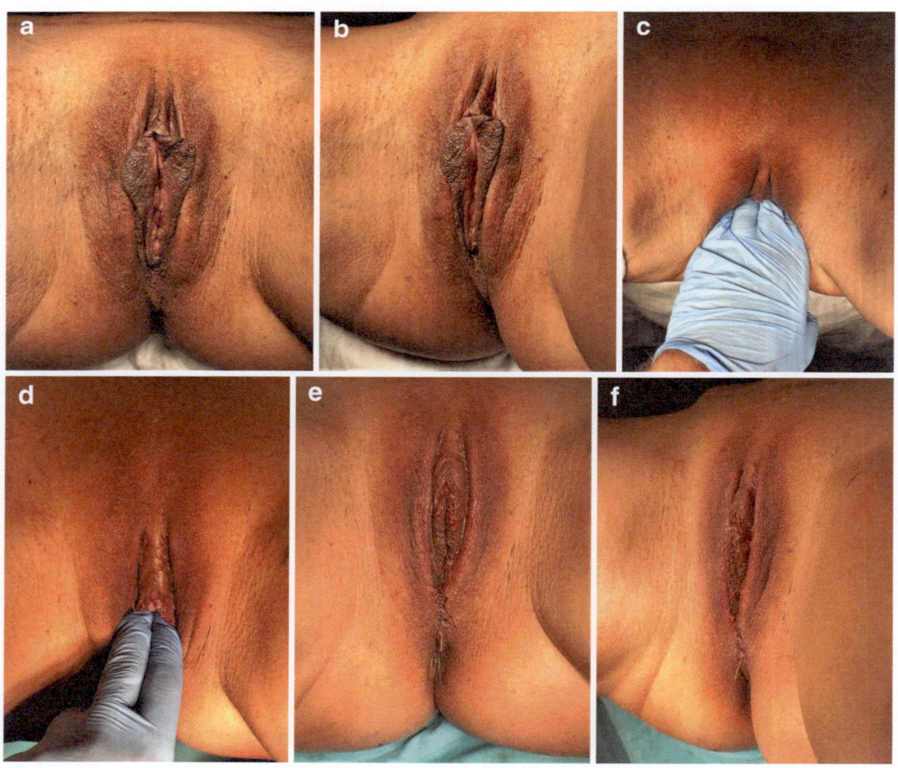

Fig. 10.3 Combined procedures of labiaplasty by trimming method, hoodoplasty by classical incision, perineoplasty, and vaginoplasty. Before (**a–c**), tightened vaginal entry after the procedure (**d**), just after views (**e**, **f**). Note that the labia majora also became more regular after the operation

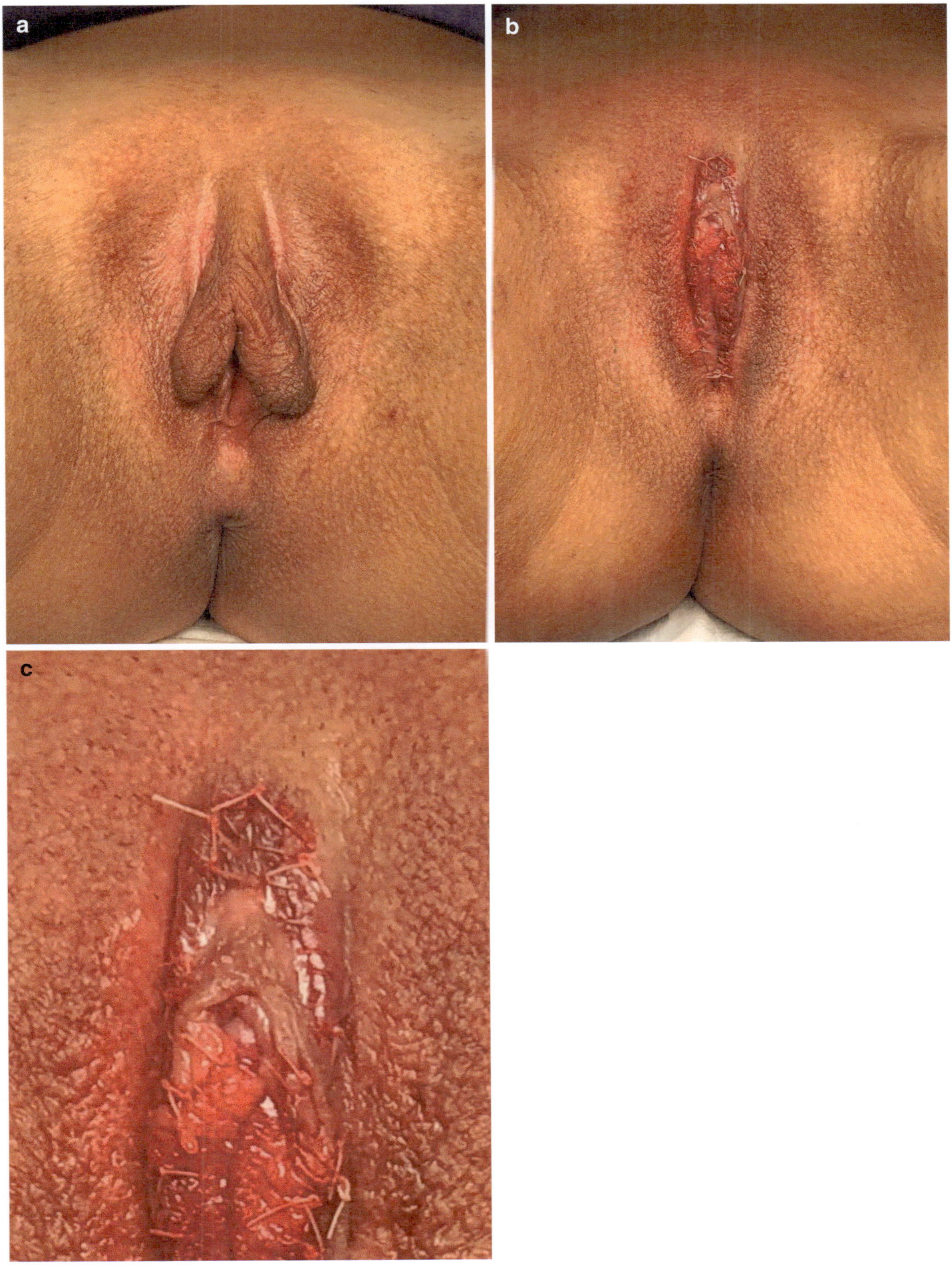

Fig. 10.4 Labiaplasty and inverted-v clitoral hoodoplasty Views before (**a**) and just after surgery (**b**, **c**)

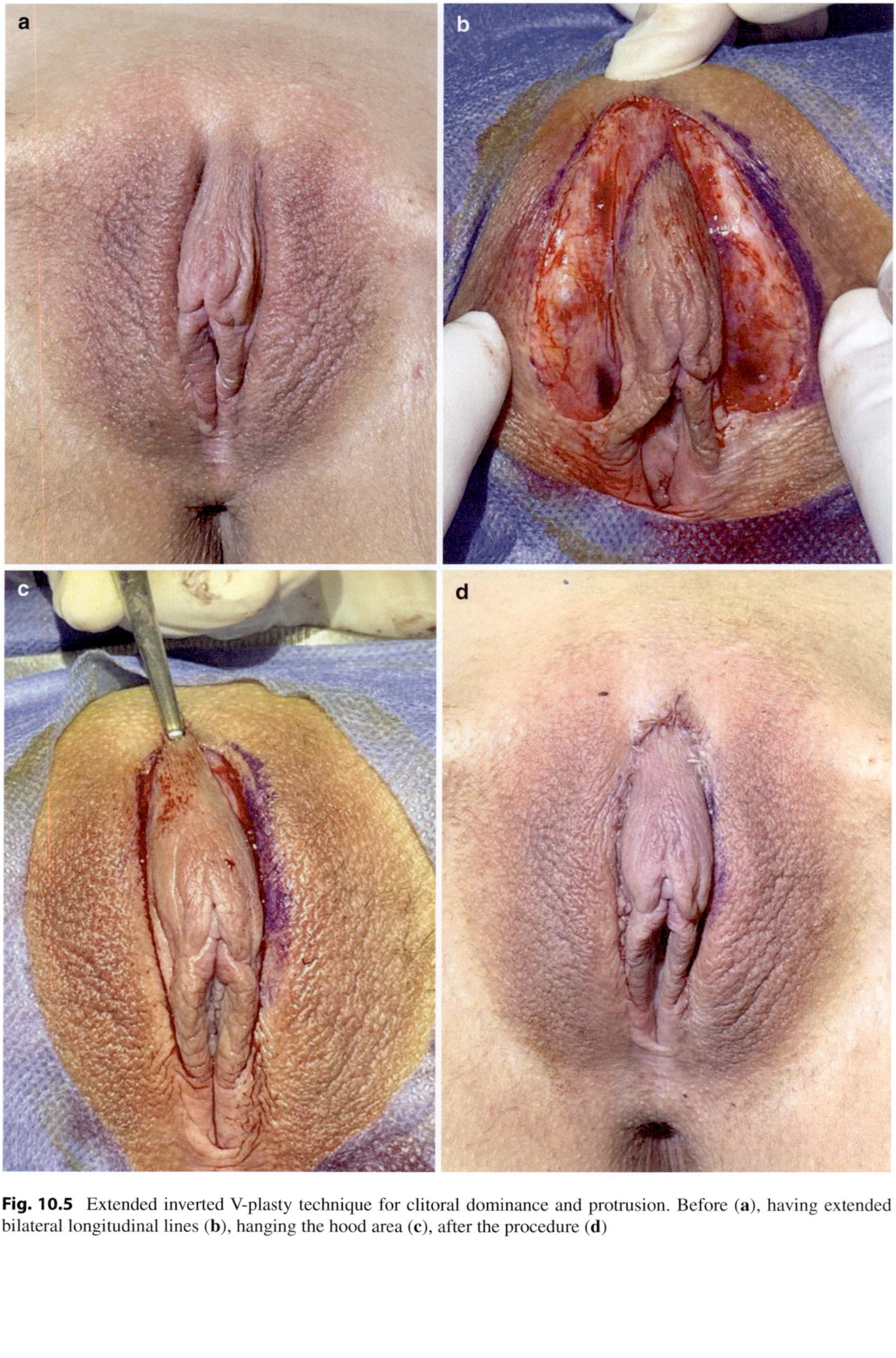

Fig. 10.5 Extended inverted V-plasty technique for clitoral dominance and protrusion. Before (**a**), having extended bilateral longitudinal lines (**b**), hanging the hood area (**c**), after the procedure (**d**)

10.4.3 Hydrodissection with Inverted V-Plasty

This is a two-step technique recommended especially in clitoral phimosis conditions such as lichen sclerosis. In the first stage, sterile saline is injected into the space between the clitoris and the preputium, debris due to the accumulated smegma is drained, and the adhesions in between are opened. In the second stage, the 45 degree-angulation of the flap to the frenulum created by making a 5 mm incision in the dorsal midline after cutting the adhesions with fine scissors is performed to make an inverted V-plasty. The incision site is closed with 6/0 rapid absorbable vicryls.

Buried glans clitoridis can be re-exposed by different methods (Fig. 10.6).

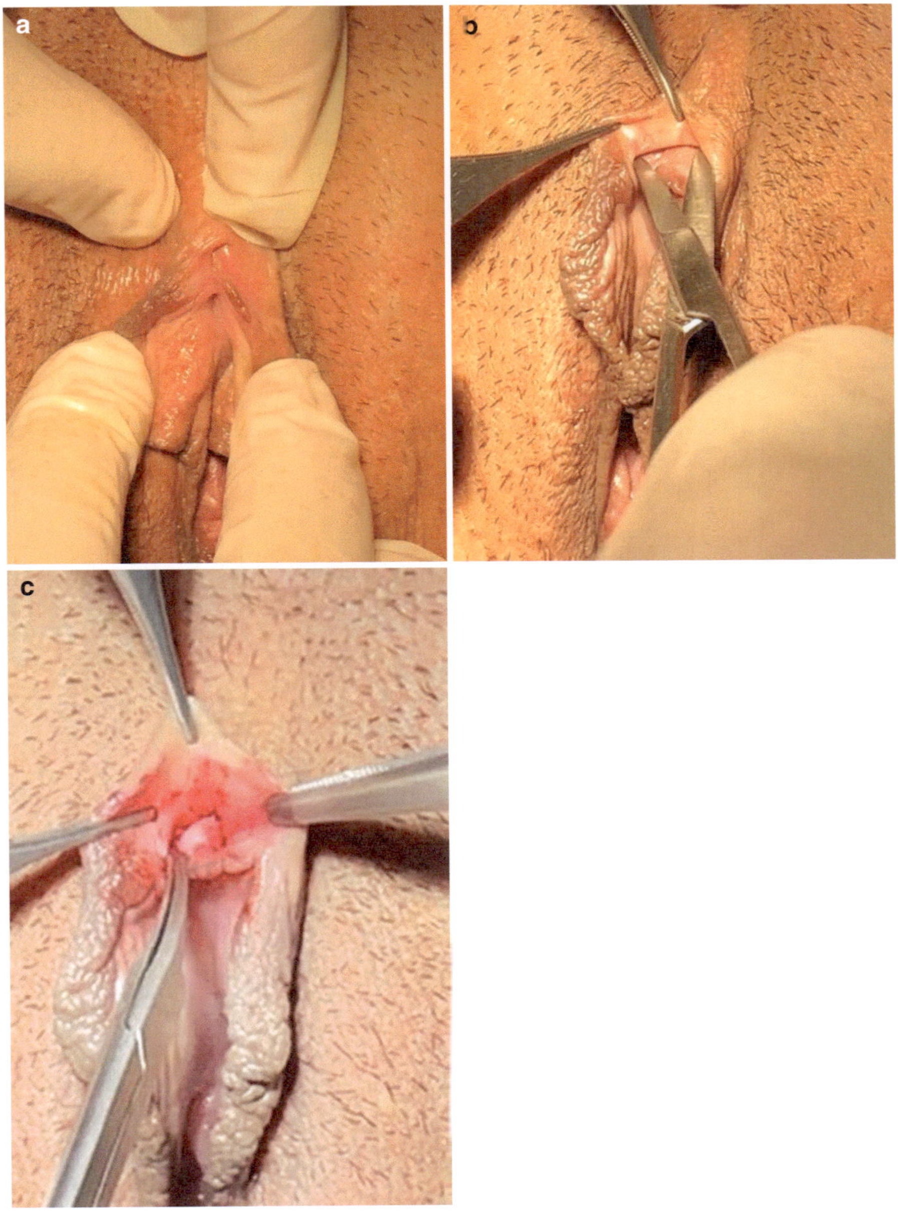

Fig. 10.6 Re-exposure of the buried glans clitoridis by blunt dissection with fine scissors. Before (**a**), scissors dissection (**b**), re-exposition of the glans (**c**)

10.4.4 Inverted-Y Plasty (Eserdag Technique)

Clitoral hoodoplasty can be added to almost all patients undergoing labiaplasty. The most common method used is the inverted Y-shaped incision on the hood by continuing the partial labial excision (Fig. 10.7). The advantages of this technique are that it allows maximum tissue removal and the desired level of clitoral lifting in the hood [5].

In the operation, in the inverted-Y incision, the bilateral skin folds starting from the edges of the labia and continuing on the hood are completely excised, and both incision lines are joined in the middle over the hood (Inverted-V appearance). With a longitudinal central incision above this junction, the excess tissues in the central area are removed by advancing to the anterior commissura and sometimes even higher (tail of the letter Y). The central incision may be long or short depending on the excess tissue of the patient. If it is below 1 cm, we call it "short-tailed Y"; if it is above 1 cm, we call it "long-tailed Y."

The clitoral area is rich in capillaries. After subcutaneous hemostasis is achieved with bipolar cautery, the subcutaneous layer is gently closed with one or two layers of 4/0 rapid absorbable sutures and the skin with 5/0 rapid absorbable sutures. In order for the wound healing process to be rapid, the skin sutures should be placed perpendicular to the skin and without excessive stretching.

A proven superiority of any hoodoplasty technique mentioned above has not yet been determined. Prospective and controlled studies on this subject are also very few.

In clitoral hoodoplasty operations, it is recommended to use only scissors or a scalpel while making the incision. Monopolar cautery or laser incisions are not recommended as they may cause tissue damage in adjacent areas. In addition, cautery and laser can increase the risk of scarring. Tight lifting and excessive tissue removal should be avoided in order to prevent the glans from being exposed outwardly.

Anterior commissuroplasty procedure with extended inverted-Y can be applied, especially in patients who demand reduction of the aperture in the clitoral hood area (Fig. 10.8).

Excision of some tumors in the clitoral hood area (Fig. 10.9) and excision of small fistulas (Fig. 10.10) can also be done with inverted-Y plasty technique as well.

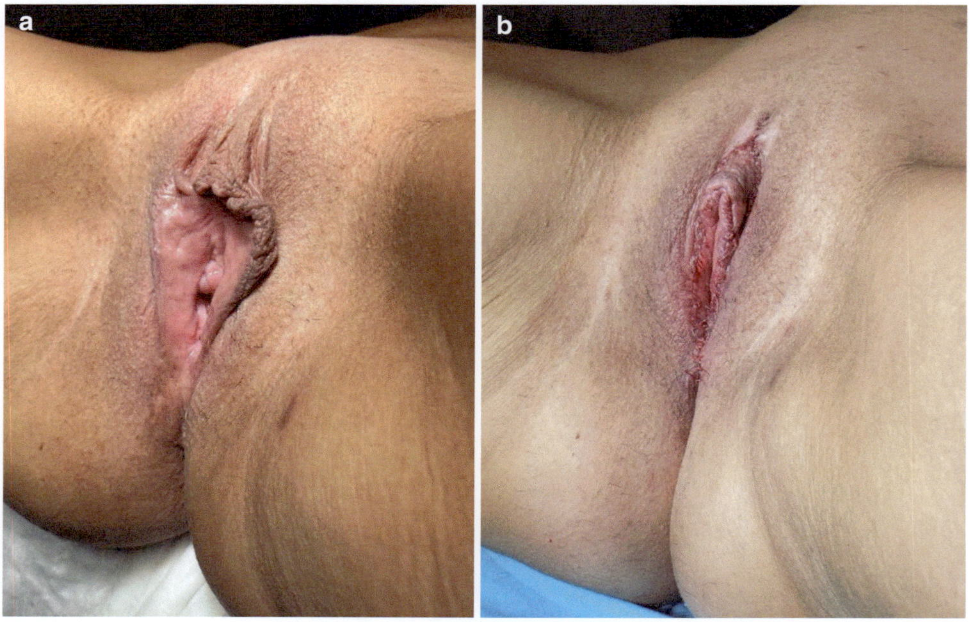

Fig. 10.7 Labiaplasty by trimming, hoodoplasty by inverted-Y technique, perineoplasty, and vaginoplasty combined surgery. Pay attention to slight "clitoral lifting" in inverted-Y hoodoplasty. Before (**a**), After (**b**)

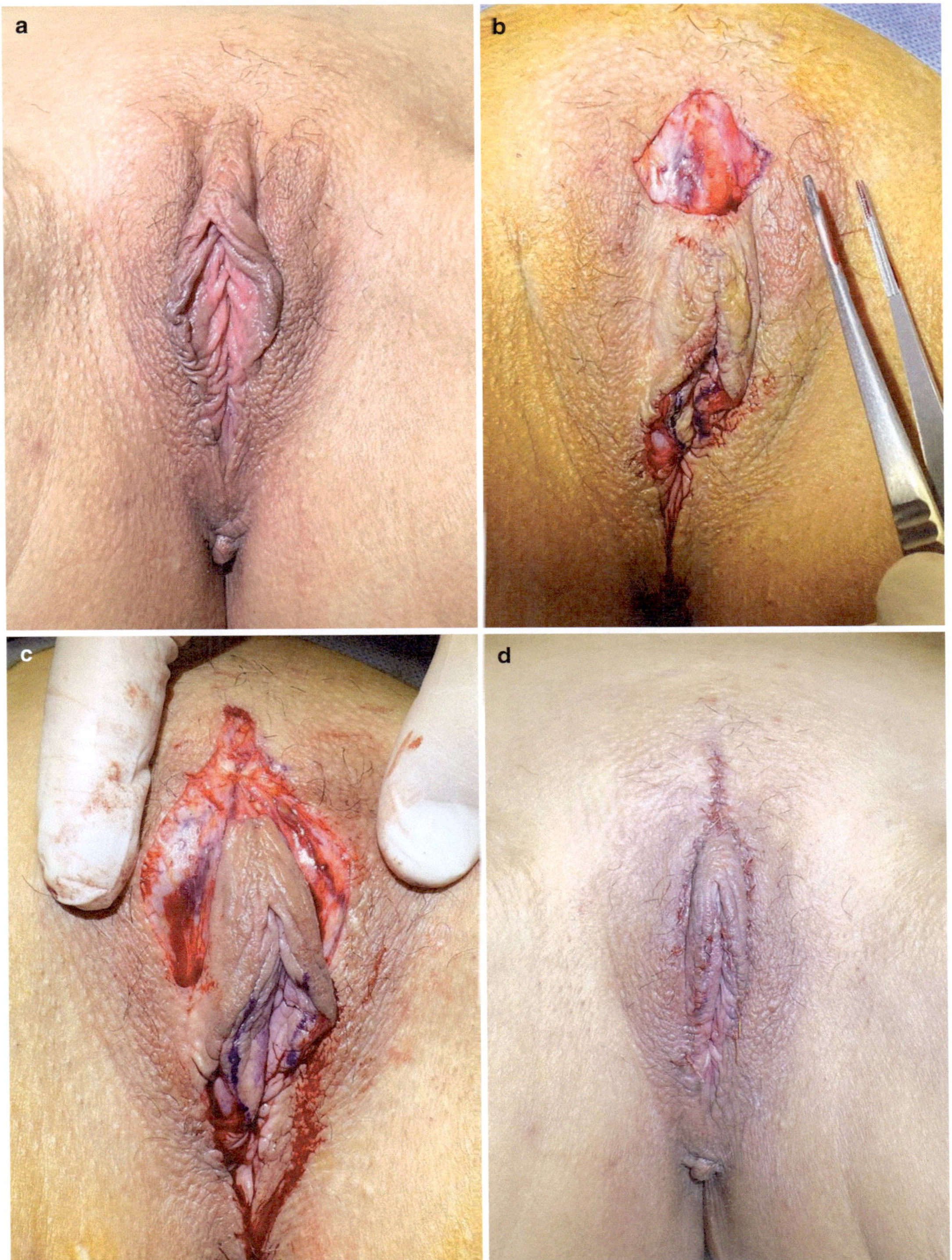

Fig. 10.8 Labiaplasty and extended inverted-Y h(*Eserdag*). Before (**a**), diamond incision are made on the hood (**b**), legs of the diamond are extended downwards (**c**), after (**d**)

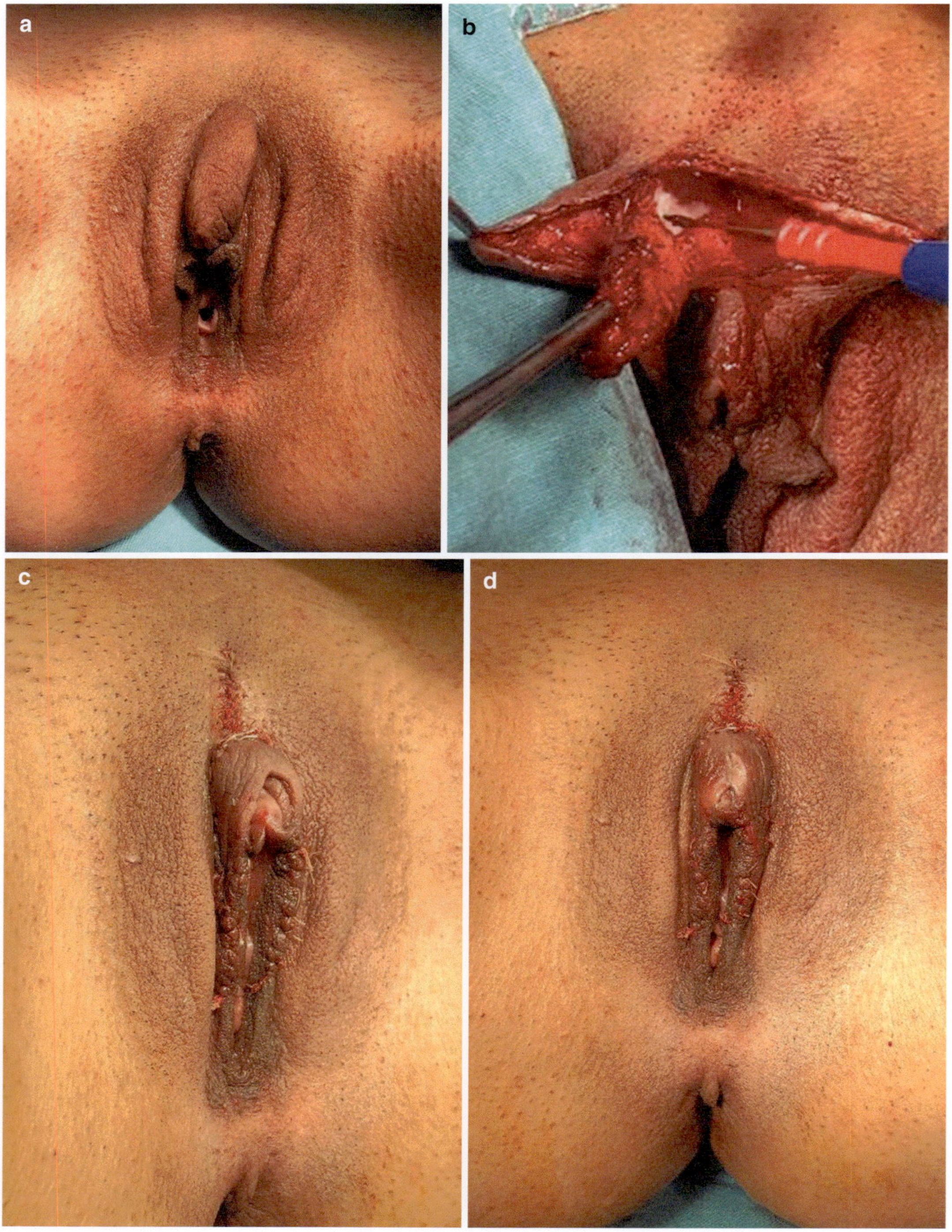

Fig. 10.9 Clitoral hood tumor excision. The pathology confirmed "epidermal infundibular inclusion cyst." Before (**a**), removal of the tumor with the Inverted-Y plasty technique (**b**), and after the primary closure (**c**, **d**)

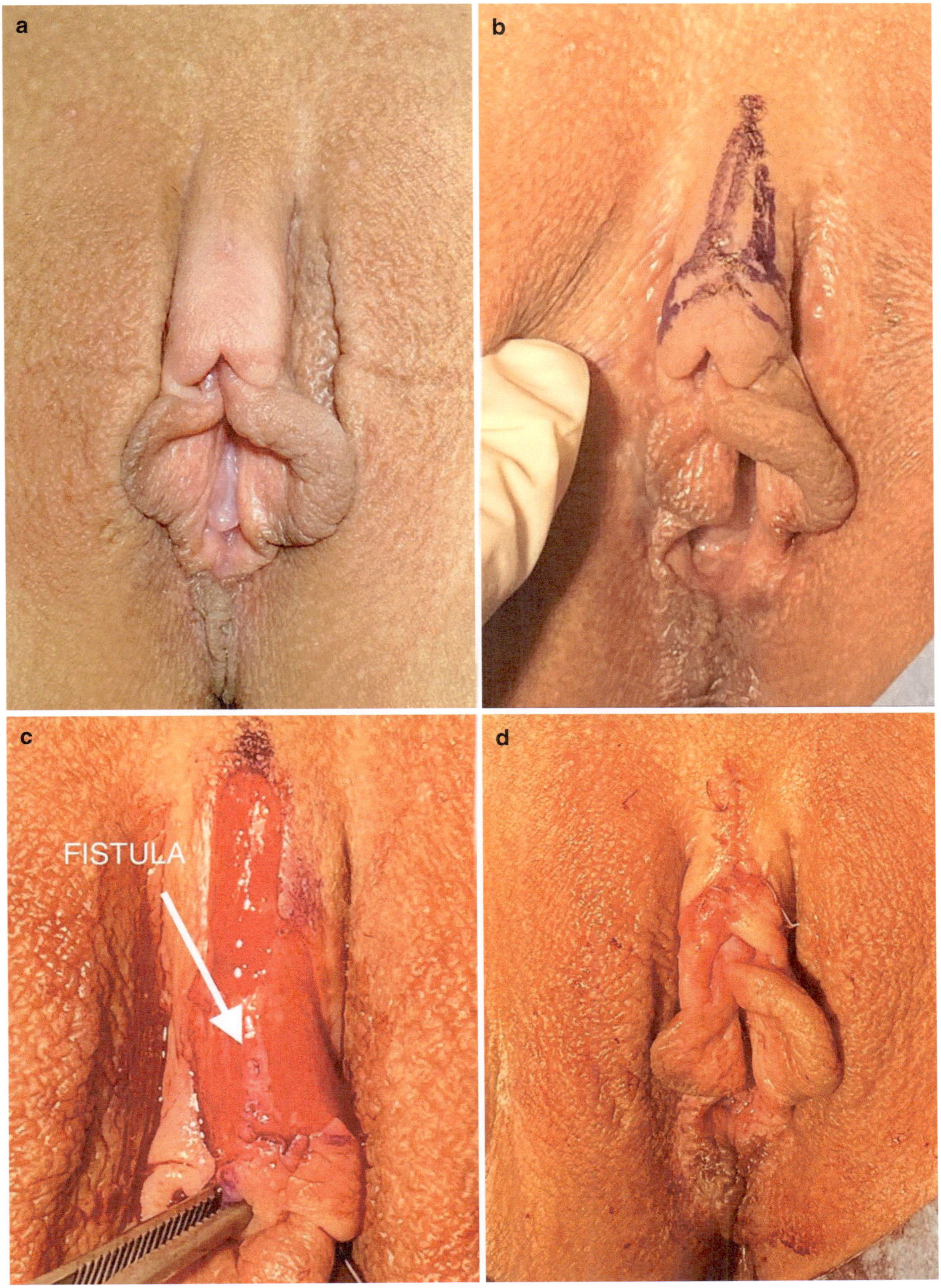

Fig. 10.10 Thin fistula between the clitoral hood and the space around the glans. Probably, the fistula has been occurred as a result of smegma collection, followed by the infection and then abscess formation. Before (**a**), marking (**b**), removal of the fistula with inverted Y-Plasty technique (**c**), and reconstruction of the hood area (**d**)

10.4.5 Inverted-U Extended Hoodoplasty (Eserdag)

Another hoodoplasty technique is in the form of an inverted-U incision. In this procedure, the hood area can be flattened and some stretching can be obtained on the superior labia majora (Fig. 10.11).

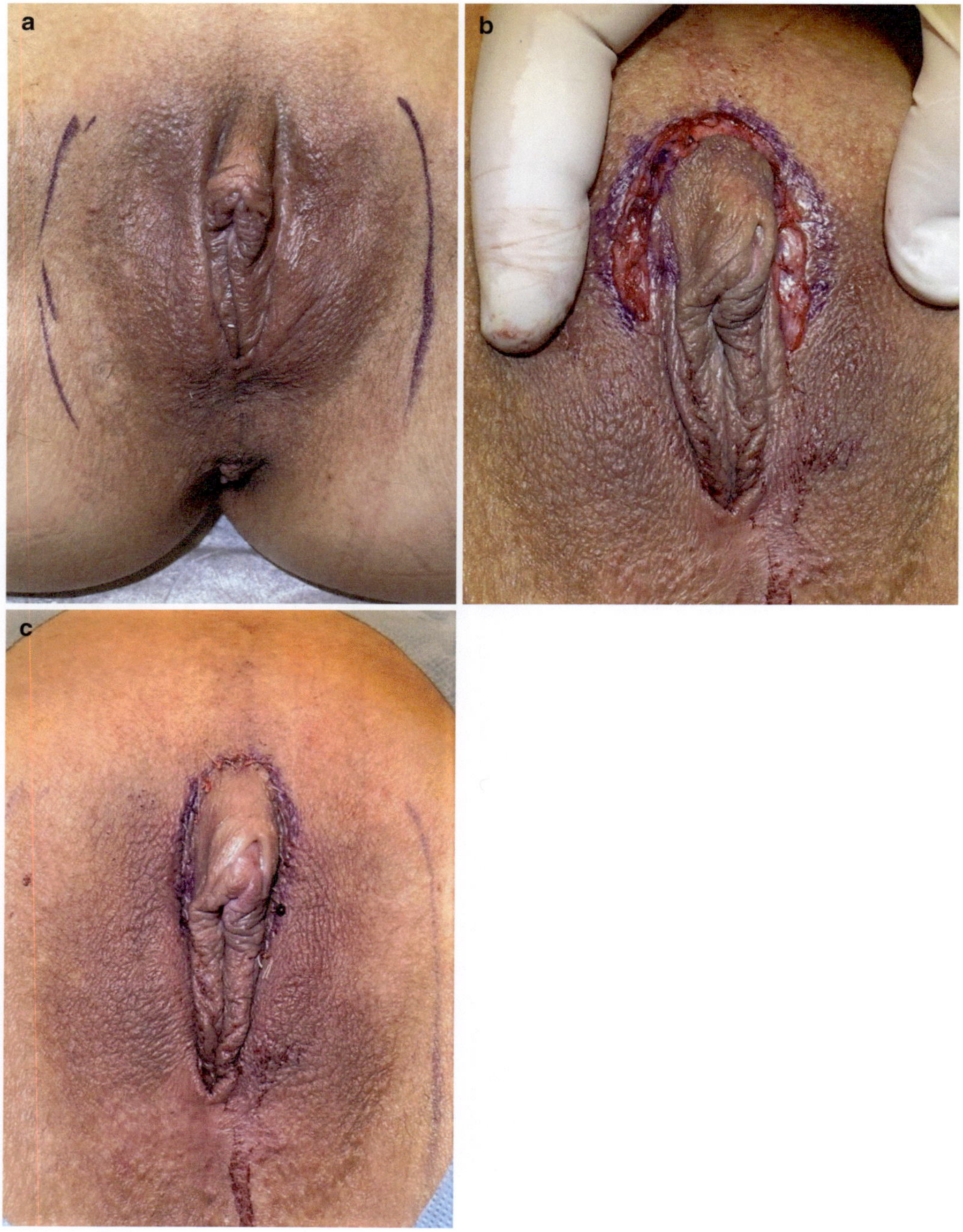

Fig. 10.11 Inverted-U extended hoodoplasty, (*Eserdag*). This allows the prominent hood region to be taken in and also ensures some tension to the superior labia majora. Before (**a**), excision of the tissue as inverted-U shape (**b**), after (**c**)

10.4.6 Hat Trimming (Eserdag)

A new technique that I can suggest among hoodoplasty techniques is the removal of excess skin tissue covering the glans clitoris, which I call *"hat trimming"* (Fig. 10.12). This management is only a suitable method for patients who have excess skin on the glans clitoris, who do not have clitoral hypertrophy, whose glans is embedded inside, and who express that they cannot sufficiently feel clitoral stimulation during sexual intercourse.

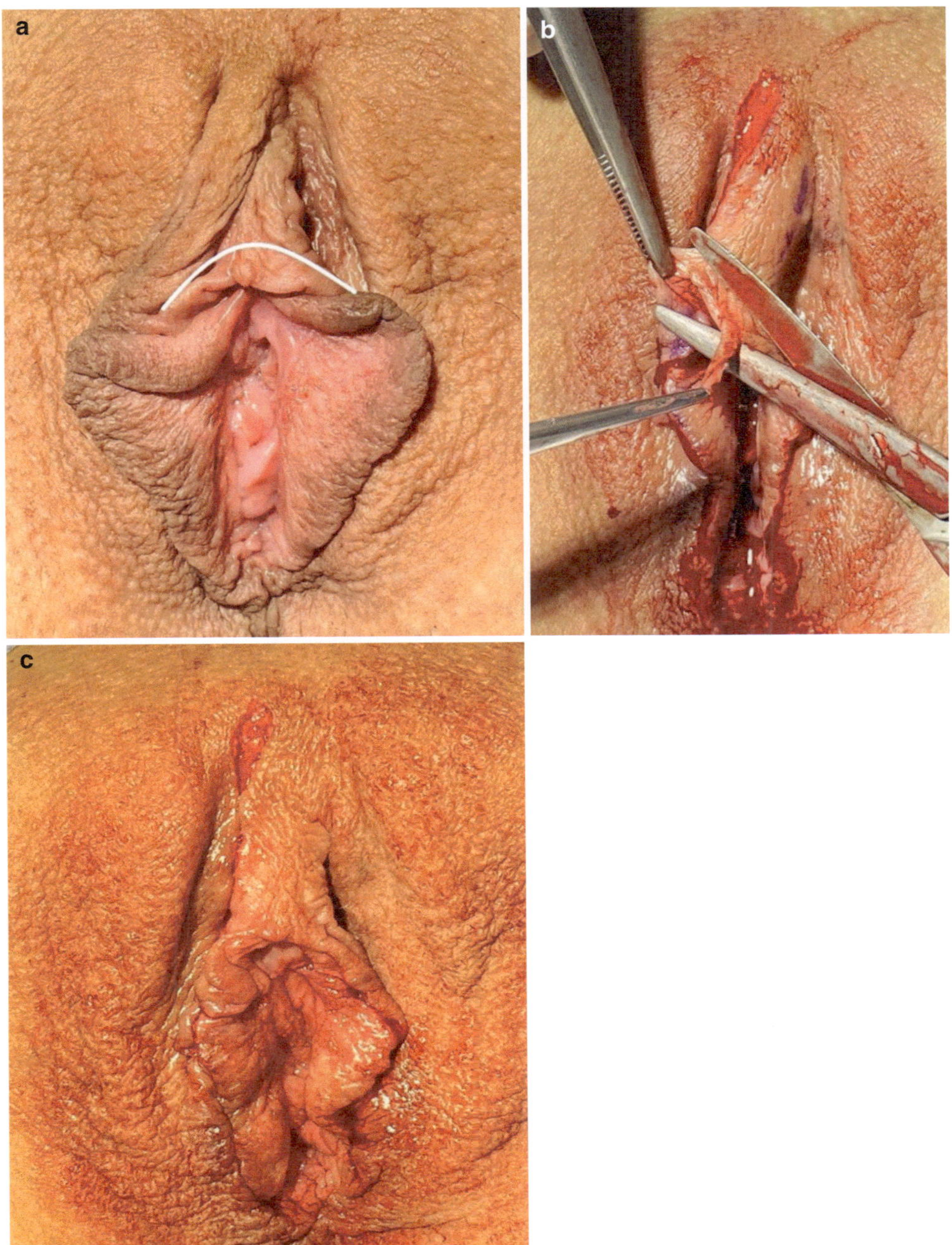

Fig. 10.12 Bilateral partial resection of the right clitoral skin fold, triangular frenuloplasty, and hat trimming operations in a case of labial asymmetry. Before (**a**), hat trimming (**b**), after closure of subcutaneous tissue (**c**)

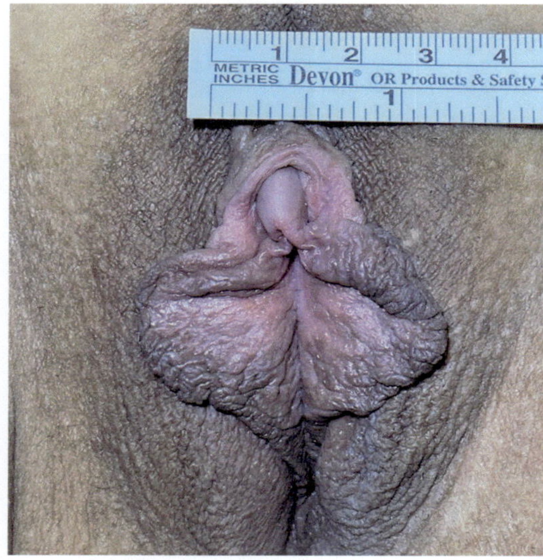

Fig. 10.13 Increased clitoral index and hyperpigmentation due to polycystic ovary syndrome

10.4.7 Subepithelial Hoodoplasty

This is a technique described by Ostrzenski in 2010, recommended for cases of asymmetry in the hood area. In this technique, subcutaneous excess areas in thick and asymmetrical hood areas are excised.

10.4.8 Edge-Wedge Labiaplasty (Edge-Wedge Technique)

In this technique, while labiaplasty is performed as partial resection (Edge), the clitoral hood is removed as a wedge (Wedge).

10.5 Complications

In clitoral hoodoplasty, complications such as bleeding, hematoma, severe pain in the operation area, and edema may occur in the acute period. In the late period, there is a risk of scar formation. Delay of wound healing process, infection, and dehiscence are factors that increase the risk of scarring. In addition, loss of sensation can be seen due to damage to the neurovascular tissue. This is an area that needs to be operated very carefully. Excessive removal of the preputium skin causes irritation due to the protrusion of the glans to the outside.

10.6 The Postoperative Term

Postoperative practices in hoodoplasty are the same as in the labiaplasty operation. In addition, sexual sensitivity during masturbation and coitus can be inquired periodically.

10.7 Clitoromegaly

The clitoris may be thicker and larger than normal size due to congenital, idiopathic, or acquired causes. This condition is known as "clitoromegaly" or "macroclitoris." Clitoromegaly may occur due to androgen exposure during the fetal, infant, or adolescent periods. Hypertrichosis is another accompanying finding in these cases [8].

In clitoromegaly as shown in Fig. 10.13, the "clitoral index" obtained by multiplying the length and width of the glans clitoridis anatomically is greater than 35 mm^2.

Clitoromegaly is a finding seen with hypertrichosis in polycystic ovary syndrome (PCOS). It can also be observed in congenital adrenal hyperplasia (CAH), use of norethisterone during pregnancy, and Fraser syndrome, an autosomal recessive disease. In some cases, isolated idiopathic clitoromegaly can also occur without any additional pathology [9]. In addition, it may rarely occur in Sertoli-Leydig cell tumors, neurofibromatosis, lymphangioma, chronic vulvar irritation, and some clitoral cysts. Acquired clitoromegaly may occur due to androgenic drugs used for bodybuilding, performance enhancement while doing sports, increasing libido, or for the treatment of sexual desire problems.

"Pseudoclitoromegaly" is a condition that can develop due to the enlargement of the labia minora and clitoral hood as a result of the mechanical effect of frequent masturbation in young girls, when in reality there is no clitoromegaly.

In case of clitoromegaly, clitoroplasty can be performed for reduction.

Complete agenesis of the clitoris is a rare condition. Bifid or duplicated clitoris can also be seen in girls with exstrophy-epispadias complex.

10.8 Clitoral Protrusion

It is the protruding position of the clitoris. While this group of patients may have clitoromegaly, in some cases, the clitoral body and glans stand out structurally. Lack of fat in the labia majora will also reinforce this appearance.

For the correction of protruded clitoris, after the dissection of clitoris, a hole is made under the clitoral body, some soft tissue is removed, and then the body is pulled inferiorly by sutures as shown in Fig. 10.14. Care should be taken not to have angulation of the clitoral body that can cause pain during orgasm. This invasive intervention has the risk of bleeding and should be preferred only in selected cases (Fig. 10.15).

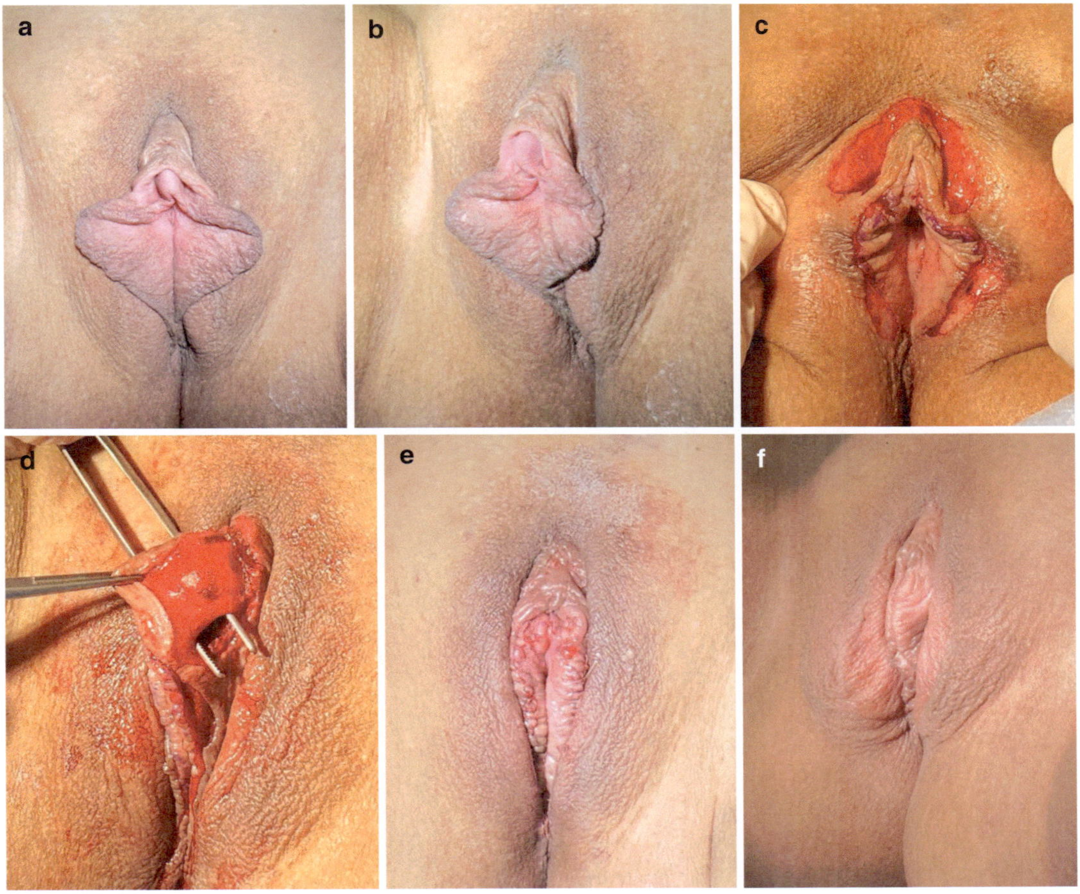

Fig. 10.14 Late onset adrenal hyperplasia, associated labial hypertrophy, mild clitoromegaly, and clitoral protrusion. Before (**a**, **b**), partial labial excision and inverted-V hoodoplasty incisions (**c**), making a hole under clitoral body, and then the body withdrawn by vicryl sutures (**d**), just after (**e**), and postop fourth month (**f**)

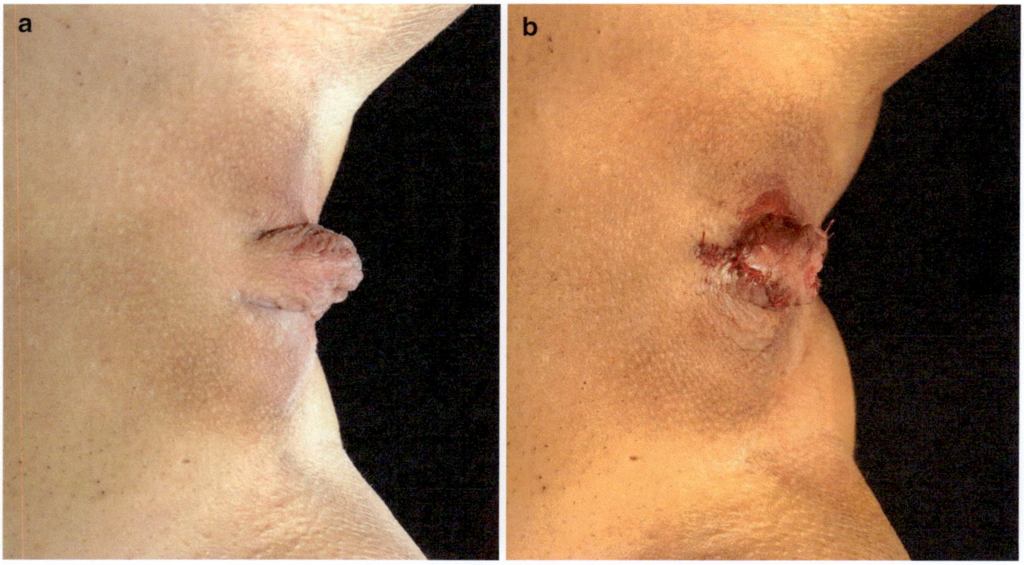

Fig. 10.15 Hood withdrawal technique *(Eserdag)* and inverted Y-Plasty procedures in a patient with clitoral protrusion. Panoramic views before (**a**) and just after the surgery (**b**)

10.9 Frenulaplasty

The frenulum is the thin skin folds that connect the labia minora to the glans clitoridis, rich in vascular circulation and nerve innervation. In some patients, it may be in the form of a very thin and small band, while in others it is quite thick and long.

Concomitant with labiaplasty and clitoral hoodoplasty, frenulum reduction is also required in patients with frenulum hypertrophy to achieve a better aesthetic result. The reduction of the frenulum by excising it surgically is mostly called "frenulaplasty," but might be better if we use the plural term "frenulaplasty."

In the frenulaplasty operation, hypertrophic tissue is removed by direct excision or triangular incision (Fig. 10.16). Due to the vascular structure of this area, there is a high tendency to bleed during the operation. Cautery should not be used as much as possible in hemostasis to avoid the risks of sensitivity, enduration, and scar formation. Suturing is usually done with a single layer and 5/0 or 6/0 rapid absorbable sutures. The healing process of this area is more troublesome than the

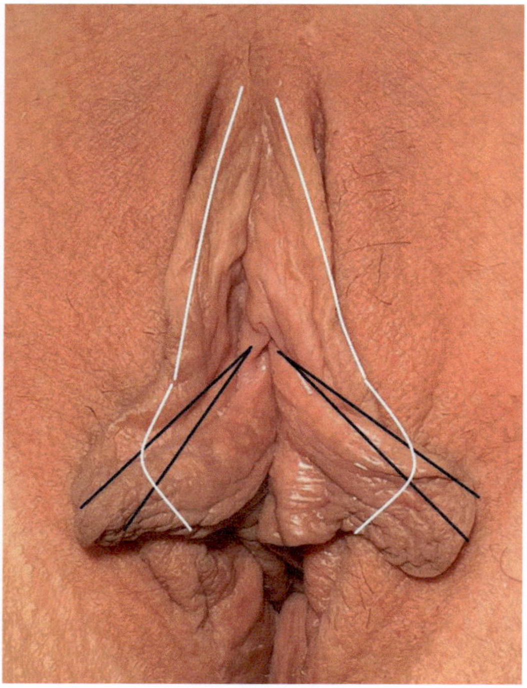

Fig. 10.16 Surgical incision lines for a combined operation. Triangular excision (black lines) for frenulaplasty and longitudinal incision for labiaplasty-hoodoplasty (white lines) are shown. The frenula attached to the clitoridis are hypertrophic so much that can mimic the labia

labia. Sutures placed in the frenulum may cause irritation in the clitoris during the healing period.

Sometimes labiaplasty, hood reduction, and frenulaplasty should be performed concomitantly to provide a whole aesthetic satisfaction (Fig. 10.17).

The technique applied in labiaplasty, frenulaplasty, and clitorohoodoplasty combined surgeries can be called as *"pine tree incision."* It is described below with the images (Fig. 10.18).

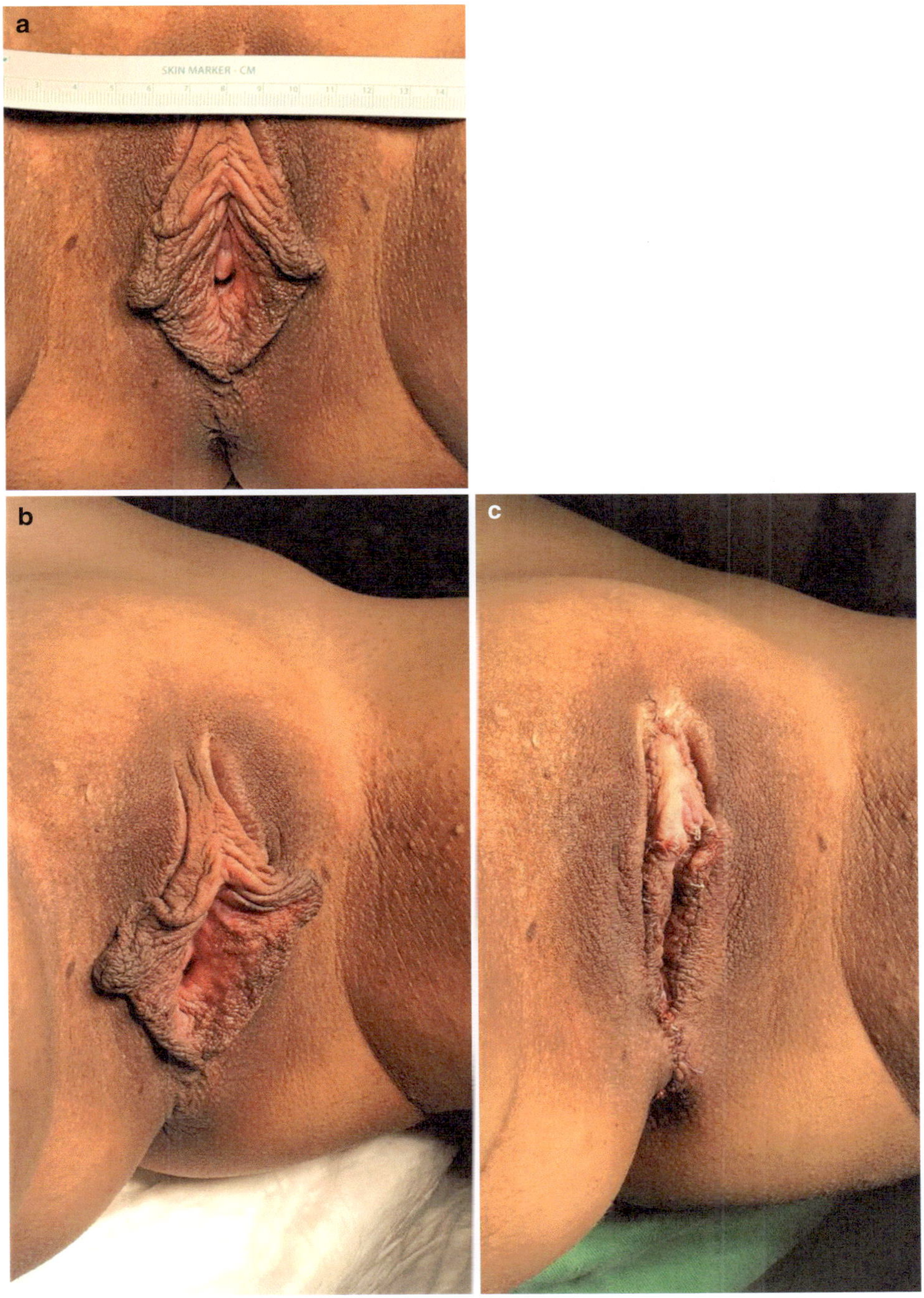

Fig. 10.17 Labiaplasty, hoodoplasty, and frenulaplasty operations of a patient with severe labial and frenular hypertrophy. Before (**a**, **b**), just after (**c**)

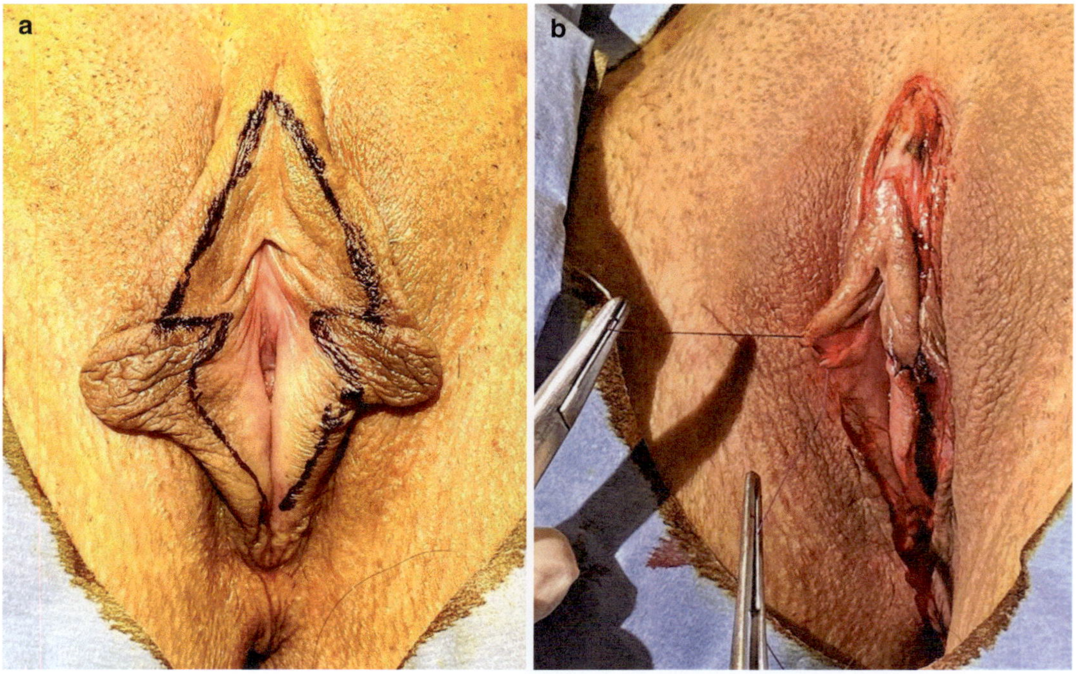

Fig. 10.18 Pine Tree Incision *(Eserdag)*. It can be preferred in the composite labiaplasty for the patients with hypertrophic labia, frenula, and hood area. Marking (**a**) and excision (**b**)

Appendix

With the purchase of this book, you can use our "SN Flashcards" app to access questions free of charge in order to test your learning and check your understanding of the contents of the book.

To use the app, please follow the instructions below:

1. Go to https://flashcards.springernature.com/login
2. Create a user account by entering your e-mail address and assigning a password.
3. Use the following link to access your SN Flashcards set: ▶ https://sn.pub/tvlq7Q

If the link is missing or does not work, please send an e-mail with the subject "SN Flashcards" and the book title to customerservice@springernature.com.

References

1. Zeplin PH. Clitoral Hood reduction. Aesthet Surg J. 2016;36(7):NP231.
2. Ostrzenski A. Selecting aesthetic gynecologic procedures for plastic surgeons: a review of target methodology. Aesthet Plast Surg. 2013;37(2):256–65.
3. Alter GJ. Aesthetic labia minora and clitoral hood reduction using extended central wedge resection. Plast Reconstr Surg. 2008;122(6):1780–9.

4. Ostrezenski A. A new, hydrodissection with reverse V-plasty technique for the buried clitoris associated with lichen sclerosis. J Gynecol Surg. 2010;26:41–8.
5. Eserdağ S, Anğın AD. Surgical technique and outcomes of inverted-Y Plasty procedure in clitoral Hoodoplasty operations. J Minim Invasive Gynecol. 2021;28:1595.
6. Ostrzenski A. Clitoral subdermal hoodoplasty for medical indications and aesthetic motives. A new technique. J Reprod Med. 2013;58(3–4):149–52.
7. Devgan L. Abstract: the edge-wedge labiaplasty: a novel technique for female genital rejuvenation. Plast Reconstr Surg Glob Open. 2017;5(9 Suppl):87–8.
8. Iezzi ML, Lasorella S, Varriale G, Zagaroli L, Ambrosi M, Verrotti A. Clitoromegaly in childhood and adolescence: behind one clinical sign, a Clinical Sea. Sex Dev. 2018;12(4):163–74.
9. Copcu E, Aktas A, Sivrioglu N, Copcu O, Oztan Y. Idiopathic isolated clitoromegaly: a report of two cases. Reprod Health. 2004;1(1):4.

11 Vaginoplasty

The end of path not leading science is dark. Science is the light illuminating roads towards the reality.

Haji Bektash Wali

Vaginal enlargement and sagging are often due to connective tissue weakness or fascia defects. The most important factor in the structure of collagen connective tissue in the whole body is our genetic features. Loosening (relaxation) due to vaginal collagen reduction generally develops due to difficult births, pregnancy, smoking, old age, menopause, collagen tissue diseases, and estrogen deficiency.

Vaginoplasty is a surgical tightening and reconstruction of the vagina, and it is a classical colporrhaphy operation. Tightening is often done through the posterior vaginal wall, sometimes through the anterior and lateral walls. Terminologically, the term "surgical vaginal rejuvenation" can also be used with some medical marketing thought.

In Turkey in the early 2000s, genital aesthetic operations started to appear in the media for the first time under the name of "vaginal aesthetics," and this misuse statement still continues. The vagina is an internal organ and there are no aesthetics of internal organs! Vaginal tightening operations are reconstructive surgeries. What is usually meant by vaginal aesthetics is vulva aesthetics because the word "vagina" is often used by the public to describe the vulva: "*I am not satisfied with the color of my vagina, I want to have vagina bleaching, I do not like the appearance of my vagina, my vagina hurts.*"

11.1 Ideal Vagina Concept

Five distinct features are important for the "ideal vagina": narrowness, ruga structure, mucosal integrity, elasticity, and vaginal axis (Fig. 11.1). The vaginal canal should be narrow, the ruga structures plentiful, the mucosal integrity should be complete, the elasticity should be good, and the axis should be straight. All surgical and nonsurgical procedures applied to the vagina aim to improve these properties.

Vaginal relaxation is closely related to physiological processes such as aging, menopause, pregnancy, and birth. There are also those who consider this situation to be a precursor of future pelvic prolapse.

Vaginal enlargement and impairment of mucosal integrity bring along sexual dysfunctions in the patient and her partner due to the decrease in sensation.

S. Eserdağ, *Aesthetic and Functional Female Genital Surgery*,
https://doi.org/10.1007/978-3-031-16019-6_11

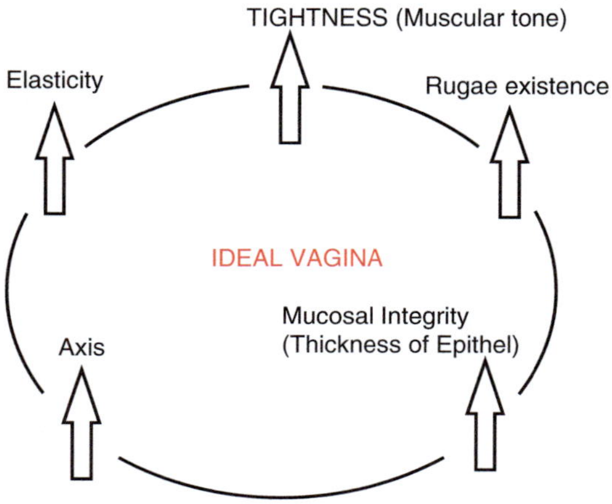

Fig. 11.1 Ideal vagina features

11.2 Juicy Vagina Syndrome *(Eserdag)*

Some patients complain of hyperlubrication and decreased sensation during intercourse. Some of them even complain of the irritating, physiological looking but excessive amount of wetness that continues outside of sexual intercourse. There are three main sources of lubrication due to sexual stimulation in women: vestibular glands (Bartholin's and Skene's glands), vaginal venous transudation, and endocervical glands. Although vaginal dryness is a subject that has been discussed extensively, "hypermucosis" or so-called by us "Juicy Vagina Syndrome," which has not yet found its place in the literature, is a subject open to research in all aspects. For treatment of this complaint, it is recommended to ablate endocervical glands by electrocautery or laser.

11.3 Vaginal Wind (Flatus Vaginalis, Queef)

This is the sound of air leakage during or immediately after sexual penetration. Air leakage from the vagina is also known as "Flatus Vaginalis" or "Vaginal Wind." Most patients state that their concentration is impaired during coitus due to this unintended sound they hear, they feel shame in front of their partners, and therefore they cannot focus on pleasure. There are even those who reject sexuality for this reason alone.

Uncomfortable sounds due to odorless vaginal air leakage can also be seen with increased intra-abdominal pressure such as yoga, fitness, and weight lifting, as well as intercourse. It has been reported to occur even in a 17-year-old, thin, nulliparous girl with a narrow vagina. In this patient, the problem was solved with the use of vaginal tampons, as the problem did not respond to many physical therapies applied by a private therapist [1].

Most women associate these coital sounds that decrease the quality of life with vaginal width and come to the physician for vaginal tightening surgeries. Yes, it is true that the vaginal canal expands like a balloon due to arousal during sexual intercourse. However, "Juicy Vagina Syndrome" also plays an important role in this. In a review article, it was stated that the prevalence of vaginal air leakage is around 20%. It is due to the enlargement of the vaginal hiatus as a result of vaginal laxity due to weakness of the pelvic floor muscles. Vaginal laser is promising for its treatment [2]. The effects of vaginoplasty operations on hyperlubrication and flatus vaginalis are not yet clear.

11.4 Vaginal Gaping

This is the state of the vaginal entrance being open (gaping) (Fig. 11.2). It causes aesthetic and functional problems for many patients. Flatus due to air exit from the vagina, frequent vaginitis due to flora deterioration, inability to feel during sexual intercourse, and an aesthetically unpleasant appearance are the most common complaints of patients. Vaginal gaping, which usually occurs after birth, is mostly due to the hypotonicity of the bulbocavernosus muscle. Vaginoplasty and

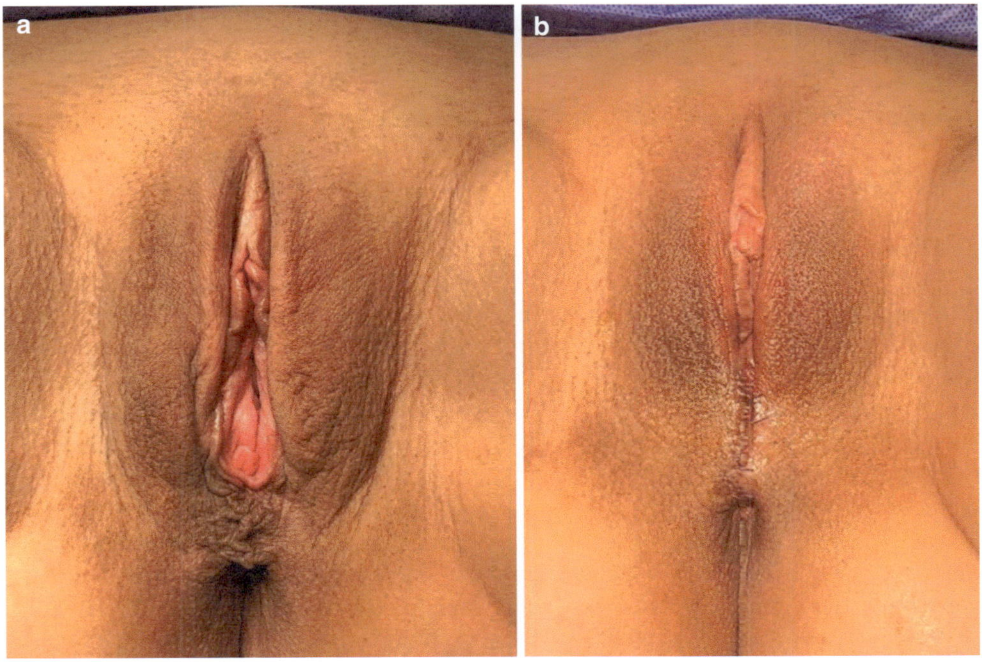

Fig. 11.2 Vaginal gaping and laxity (38 years old). Notice that the problem of laxity in the labia majora seems to have been resolved considerably even though no procedure was performed on this area. Before (**a**), after (**b**)

perineoplasty operations are performed to eliminate the problem.

11.5 Lost Penis Syndrome

Inability to feel during sexual intercourse due to excessive enlargement of the female vagina is known as "Lost Penis Syndrome." The problem is characterized by the fact that the partner does not feel anything in the vagina during sexual intercourse due to hypotonicity in the vaginal muscles of the woman. The solutions are vaginal muscle trainings, energy-based technologies, and vaginoplasty.

11.6 Vaginal Relaxation Syndrome (VRS)

Although there is no organ prolapse in the gynecological examination of many patients who apply to the physician for vaginoplasty due to complaints such as vaginal enlargement, insensitivity, and difficulty in reaching orgasm, there are findings such as vaginal hypotonus, reduced rugae, and increased hiatus width. All these complaints are collected under the name of "Vaginal Relaxation Syndrome" (VRS), which is a new term.

VRS generally includes changes in the vaginal wall as a result of the age-related reduction in connective tissue. Pregnancy and birth(s), menopause, and decreases in hormone levels due to menopause increase the symptoms of VRS. According to some authors, VRS is considered as a preliminary stage of organ prolapse that may develop in the future.

Ablative CO_2 lasers, smooth pulse mode and non-ablative Er:YAG lasers [3], and vaginoplasty operations can be applied for VRS treatment.

Vaginoplasty for tightening can be performed in the forms of anterior colporrhaphy, posterior colporrhaphy, and lateral colporrhaphy. The most common procedure is posterior colporrhaphy. Posterior colporrhaphy is often performed simultaneously with perineoplasty and is called "colpoperineoplasty" (vaginoperineoplasty).

11.7 Surgical Vaginoplasty Techniques

Surgical vaginal tightening operations are named according to the area where they are performed. These include:

- Anterior colporrhaphy,
- Posterior colporrhaphy, and
- Lateral colporrhaphy.

Sometimes several walls can be tightened at the same time. Here, the more commonly preferred posterior vaginoplasty technique will be explained in detail.

11.7.1 Posterior Colporrhaphy Technique (Posterior Vaginoplasty)

First, the type and extent of the operation to be applied should be determined. At this point, the age of the patient, their menopausal status, sexual activity, chronic diseases, and whether they have undergone prior surgery are important. In addition, POP, region-specific defects, presence of incontinence, and presence of rugae are other issues that should be examined.

Although there are several techniques in labiaplasty, there are fewer options in vaginoplasty operation. Nevertheless, small tips will allow both the operation to be safer and have better results. ACOG stated that the term vaginal rejuvenation is a modification of traditional vaginal procedures. In one of his articles, Ostrzenski divided the "wide-soft vagina," in his own words, which causes sexual numbness, into four groups [4].

Before the operation, the vaginal opening can be evaluated simply by "finger breadth." But everyone's fingers are different from the other and the patient's involuntary contraction during gynecological examination causes a subjective evaluation. In order not to be misleading, it is important to relax the patient first with suggestions, to eliminate involuntary contractions, and to perform the measurement later. Afterward, photographs are taken from different directions in the lithotomy position, and the operation area is cleaned with iodine solutions and covered with sterile drapes. It is recommended that a local anesthetic containing epinephrine diluted with 50–60% isotonic be injected into the perineum after marking the skin in the form of a rhombus. Injection can be made into the subcutaneous areas of the entire operation area with fine-tipped dental injectors. Local anesthetic infiltration into the tissue provides three important advantages:

- The amount of bleeding is reduced due to the epinephrine content,
- Mucosal dissection becomes easier,
- Postoperative pain is not felt or minimally felt.

Perineoplasty surgery should be performed simultaneously with vaginoplasty due to gaping in the vaginal entrance, atrophic or hypertrophic episiotomy scars, or unsightly perineal skin excess in many patients. Therefore, the incision usually starts from the perineum area. The perineoplasty component is the aesthetic aspect of this operation.

Vaginoplasty operations can be performed under local, regional, or general anesthesia in a hospital or office conditions. In classical posterior vaginoplasty, after the incision starting from the perineum and advancing 6–8 cm above the hymen along a vertical line, mucosal dissection is performed toward both laterals. After dissection, the vaginal mucosa is cut out in a diamond shape, hemostasis is achieved with electrocautery, and primary repair of the rectovaginal fascia is started. In order to avoid excessive

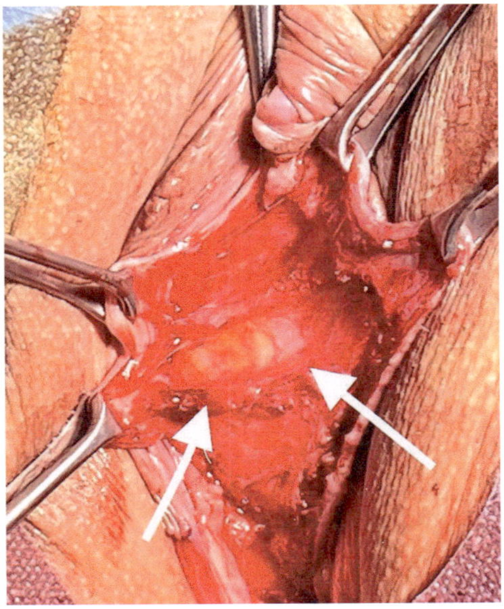

Fig. 11.3 Fascia defect in the posterior vaginal wall. In these cases, fascial defect should be repaired first, and then muscles can be approximated

bleeding, it is important to make the dissection thin, not to extend the dissection area to the lateral vaginal walls, and to ensure good hemostasis.

The amount of tissue to be removed in the operation is adjusted according to the width of the vagina: *the larger the width, the greater the amount of tissue removed*. In another technique, tissue dissection is performed after a horizontal incision is made in the vagina, and then reconstruction is performed by repairing fascia and muscles, and then mucosa is closed without any resection (Fig. 11.3). Generally, 2/0 delayed absorbable sutures or special suture materials with barbs facing the same direction can be used for the repair. FDA-approved spiral knotless barbed sutures (Stratafix™, V-lock 90™) are very safe but expensive.

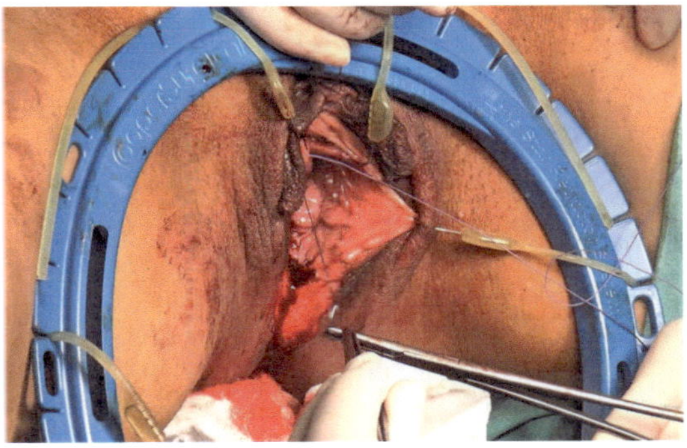

Fig. 11.4 Lone Star™ retractor may be preferred for vaginal and abdominal surgeries and provides atraumatic retraction

If there is a rectocele, the levator muscles are approximated to each other with sutures made with the dominant hand while the forefinger of the passive hand is in the rectum, and fascia defects are repaired. However, due to the risk of dyspareunia, it is recommended to avoid excessive narrowing and levator suture in patients without fascia defects. In the presence of enterocele, hanging to the sacrouterine ligament can be applied.

In order to facilitate the operation, a "Lone Star™" retractor can be used instead of the classical vaginal retractor. Thanks to its blunt end hooks, Lone Star retractor can be easily retracted (Fig. 11.4).

Laser, monopolar needle-tipped radiofrequency, or monopolar electrocautery can also be used for wall dissection and cutting procedures (Table 11.1).

The stages of vaginal tightening surgery are shown below (Fig. 11.5).

In vaginal tightening operations, only cutting and repairing the vaginal mucosa without fascia defect repair will not provide sufficient benefit. Fascia and muscle defects must be repaired.

Table 11.1 General stages of the posterior wall colporrhaphy operation

• Take pre-op images
• Make a diamond marking from the perineum to inside the vagina
• Inject the local tumescent anesthetic solution to the entire area subcutaneously
Tumescent recommendation (Eserdag):
– 6 cc ampoule of lidocaine (20 mg/mL) + epinephrine (0.0125 mg/mL)
– 4 cc isotonic serum
– 2 cc tranexamic acid (100 mg/mL)
• Proceed longitudinally toward the distal of the vagina by dissecting with Metzenbaum scissors between the two Allis clamps and then dissect the vaginal tissue from both sides
• Excise the tissue you have dissected
• Wash the area with H_2O_2
• Provide hemostasis by cauterizing open-ended vessels (bipolar cautery may be preferred)
• Repair the fascia and approximate the bulbospongiosus muscles, if necessary (2/0 vicryl). In the meantime, the forefinger of the passive hand should be placed in the rectum so that no sutures pass through the rectum
• Suture the mucosa (2/0 vicryl)
• Repair the subcutaneous and skin tissue of the perineum (4/0 vicryl or monocryl)
• Take postop images
• Cover the operation area by dressing with antibiotic creams and take the patient to rest

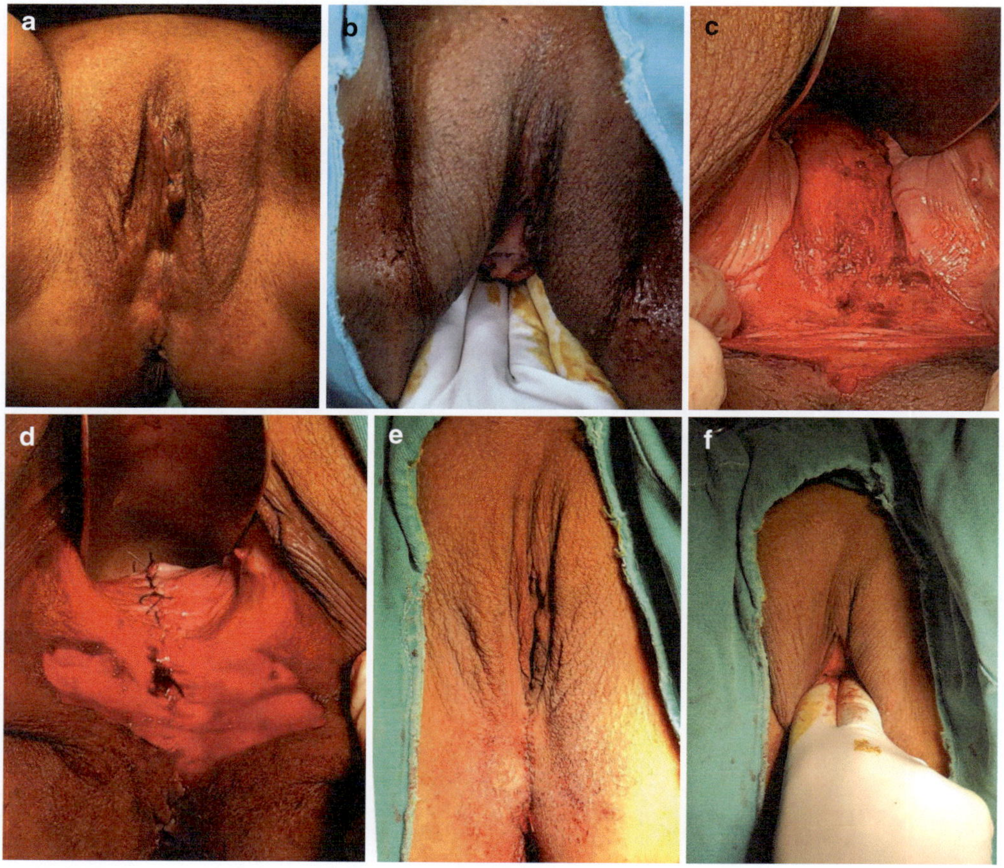

Fig. 11.5 Step-by-step vaginoplasty operation. A 44-year-old patient with severe deformations due to multiple vaginal deliveries. Before (**a**, **b**), dissection and removal of vaginal mucosa (**c**), closure of mucosa after repair of fascia and muscular re-approximation (**d**), Just after (**e**, **f**)

11.8 Surgical Results

Vaginal tightening operations aim to increase the pleasure of both men and women with the increase of mechanical effect during sexual intercourse. Vaginal tightening operations also provide a secondary benefit by correcting the angulation of the vaginal axis after birth. As a matter of fact, distortion of the vaginal axis reduces the contact of the penis with the anterior wall, which is the most sensitive area of the vagina.

In a study involving 53 women in whom the vaginal diameter was tightened by 2/3 with surgical colporrhaphy, 66% of the patients stated that their sexual life was much better, 24% stated that their sexual life was significantly better after surgery, and 10% stated that there was a slight or no change in their sexual life [5].

Goodman et al. concluded in a large multicenter study of 258 women, including 47 vaginoplasty patients, that vaginoplasty/perineoplasty operations increased sexual function in both men and women [6].

Abedi et al. demonstrated a general increase in FSFI (Female Sexual Function Index) scores of 79 women who underwent colpoperineoplasty [7]. In another study involving 39 patients, FSFI scores increased from 19.5 to 27 [8]. In the same study, 81.6% of the patients were very satisfied with the operation, 14.5% were satisfied, and 3.9% were not satisfied in the postoperation survey.

Before and after vaginoplasty, the hiatus diameter can be measured simply with the fingers (Fig. 11.6). When the entry diameter is reduced by half, the hiatus circumference will also be reduced by half (Circumference = $\pi \times$ Diameter). But the area decreases by ¾ ratio (Area = $\pi \times \text{Radius}^2$).

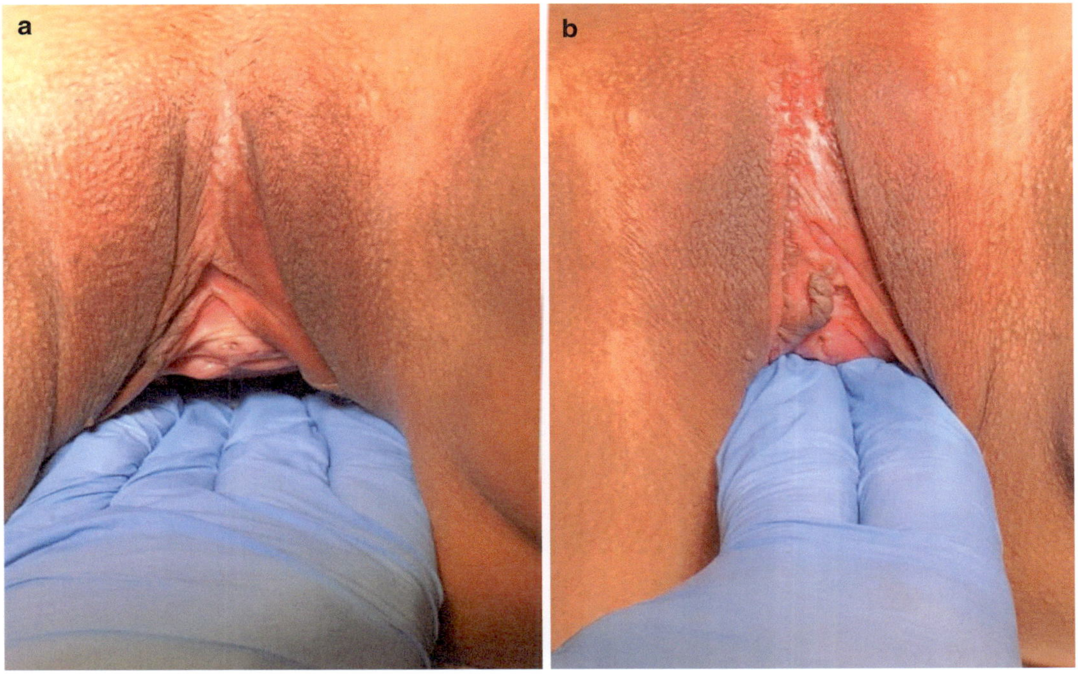

Fig. 11.6 Hiatus measurement by finger. Before (**a**), after (**b**)

11.9 Combined Procedures

Vaginoplasty–perineoplasty operations can be performed simultaneously with labiaplasty, labia majora fat transfer, HA injections, genital bleaching, and genital PRP applications (Figs. 11.7, 11.8, and 11.9). Posterior colporrhaphy and anterior laser resurfacing can be performed simultaneously in patients who have vaginal relaxation on examination but who have incontinence problems without any sign of POP. Most such initiatives yield successful results.

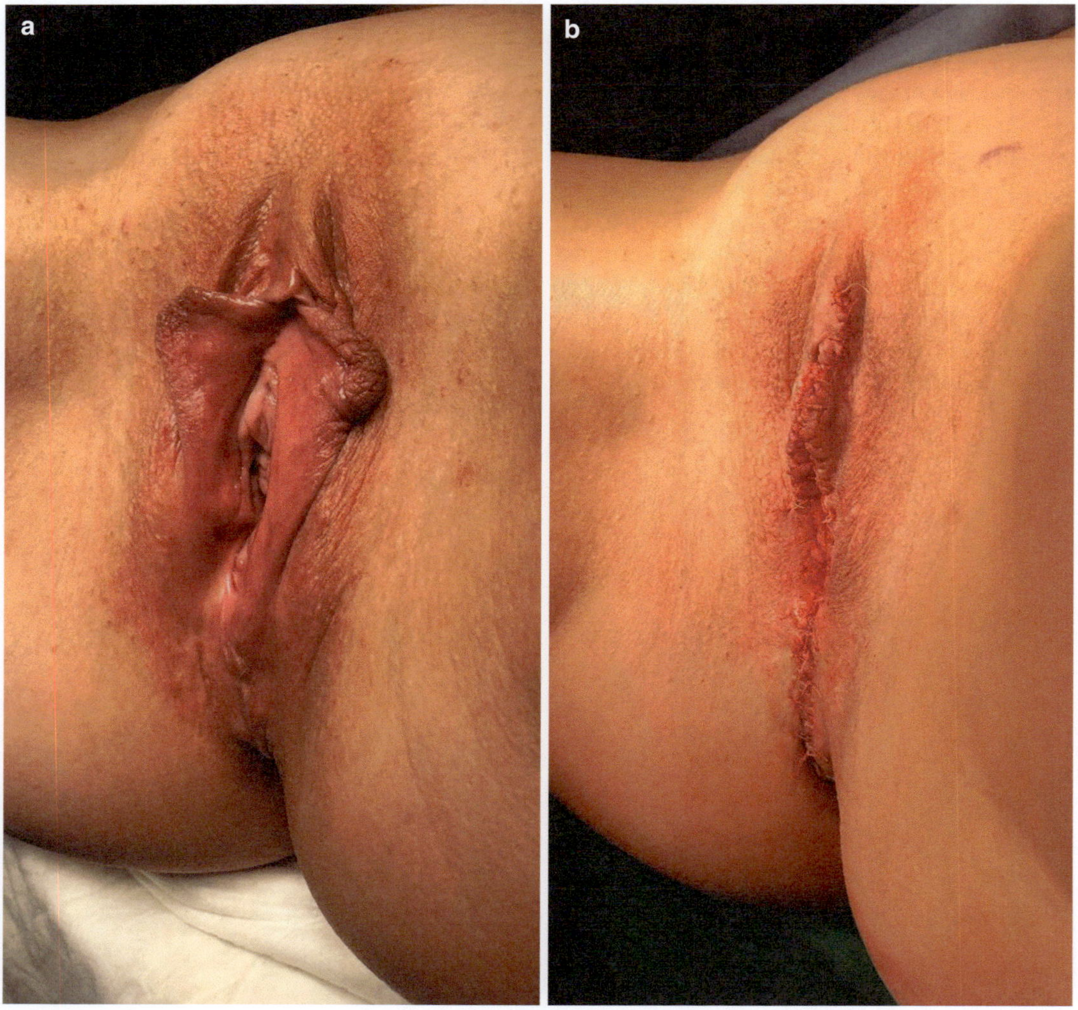

Fig. 11.7 Combined surgery. Before (**a**), after (**b**)

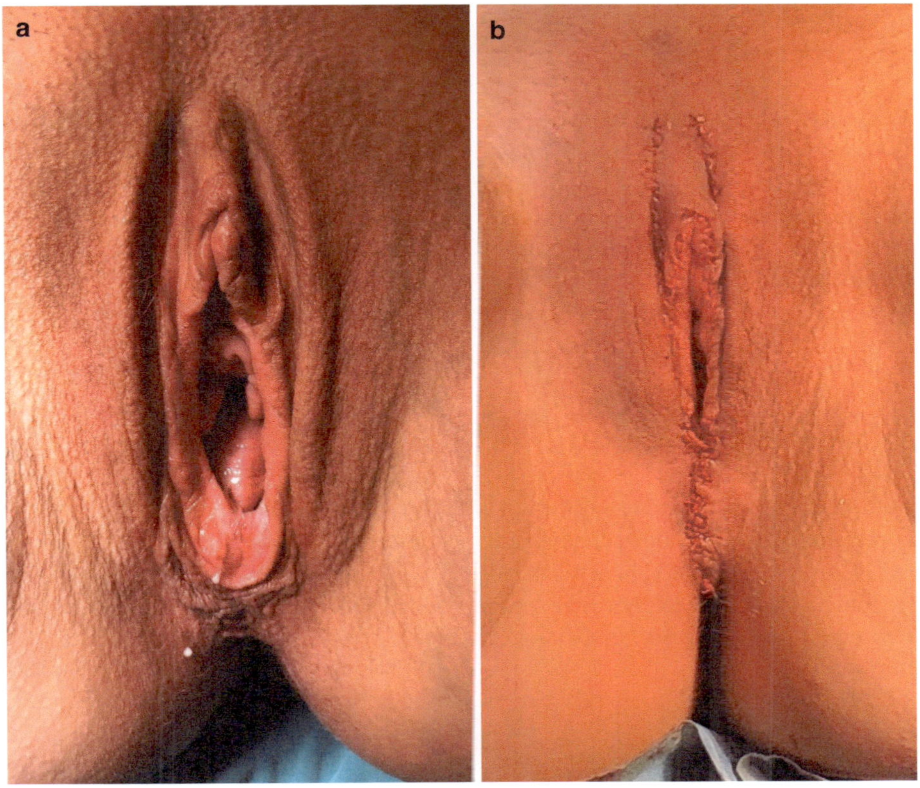

Fig. 11.8 Combined surgery. Four operations of another patient: vaginoplasty, perineoplasty, labiaplasty, and hoodoplasty. Before (**a**), after (**b**)

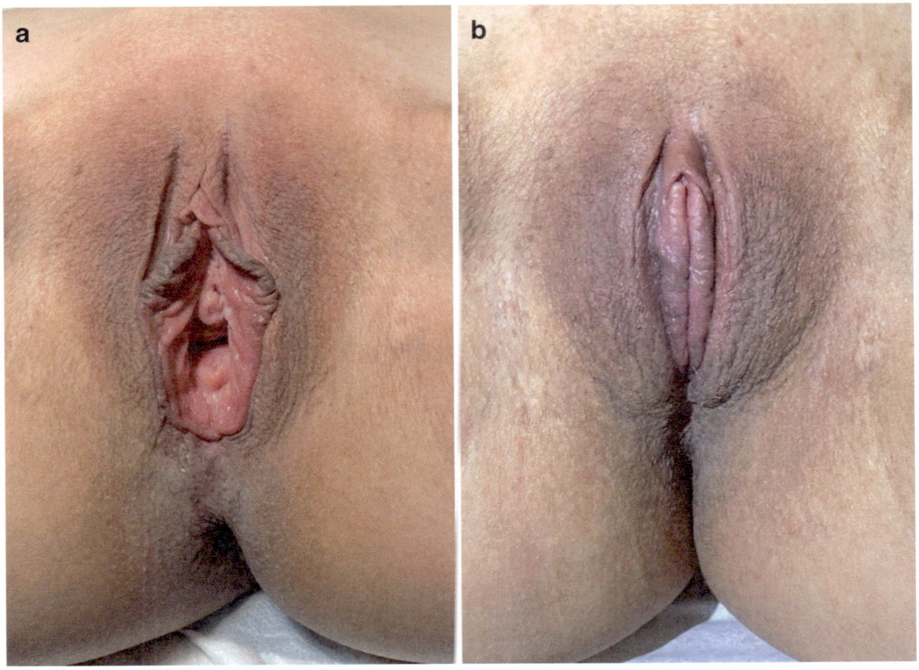

Fig. 11.9 Combined AGS. Before (**a**), 4 months after (**b**)

11.10 Common Complaints After the Operation

Although vaginal tightening operations are generally performed in hospital operating rooms, they can also be performed in a clinical setting under local anesthesia or mild sedation under appropriate conditions. Preoperative patient selection and detailed consent forms are important. Common complaints after the operation are listed below.

11.10.1 Vasovagal Reflex

Syncope attack due to vasovagal reflex during or after the operation usually develops due to bradycardia and hypotension. Fluid support is important. The patient should be accompanied by a health care professional when first standing up after the operation.

11.10.2 Bleeding

Although bleeding in the form of mild leakage is accepted as normal, the patient should be informed about how to reach the physician in cases of gradually increasing bleeding or onset of massive bleeding.

11.10.3 Pain

It is considered normal to have pain within the first 3 days and for the pain to spread in a throbbing manner, especially pressing on the rectum. The pain should subside over time. The throbbing pain leaves in its place pricking, burning, and stinging over time.

11.10.4 Itching

Itching during the recovery period can be very uncomfortable for some patients. Antihistamine drugs or non-potent topical corticosteroids can also be used during this period.

11.10.5 Edema

Edema can occur, especially in the first week. It is a good idea for the patient to not stand for too long and especially to apply the recommended ice compressions in the first 3 days.

11.11 Complications

11.11.1 Acute Term

Bleeding and hematoma are among the most important complications that can occur in the acute period in vaginoplasty operations. Particularly, care should be taken in patients with submucosal varicose veins.

Patients with diffuse varicose veins on the vulva and legs are also rich in vaginal varicosities (Fig. 11.10).

Prolonged bleeding in the form of leakage can also be seen due to the activation of subcutaneous open vessels. Massive bleeding that drains outside or accumulates under the skin and may lead to hematoma is rare but important complications that can cause shock. Hematomas between the rectum and vagina are clinically manifested by the patient's description of extreme pain radiating to the rectum in the postoperative period. There is a palpable hard mass in vaginal or bimanual rectovaginal examinations. In this situation, it is important to immediately open the incision line, ligate the open vessels, and close the wound site without leaving a dead space. In patients with greater than normal bleeding during the operation, platelet-rich plasma (PRP) and platelet-rich fibrin (PRF) can be applied to the operation area. In addition, after the surgery, vaginal packing with gauze or absorbable hemostatic gelatin sponge can be applied. In order to reduce bleeding, 1000 mg IV tranexamic acid injection is also recommended during the operation.

The preventative measures to reduce bleeding in vaginoplasty are listed in Table 11.2.

Other complications include allergic reactions to drugs or anesthetic agents used in the acute period and hypotension due to vasovagal reflex and/or temporary loss of consciousness if the

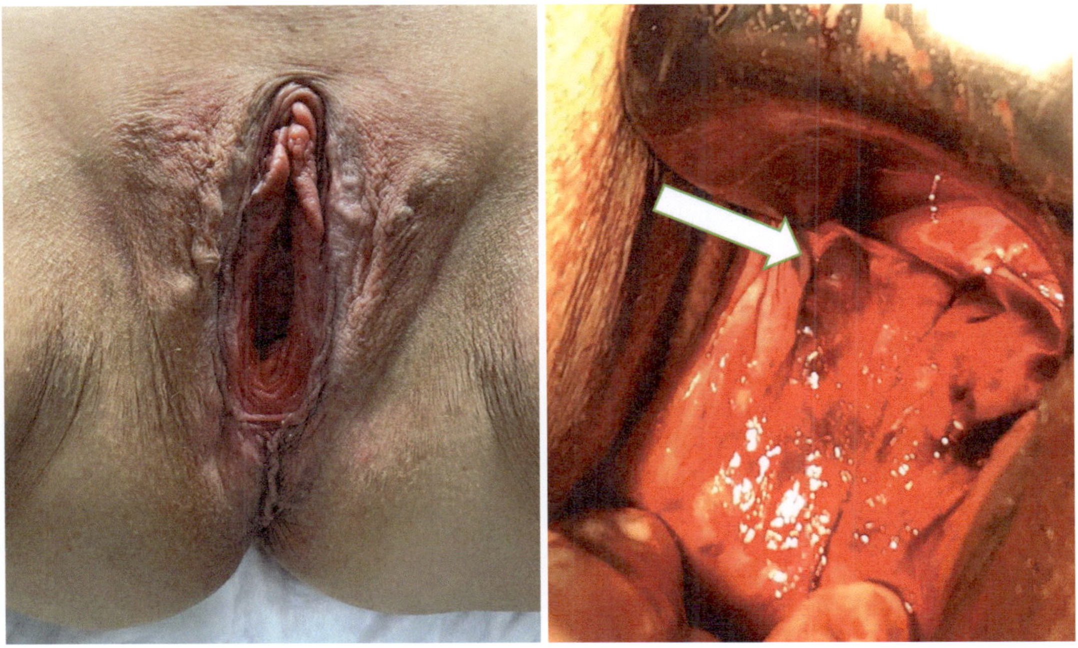

Fig. 11.10 Diffuse genital and vaginal varicose veins in the same patient

Table 11.2 Precautions to reduce the risk of bleeding in vaginoplasty

• Patient should stop omega 3, aspirin, and coumadin-derivatives before the operation
• Question the amount of bleeding during menstruation, previous births, or surgeries in the anamnesis
• Preoperative measurement of INR, especially in patients with chronic disease or a history of bleeding
• If the patient has diffuse varicose veins on physical examination, perform vaginal dissection more carefully
• Injection of local anesthetics containing epinephrine into the vaginal walls, subcutaneous infiltration before the procedure (it is recommended even if surgery will be performed under general anesthesia; it will also facilitate dissection). 250 mg tranexamic acid can also be added in local anesthetic solution
Tumescent recommendation (Eserdag):
– 6 cc ampoule of lidocaine (20 mg/mL) + epinephrine (0.0125 mg/mL)
– 4 cc isotonic serum
– 2 cc tranexamic acid (100 mg/mL)
• After the local anesthesia injection, wait for 15–20 min before the incision is made
• Thin dissection and do not extend to the lateral walls unless necessary
• In cases where very good dissection cannot be achieved, make incision with RF or laser
• Provide good hemostasis with unipolar/bipolar cautery in excessive bleeding
• If there is excessive hypotension under general anesthesia, this may prevent open vessel ends from being activated. In this case, the anesthetic gases are reduced a little, so the blood pressure will elevate slightly, and then the tissue will be closed after bleeding is controlled
• Injection of local PRP in heavy bleeding (this can also accelerate wound healing)
• 500–1000 mg IV tranexamic acid administration may be done routinely in patients without hypercoagulopathy
• Insertion of gauze into the vagina postoperatively for the compression. When necessary, absorbable hemostatic gelatin sponges can also be used for this purpose

procedure is performed in the office and under local anesthesia. There are risks such as rectal injury in posterior colporrhaphy and bladder injury in anterior colporrhaphy. It should not be forgotten that the posterior wall of the vagina is thinner than the anterior wall, and the thickness of the vaginal posterior wall is only 3 mm in some parts.

11.11.2 Subacute Term

In the subacute period, complications such as severe pain radiating toward the rectum, widespread edema, wound infection, and especially dehiscence of perineal sutures may occur. Dehiscence is generally more common in the perineum where the tension is highest. Sometimes annoying bleeding in the form of slight leakage can be observed for up to a week.

11.11.3 Chronic Term

Fistulas and poorly healing perineal and vaginal scars are among the complications seen in the late period (Figs. 11.11 and 11.12).

Bartholin's gland cysts may also occur if sutures block their ducts. Therefore, the incision area in the vestibulum should not be so lateral.

Inclusion cysts may also develop due to the implantation of the epidermis into the dermis during surgery (Fig. 11.13). These subcutaneous cysts, which are synonymously known as "epidermoid cysts," "epidermal inclusion cysts," "infundibular cysts," and "keratin cysts," can often survive for years without symptoms or may become abscessed if infected.

Avascularization of the tissue can lead to necrosis and fistulas (Fig. 11.14).

Some patients may state that they are not satisfied with the vaginal tightening in the postoperative period. This is due to the inadequate tightening of the vagina (insufficient surgery) or the high expectations of the patient. I have encountered patients who have undergone vaginal tightening operations four times before but are still not satisfied with the results. The operation requests of patients who come with extreme expectations or have no indications should be politely rejected.

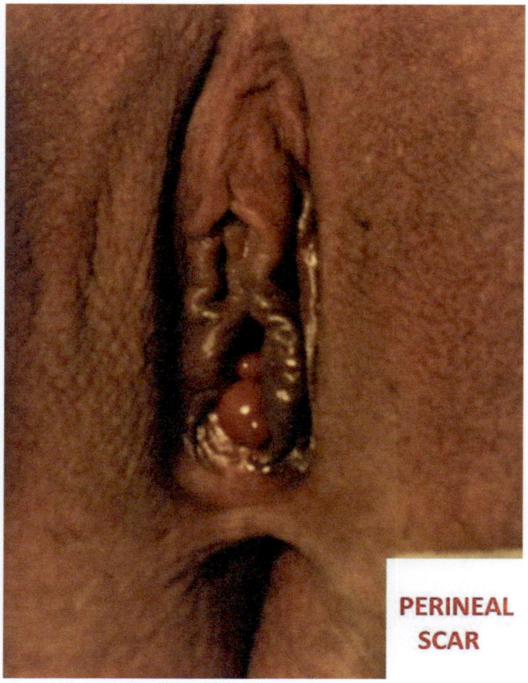

Fig. 11.11 Scar tissue in the perineum causes dyspareunia; however, the problem of vaginal relaxation continues in a patient who had prior vaginal tightening and perineoplasty

One of the common mistakes is to narrow the vaginal entrance with an excessive elevation of the perineum. The wider the transverse incision made in the perineum in the first stage of the surgery, the higher the perineum will elevate. In this case, the problem of dyspareunia can make sexual penetration extremely painful, sometimes even impossible. Depending on the negative conditioning, it may cause an "iatrogenic vaginismus" problem, which manifests itself with involuntary vaginal contractions over time.

Pain and pleasure in sexual intercourse are like two panes of a scale. As the pain increases, pleasure will decrease, arousal will decrease, and vaginal lubrication will be replaced by dryness, which will further increase the pain in a vicious cycle. In time, it will be inevitable that the sexual desire problems will arise due to negative conditioning.

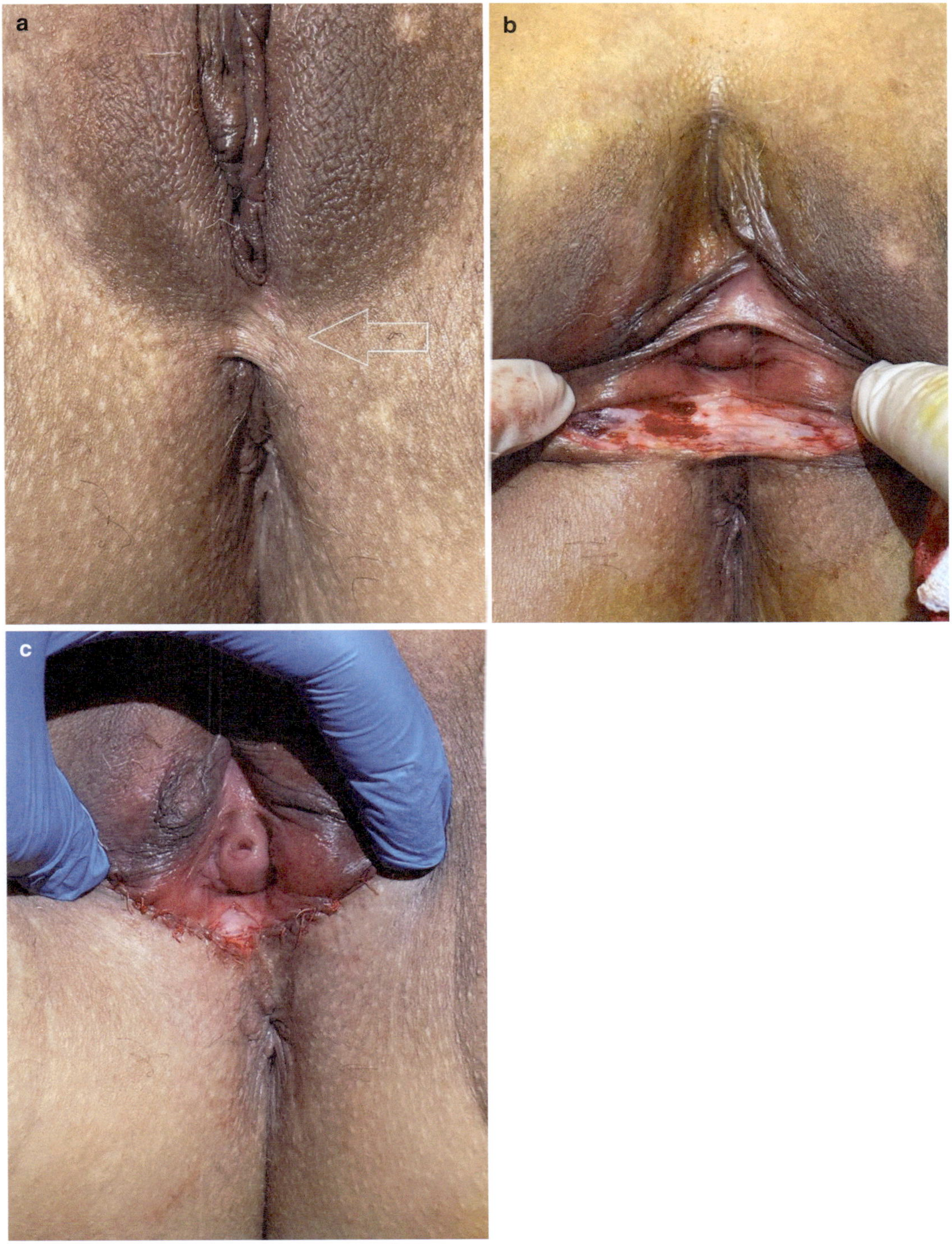

Fig. 11.12 Dyspareunia due to scar tissue in a patient who had undergone vaginoplasty and perineoplasty 6 years ago. Before (**a**), scar removal (**b**), and transverse suturing (**c**)

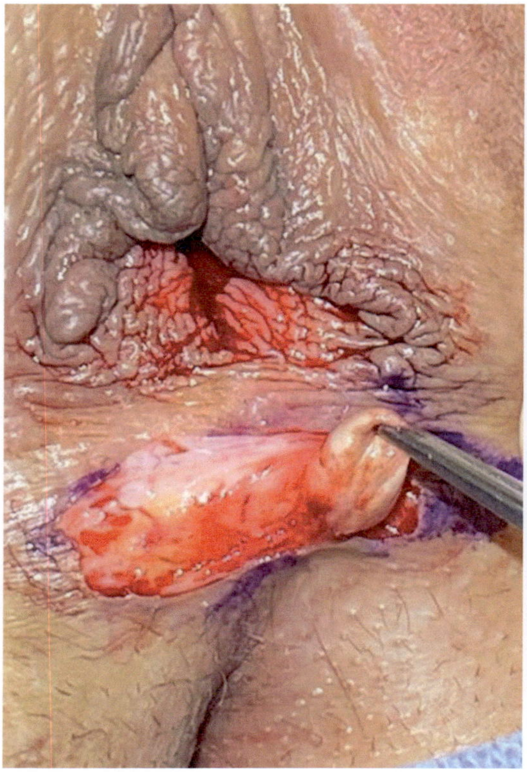

Fig. 11.13 Perineal inclusion cyst. Inclusion cyst in the perineum of a patient who had undergone vaginoplasty and perineoplasty twice before

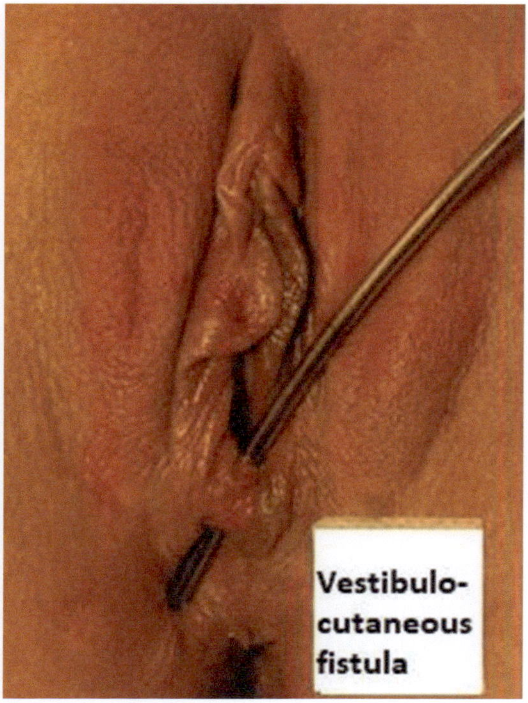

Fig. 11.14 Vestibulo-cutaneous fistula that developed after vaginal tightening surgery

The perineum is a very sensitive and delicate area; therefore, it should not be stretched excessively or elevated and blood circulation should not be impaired with frequent sutures or electrocauterization. The same is also true for the excision of the perineal skin tags performed simultaneously in labiaplasty operations.

The amount of tightening will be determined by the demands of the patient and her tissue conditions. The amount of tightening should be greater in those with too much laxity and less in cases with less enlargement. The anamnesis given by the patient is also important in this regard. In fact, the penis width of the partner is also a determining factor. One of the common mistakes is that tightening only the introitus without providing sufficient tightness in the width and length of the entire vaginal canal. The other common mistake in vaginoplasty is embedding mucosal tissue in the subcutaneous tissue during the operation. Accordingly, inclusion cysts can develop over time. In a patient who applied to our clinic with the complaint of dyspareunia, we encountered many abscesses in the perineal and rectovaginal areas during the revision operation of this patient who had vaginoplasty at an external center 10 years ago.

Pardo et al. reported a complication rate between 2 and 3.77%. The most common complications reported were dyspareunia, lack of lubrication, constipation, wound infection, bleeding, dehiscence (especially in the perineum), hip pain persisting for weeks, and rectal mucosal perforation [5].

11.12 The Postoperative Term

After vaginoplasty, patients can be discharged home on the same day. There is no need for urinary catheterization after posterior or lateral vaginoplasty operations. It is recommended that they spend the first 3 days at home resting as much as possible and regularly use prescribed NSAI and antibiotic drugs. Intermittent ice application for 3 days after the operation using ice wrapped in a cloth will reduce pain, edema, and bleeding complaints. Compliance with hygiene rules, especially when using the toilet and dressing with antiseptic creams for 7 days reduces the risk of infection. It is also important that the patient not experience constipation for at least 5 days and to eliminate this situation with diet and laxatives.

Until 1 month after vaginoplasty, heavy sports exercises, fitness, hair removal, yoga and Pilates, cycling, and horse riding should be avoided. Sexual intercourse should be avoided for at least 1.5 months; in some cases the prohibition on penetrative sexual intercourse can be extended for up to 2 months. In addition, it is important to start Kegel exercises during this recovery process in order to strengthen the pelvic muscles. Patients should be informed that some pain and slight bleeding may occur in the first coitus after the operation. It is also recommended to use lubricant gel in the first instances of sexual intercourse due to fear and involuntary contractions and lack of lubrication.

Giving all this information in writing to the patients reduces postoperative anxiety and prevents the patient from occupying the physician with questions unnecessarily. Therefore, normal and abnormal situations that may be encountered in the postoperative period, and what to do and what to avoid should be given in writing to all genital aesthetic patients.

After vaginal tightening, some patients may experience anxiety about having sexual intercourse with their partners. These patients can reduce their anxiety by performing finger dilatation exercises recommended to be done a few days before sexual intercourse. Some patients may encounter dyspareunia. In the examinations of these patients, only anxiety-related contractions are detected. If it is thought that dyspareunia is caused by these contractions, the problem can be easily overcome with pelvic rehabilitation exercises and verbal suggestions. Perineum stretching exercises with the fingers or dilators may also be recommended. However, if it is determined that the perineum is raised too much and prevents the entry of the penis, the vaginal entrance should be surgically enlarged. Perineal and vestibular enlargement can also be done with laser incision.

Routine checks after vaginoplasty are on the second day, 1 week after surgery, and before intercourse (1.5 months). However, these follow-up visits may not be suitable for patients coming from outside of the city. Obtaining written and verbal consent and taking postoperative photos are important in terms of following the healing process of the patients.

Finally, a significant number of patients who apply for vaginoplasty may also experience sexual dysfunction disorders or some marital problems. Sexual therapy and/or marriage therapy can also be recommended to these couples.

11.13 Vaginoplasty Revision Surgery

Patients who are not satisfied after the operation, who state that they cannot get the desired results, or who encounter different problems apply to physicians for vaginoplasty revision surgeries (Fig. 11.15).

The most common problems after vaginoplasty that need revision procedures are listed in Table 11.3.

We also observed that some patients who had anterior vaginal wall repair or TOT surgery applied to us with acute onset insensitivity during penetration and orgasm problems postoperatively. Anterior vaginal wall is the most sensitive region in the vagina.

In patients who develop dyspareunia due to fibrotic band formation in the posterior vestibulum and perineum after vaginal surgery or interventions, or who cannot achieve sexual penetration, laser incision can be made in this area along the vertical line and left for secondary healing. The area will renew itself with fresh granulation tissue formed within a month. In some cases, it may be necessary to completely remove the scar tissue. In addition, pelvic rehabilitation and sexual therapy are also important for iatrogenic vaginismus that may develop secondarily in these patients (Fig. 11.16).

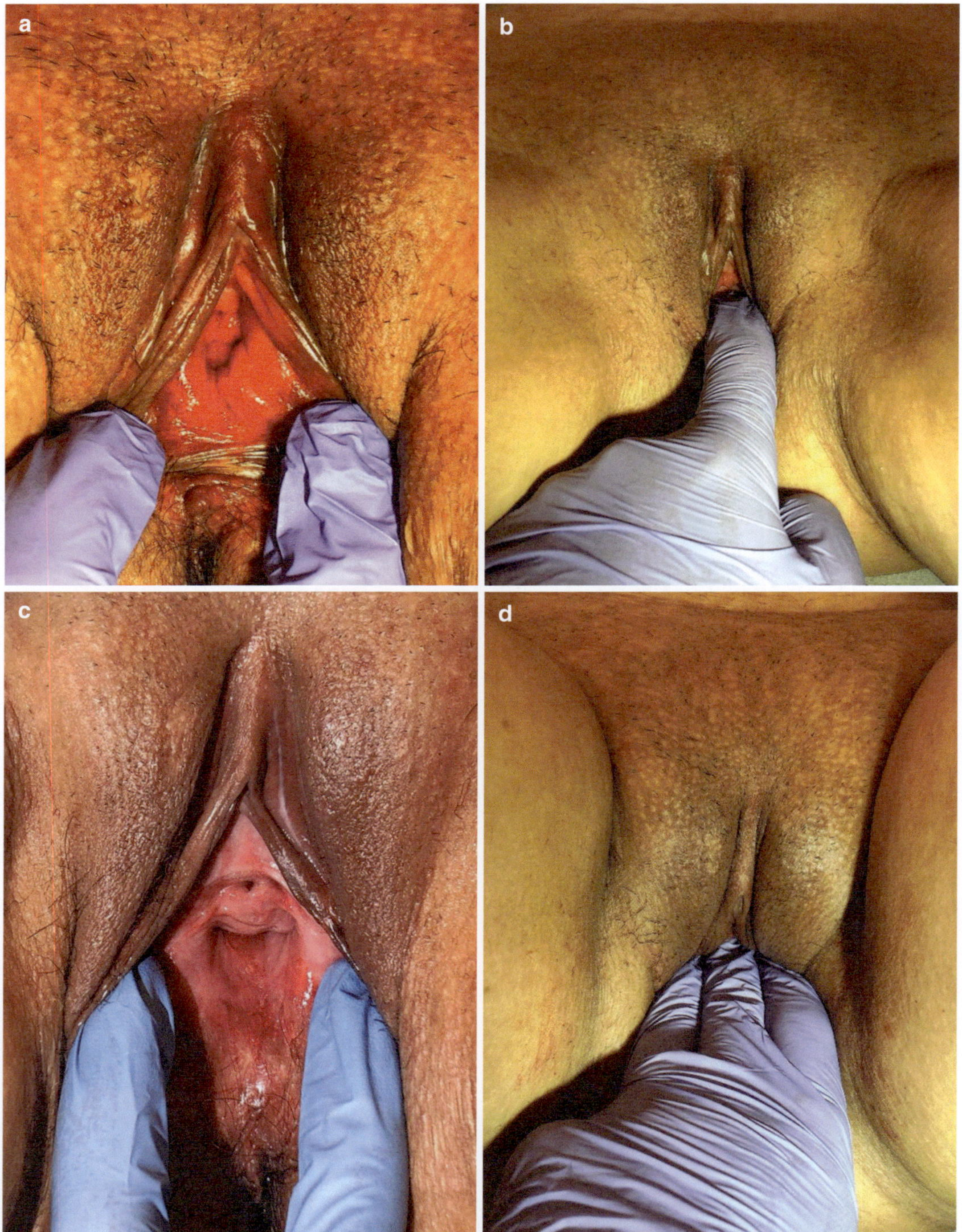

Fig. 11.15 Excessive vaginal tightening. A patient who underwent vaginoplasty and labiaplasty 3 months ago and could not have sexual intercourse due to excessive vaginal tightening (**a**, **b**). So, vaginal enlargement operation has been performed. Two months after vaginal entrance enlargement (**c**, **d**)

Table 11.3 Conditions that may require revision after vaginoplasty

• Inadequate vaginal tightening. Tightening of the introitus, not the entire vaginal canal
• Pain in sexual intercourse or problems not having intercourse due to excessive tightening of the vaginal entrance ("iatrogenic vaginismus")
• Dyspareunia due to fibrotic band formation in the posterior vestibular area
• Inclusion cysts in the vaginal wall or perineal area (these cysts may become abscessed over time)
• Scar tissue formation in the perineum

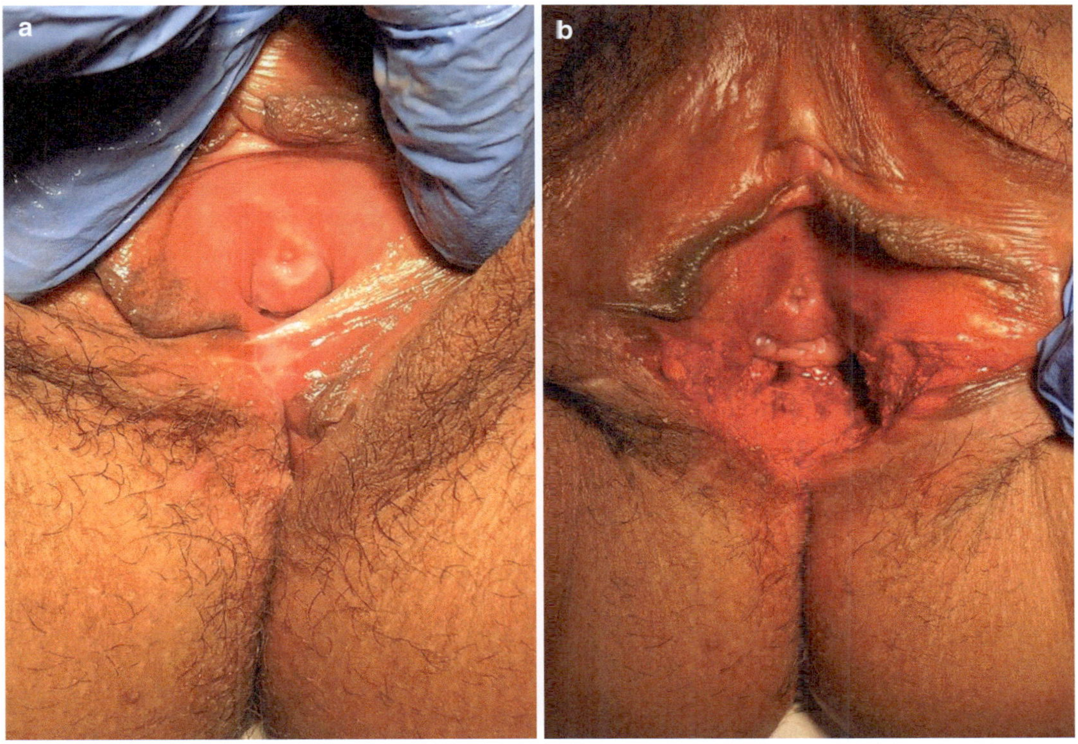

Fig. 11.16 Vaginal and perineal fibrosis due to urgent intervention in the postpartum period because of excessive hemorrhage and hematoma formation (**a**). After the healing, scar formation was not allowing sexual penetration. For the treatment, scar tissue in the vagina and perineum excised (**b**), and then the wound has left to the secondary healing. Light bath, zinc cream, and dilator exercises were recommended postoperatively

11.14 Neovaginoplasty Due to Vaginal Aplasia

Mayer–Rokitansky–Küster–Hauser (MRKH) syndrome occurs in one per 4000 to 10,000 women and is the most common cause of vaginal aplasia [9]. Usually there is no uterus or upper two-thirds of the vagina. Gynecological examination, ultrasound, and MRI play an important role in its diagnosis. The etiology of MRKH, which is the cause of 10% of cases of primary amenorrhea, is thought to be genetic. The management of these patients involves the creation of a neovagina with psychological support.

Some of these patients with normal secondary sex characteristics, normal 46 XX karyotype, and normal ovarian function have an endometrium functioning with a very rudimentary uterus. Therefore, abdominal pain complaints occur due to menstrual blood accumulation in the intrauterine cavity. In some patients, urinary system anomalies such as horseshoe kidney, unilateral renal agenesis, duplication of renal pelvis and ureter, and skeletal system and auditory system anomalies also occur. MRKH patients apply to the physician with primary amenorrhea, with the inability to have sexual intercourse, or requesting to get pregnant. However, since it is not possible for them to become pregnant, the treatments applied are directed to the problem of the inability to have sexual intercourse. Surgical and non-surgical methods are recommended for the treatment of these patients.

11.14.1 Management

Management includes non-surgical and surgical methods.

11.14.1.1 Non-surgical Methods

The Frank technique is a non-surgical technique that involves the application of dilators in the vaginal cavity. It is recommended to insert a dilator into the vaginal cavity for 30–120 min a day. By increasing the diameter and length of the dilator, an attempt to create normal-sized vagina over time is made. It has been suggested by Ingram that this dilator application should be done sitting on a bicycle saddle [10]. This method, which does not involve surgical risks, is difficult and troublesome, especially for young girls. This treatment method is suitable for patients who are afraid of surgery, whose vaginal cavity is at least 3–4 cm, and whose vaginal dome is flexible and soft.

11.14.1.2 Surgical Methods

The goal of all surgical methods is to create a vaginal canal that allows sexual intercourse. The McIndoe (or Abbe-McIndoe) operation is among the most common surgeries for this condition [11]. This technique is based on creating a space between the vagina and bladder by dissection and placing a skin graft taken from the patient into this space by wrapping it in mold. The use of amniotic tissue or cultured vaginal tissues in this field is promising. After this technique, a 6–10 cm long neovagina can be created, but it is important to apply a dilator until the woman becomes sexually active.

Another of the neovagina creation techniques is the Vecchietti operation [12]. The traction procedure takes a few days and is painful for the patient. Dilator exercises are also recommended after the procedure (Fig. 11.17).

Another technique is the Davydov operation. In this complex procedure, the patient's peritoneum is used. There are risks such as urethral damage and fistula formation [13].

Another method is an intestinal colpoplasty operation performed by removing an intestinal segment [14]. Since failure rates are higher, this treatment should not be the first-line treatment.

Another method used in creating a neovagina is Williams vaginoplasty. This technique has been modified by Creatsas. In this method, a U-shaped symmetrical incision is made starting 4 cm lateral to the external urethral meatus, reaching the perineum and then the other part of the vulva. After the perineal subcutaneous tissue is released, the transverse incision of the perineum is sutured vertically. Thus, the perineum is raised and a perineal pouch is formed. The advantages of the operation are its simplicity, short duration, low morbidity, and no need to use dilators after the procedure [15].

In some patients undergoing genital cancer treatment, adhesion, stenosis, and shortening of the vagina may occur due to vaginal irradiation. This incidence varies between 2.5% and 88% depending on the age of the patient, the type of the surgery, the dose of radiation, and whether or not a vaginal dilator is used. Vaginoplasty operations can be performed in these patients who experience sexual dysfunction after gynecological malignancy treatment, similar to Müllerian agenesis patients.

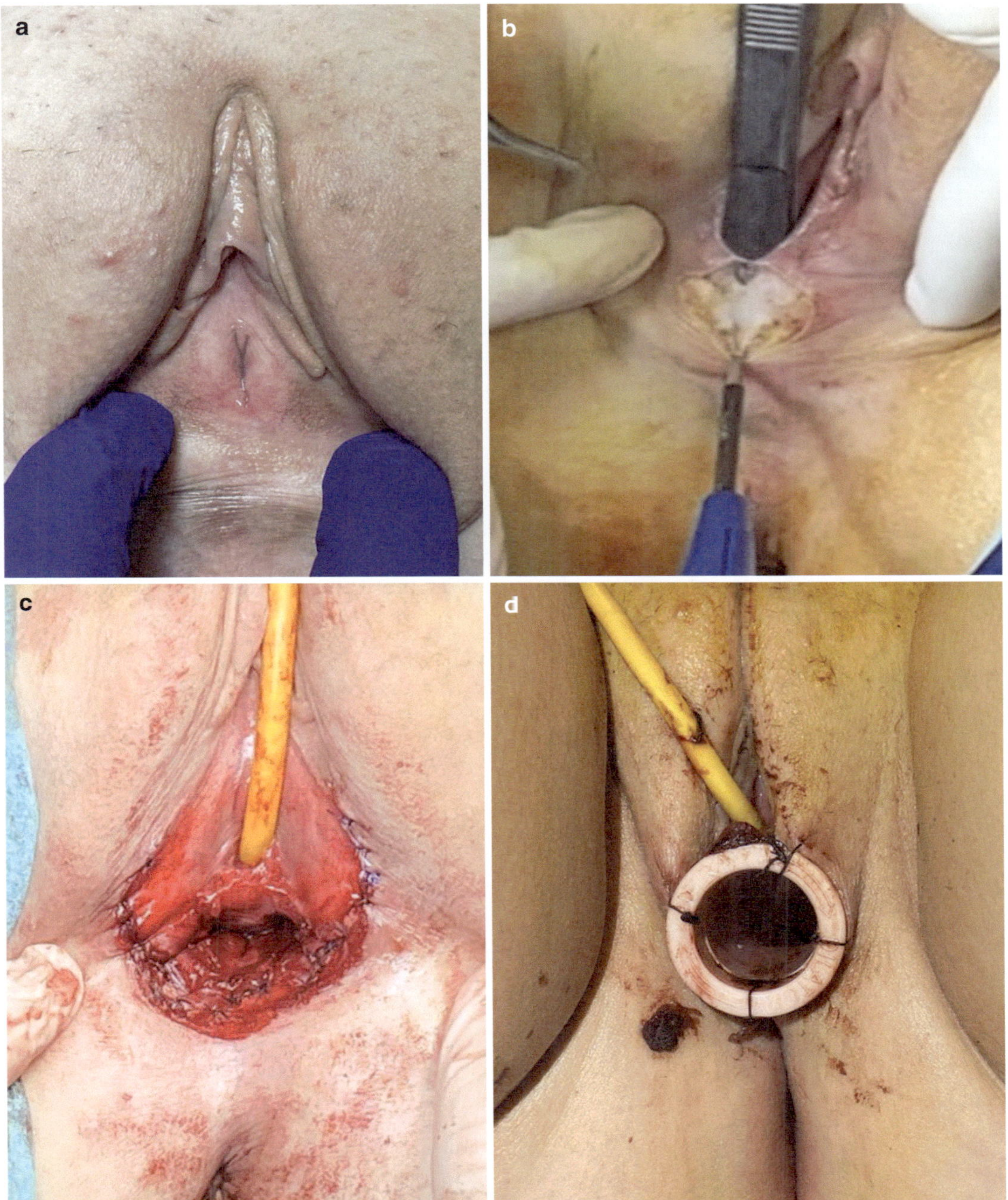

Fig. 11.17 Mullerian agenesis. Before (**a**), enlargement of perineum (**b**) and vaginal cuff, transverse suturing (**c**) and insertion of urinary catheter, insertion of a dilator into the canal for 7 days (**d**). Blind vagina has been enlarged from 3 to 10 cm length surgically

Appendix

With the purchase of this book, you can use our "SN Flashcards" app to access questions free of charge in order to test your learning and check your understanding of the contents of the book.

To use the app, please follow the instructions below:

1. Go to https://flashcards.springernature.com/login
2. Create a user account by entering your e-mail address and assigning a password.
3. Use the following link to access your SN Flashcards set: ▶ https://sn.pub/tvlq7Q

If the link is missing or does not work, please send an e-mail with the subject "SN Flashcards" and the book title to customerservice@springernature.com.

References

1. Allahdin S, Oo N, Jones C. Intractable flatus incontinence treated by percutaneous tibial nerve stimulation. Int J Color Dis. 2011;26(10):1355–6.
2. Amarenco AG, Turmel N, Chesnel C, Mezzadri M, Le Breton F, Charlanes A, Hentzen C. Gaz vaginaux : revue de la littérature [Vaginal gas: Review]. Prog Urol. 2019;29(17):1035–40.
3. Gaviria PKB, Fernandez J, Montero G. Up to 3-year follow-up of patients with vaginal relaxation syndrome participating in laser vaginal tightening. J Laser Health Acad. 2016;1:6–11.
4. Ostrzenski A. An acquired sensation of wide/smooth vagina: a new classification. Eur J Obstet Gynecol Reprod Biol. 2011;158(1):97–100.
5. Pardo JS, Solà VD, Ricci PA, Guiloff EF, Freundlich OK. Colpoperineoplasty in women with a sensation of a wide vagina. Acta Obstet Gynecol Scand. 2006;85(9):1125–7.
6. Goodman MP, Placik OJ, Benson RH 3rd, Miklos JR, Moore RD, Jason RA, Matlock DL, Simopoulos AF, Stern BH, Stanton RA, Kolb SE, Gonzalez F. A large multicenter outcome study of female genital plastic surgery. J Sex Med. 2010;7(4 Pt 1):1565–77.
7. Abedi P, Jamali S, Tadayon M, Parhizkar S, Mogharab F. Effectiveness of selective vaginal tightening on sexual function among reproductive aged women in Iran with vaginal laxity: a quasi-experimental study. J Obstet Gynaecol Res. 2014;40(2):526–31.
8. Desai SA, Dixit VV. Audit of female genital aesthetic surgery: changing trends in India. J Obstet Gynaecol India. 2018;68(3):214–20.
9. ACOG Committee on Adolescent Health Care. ACOG Committee opinion no. 355: vaginal agenesis: diagnosis, management, and routine care. Obstet Gynecol. 2006;108(6):1605–9.
10. Williams JK, Lake M, Ingram JM. The bicycle seat stool in the treatment of vaginal agenesis and stenosis. J Obstet Gynecol Neonatal Nurs. 1985;14(2):147–50.
11. Fliegner JR. A simple surgical cure for congenital absence of the vagina. Aust N Z J Surg. 1986;56(6):505–8.
12. Vecchietti G. Neovagina nella sindrome di Rokitansky-Küster-Hauser [Creation of an artificial vagina in Rokitansky-Küster-Hauser syndrome]. Attual Ostet Ginecol. 1965;11(2):131–47.
13. Davydov SN, Zhvitiashvili OD. Formation of vagina (colpopoiesis) from peritoneum of Douglas pouch. Acta Chir Plast. 1974;16(1):35–41.
14. Cai B, Zhang JR, Xi XW, Yan Q, Wan XP. Laparoscopically assisted sigmoid colon vaginoplasty in women with Mayer-Rokitansky-Kuster-Hauser syndrome: feasibility and short-term results. BJOG. 2007;114(12):1486–92.
15. Creatsas G, Deligeoroglou E. Creatsas modification of Williams vaginoplasty for reconstruction of the vaginal aplasia in Mayer-Rokitansky-Küster-Hauser syndrome cases. Womens Health (Lond). 2010;6(3):367–75.

12 Perineoplasty

Yesterday, I was clever, I wanted to change the World.
Today I am wise, so I am changing myself.
Mewlana Jalaluddin Rumi

Another operation in AGS that is performed, especially in combination with vaginoplasty operations, is perineoplasty, that is, aesthetic repair and/or reconstruction of the perineum.

12.1 Perineoplasty Indications

Congenital defects of the perineum, skin tags of the labia minora continuing to the perineum, and perineal traumas are among the main indications for perineoplasty operations.

Perineoplasty is a reconstructive operation known as "perineal repair" or "perineal reconstructive surgery." It is performed for reasons such as correcting hypertrophic or atrophic episiotomy scars, excising skin tags, extending the distance between the vaginal entrance and anus, or closing vaginal gaping. It is mostly applied in the form of colpoperineoplasty, simultaneously with posterior colporrhaphy; this forms the aesthetic and reconstructive part of the operation that is visible from the outside. Conversely, enlargement of the introitus and perineum can decrease sensitivity by reducing the mechanical pressure on the anterior wall of the vagina during sexual intercourse. For this reason, it can also be done to increase sensitivity in sexual intercourse.

Episiotomy scars generally develop due to postpartum infection, dehiscence of episiotomy sutures, or faulty technique in episiotomy suture. Especially in difficult and traumatic deliveries, lacerations are more common, and the risk of scarring increases due to delayed wound healing.

The most frequent perineoplasty indications are listed in Table 12.1.

Table 12.1 Perineoplasty Indications

• Atrophic or hypertrophic episiotomy scar revisions
• Excision of perineal skin tags
• Elimination of vaginal gaping problem
• Lack of pleasure during sexual intercourse due to introital enlargement
• Repairing perineal ruptures caused by vaginal births, coitus, or other mechanical impacts
• Making the perineal area flatter and more aesthetically pleasing in combination with colporrhaphy or labiaplasty operations

S. Eserdağ, *Aesthetic and Functional Female Genital Surgery*,
https://doi.org/10.1007/978-3-031-16019-6_12

12.1.1 Perineal Traumas

Perineal traumas can occur after hard coitus or mechanical impacts, or more often after obstetric interventions such as episiotomy or operative deliveries.

The incidence of perineal trauma reported during vaginal delivery is approximately 85%, but this rate may differ depending on the clinical practices during vaginal delivery [1]. Anal sphincter injuries, which are among the most severe perineal traumas, are gradually increasing. In recent years, population-based studies have shown that the incidence rates range from 4.1 to 16.0%.

Perineal traumas during vaginal delivery may cause maternal morbidity such as blood loss, perineal pain, and infection in the early period. Complications such as dyspareunia, flatus, fecal incontinence, sexual dysfunction, pelvic organ prolapse, and rectovaginal and vesicovaginal fistula may develop in the future.

Prevention of perineal trauma is important in women both physically and emotionally. A controlled multicenter study conducted to demonstrate the effectiveness of hyaluronidase administration in the prevention of perineal lacerations due to vaginal deliveries showed that vaginal hyaluronidase injection did not prevent perineal lacerations but was highly effective in resolving postpartum edema compared to the control group [2]. Perineoplasty operation may become essential to repair unavoidable perineal lacerations.

12.2 Perineoplasty Techniques

Perineoplasty operation can be applied with different techniques. These techniques are:

- *Diamond-shaped excision*
- *Elliptical excision (Episiotomy scar revision)*
- *Triangular excision*
- *Z-plasty*

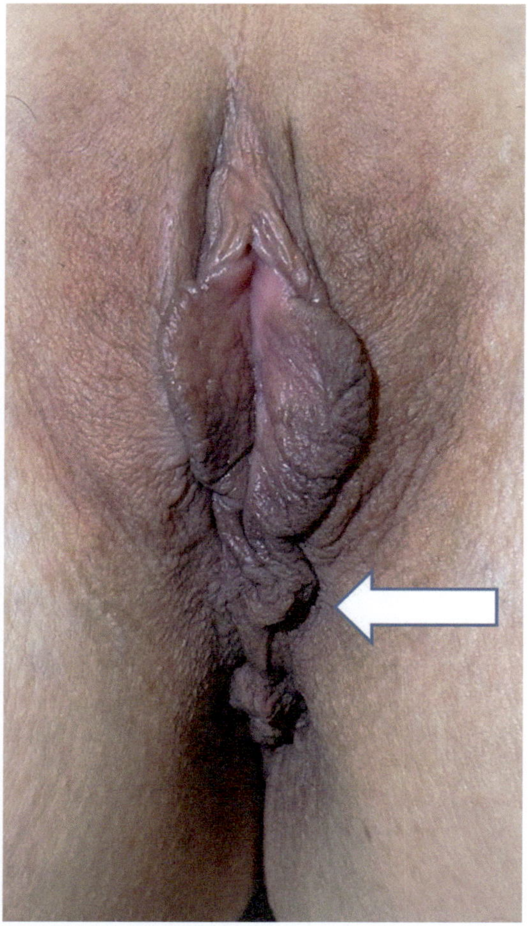

Fig. 12.1 "Rooster comb" appearance in the perineum (*Eserdag*). This perineal skin fold is an extension of asymmetrically elongated left labium minus

The excision line can sometimes be extended longitudinally up to the anus in order to eliminate the deformation.

In perineoplasty, the perineal body, vulvar vestibulum, and vaginal introitus are all reconstructed. Perineoplasty is mostly applied simultaneously with vaginal tightening surgeries. Sometimes, during labiaplasty operation, perineoplasty can also be performed due to the unification of the hypertrophic labium minus with the perineum and the skin fold in the form of a *"rooster comb"* (in our terminology) descending vertically from the posterior commissure to the anus (Fig. 12.1).

12.2.1 Diamond-Shaped Excision

Isolated perineoplasty, which is performed to reconstruct episiotomy scars, is the cutting and removal of a piece of tissue in the shape of a diamond, as in vaginal tightening. The apex of the removed tissue is at the bottom one-third of the posterior wall of the vagina, and the lower point is on the perineal region. The outer edges of the diamond extend laterally at the level of the hymenal ring. In addition to correcting the aesthetic appearance, in order to increase the stimulation in sexual intercourse, the perineum is raised a little by bringing the pelvic muscles in the vaginal entrance closer and the perineal body is strengthened. However, excessive elevation and tension should be avoided.

Sometimes, diamond and elliptical excisions can be combined. Thus, both the vaginal opening is tightened and the episiotomy scars are removed (Fig. 12.2).

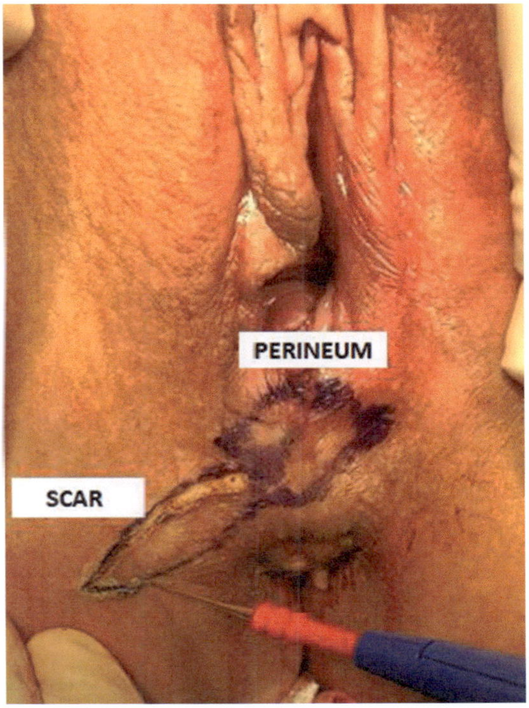

Fig. 12.2 Combined elliptical and diamond incisions

12.2.2 Elliptical Excision (Episiotomy Scar Revision)

This is an isolated elliptical excision made on the episiotomy lines of patients with normal introitus width and without vaginal gaping (Fig. 12.3).

12.2.3 Triangle-Shaped Excision

The operation area is in the perineum and in a triangular shape, without extending the perineal incision line to the introitus (Fig. 12.4).

If there is vaginal gaping and/or fecal incontinence problems related to perineal muscle separation, muscle repair is a must. In muscle repair, delayed absorbable sutures with 2/0 or 3/0 round needles are generally used. For skin closure, continuous, unlocking sutures with 4/0 sharp needle and delayed absorbable suture material are recommended.

12.2.4 Z-Plasty

In some cases, perineal repair can be performed in the form of Z-plasty. Patients with wide perineal opening and irregular deformation are especially suitable candidates for Z-plasty (Fig. 12.5).

Perineoplasty operations are sometimes a part of a combined surgery (Fig. 12.6).

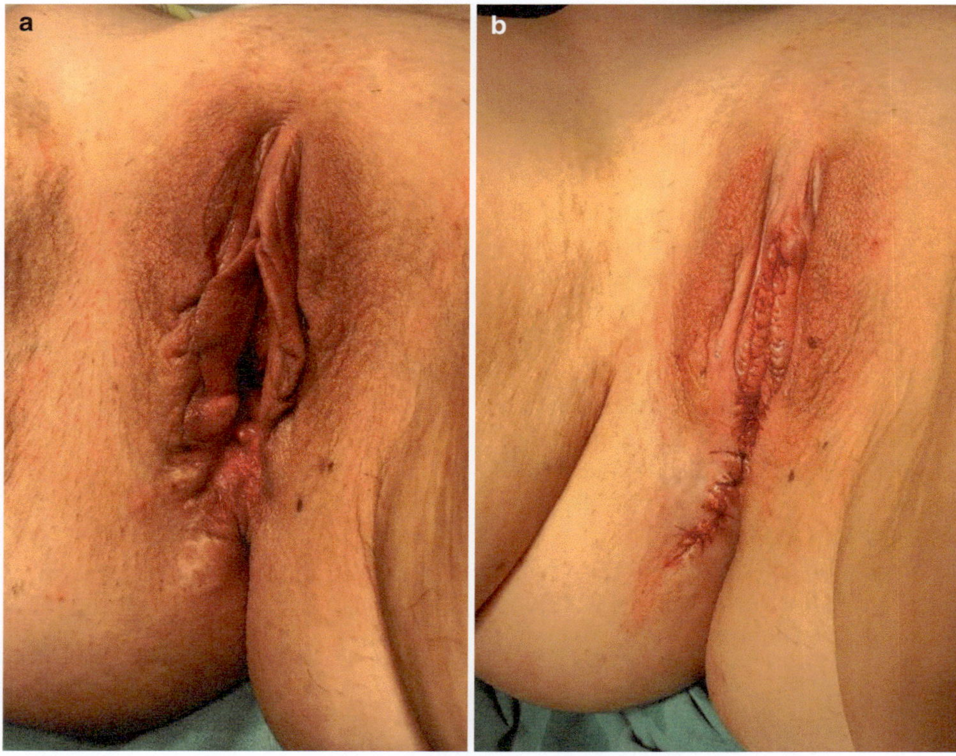

Fig. 12.3 Perineal scar revision with elliptical excision. Before (**a**), after (**b**). Labiaplasty operation was also performed

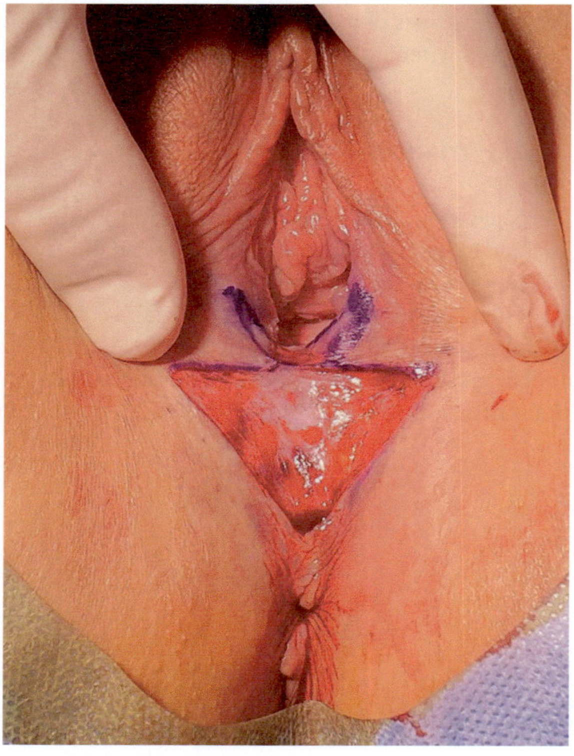

Fig. 12.4 Triangular excision

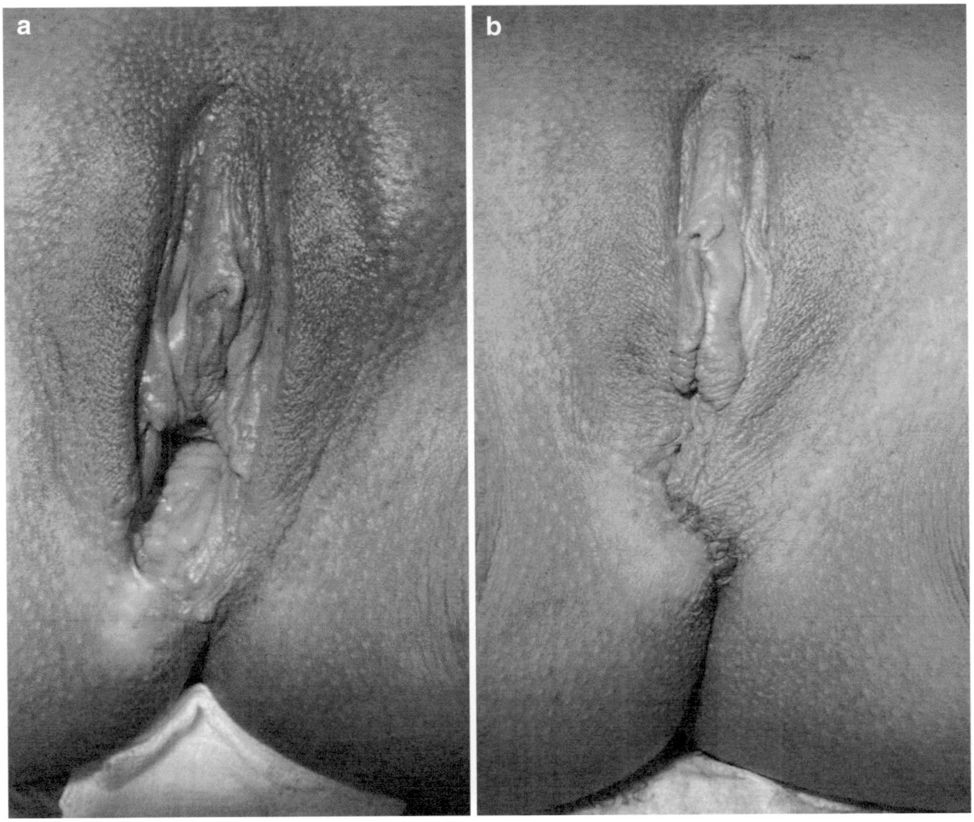

Fig. 12.5 Vaginal gaping and perineal scar. Before (**a**) and after repair with Z-plasty (**b**)

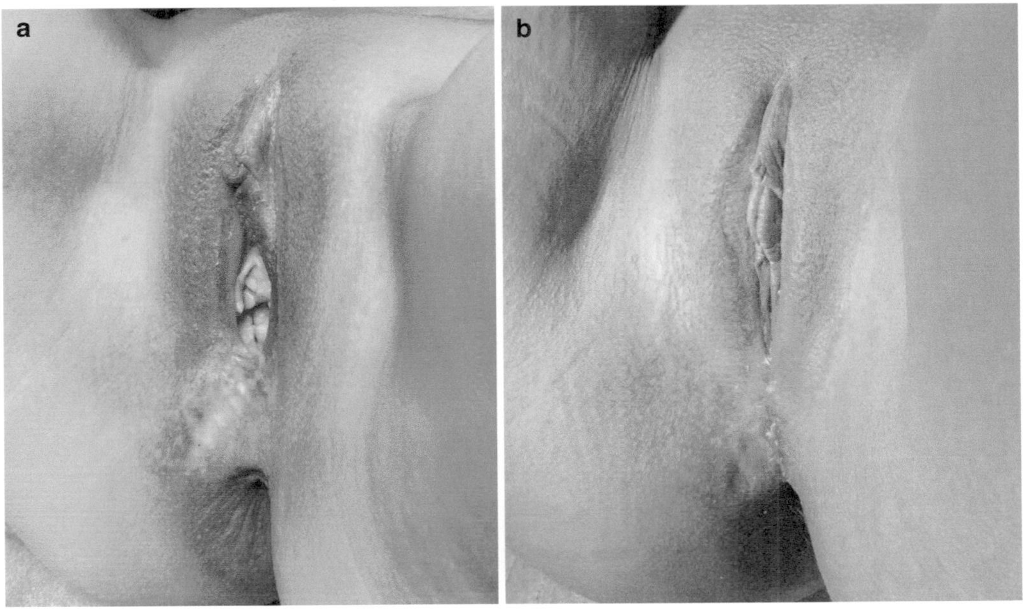

Fig. 12.6 Combined surgeries; perineoplasty, vaginal tightening, labiaplasty, and laser bleaching operations on a patient with intense scarring in the perineum. Before (**a**) and 2.5 months after (**b**)

Table 12.2 Different approaches to atrophic scar treatments

• Surgical removal of atrophic scar tissue and reconstruction of the area (elliptic excision or Z-plasty)
• Autologous fat grafting or hyaluronic acid injections to the atrophic scar
• Injection of special serums containing collagenase and hyaluronic acid

12.3 Atrophic Scar Treatments

Atrophic scars developing after episiotomy in the perineum are generally the result of the deterioration of tissue vascularization due to faulty technique. During the recovery period, an excessive increase of subcutaneous fibrosis can retract the skin down. In this case, several road maps can be followed. The first is the complete removal of the atrophic scar by performing perineoplasty with the classical method or Z-plasty. The second option is fat grafting to the atrophic scar (Table 12.2). While the adipose tissue fills the collapsed area, the mesenchymal stem cells in the tissue provide a regenerative effect. A third approach is injection of hyaluronic acid fillers used for similar purposes as fat injection or special solutions containing high-density collagenase + hyaluronic acid used in scar treatment (PBSerum™). All of these procedures are also suitable for surgical and non-surgical scar treatments after cesarean section or on different parts of the body.

12.4 Perineal Hernias

Herniation can be seen very rarely in the perineum. In such hernias, hernia repair is performed by laparoscopic or vulvar approach. To prevent the formation of a hernia, especially if adipose tissue reduction was performed in majoraplasty operations, it is important to stitch up the tunic sac properly. Conversely, a bulging can be observed in the episiotomy line, mimicking the hypertrophic scar appearance, due to improper suturing of the episiotomy layers, especially after vaginal delivery. In such cases, adipose tissue is encountered directly under the elliptical incised skin tissue. What needs to be done is to debulk the adipose tissue a little and to achieve primary repair by approximating the fascia and connective tissues from the subcutaneous part (Fig. 12.7).

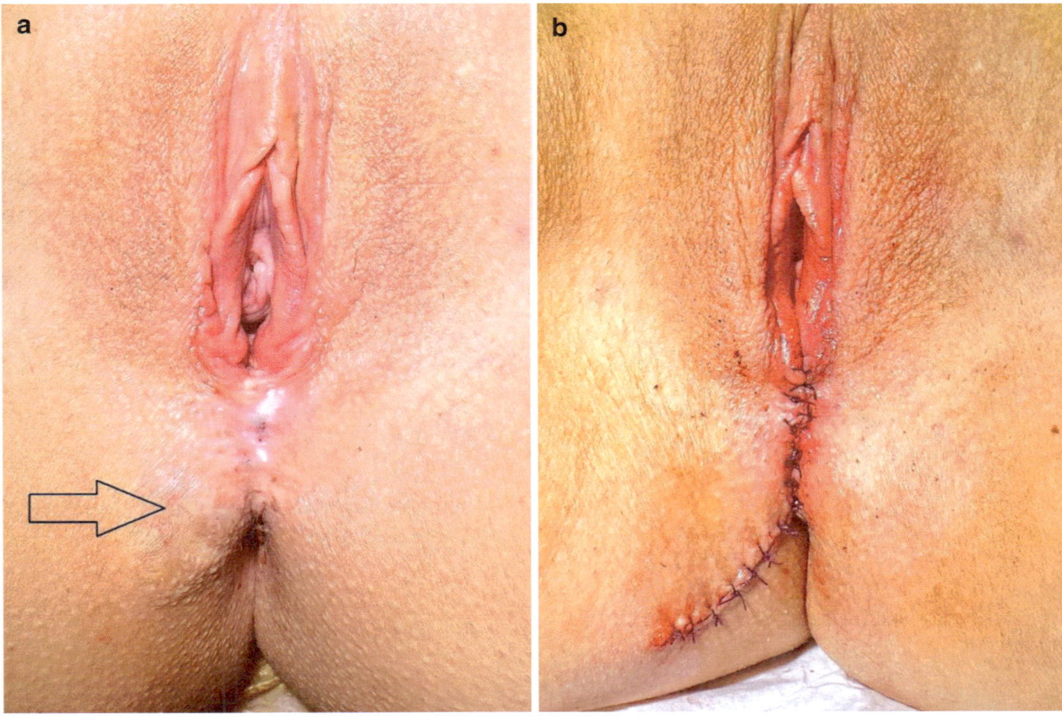

Fig. 12.7 Perineal herniation. Bulged appearance in the episiotomy line resembles a postpartum hypertrophic scar. After the dissection of the skin tissue, adipose tissue was emerged directly, because of the herniation. After the excessive adipose tissue was debulked, the dartos fascia and subcutaneous connective tissues were supported by sutures, and then primary repair was achieved. Before (**a**) and after (**b**)

12.5 Perineal Granuloma Fissuratum

“Granuloma fissuratum” is a general term describing skin injuries caused by minor and chronic traumas. It is used for different parts of the body. “Perineal granuloma fissuratum” is characterized by multiple perineal tears after the sexual penetrations due to bad wound healing and loss of tissue elasticity in the perineum (Fig. 12.8). After mechanical separation of tissue, a delicate granulation tissue will form in that area, but then it will be torn again in the next intercourse. Apart from previous perineoplasty operations and episiotomy repairs, it can also be observed in lichen sclerosus disease, menopausal atrophies, and some inflammatory diseases of the vulva. Chronicle tears, dyspareunia, and tissue separation can lead to psychological mood impairment, sexual arousal, and desire problems in women.

For the management, PRP or regenerative HA injections can be applied to improve collagen remodeling in the perineal region. The last resort is surgical excision of the scar tissue. In resistant cases, rotating a flap from the posterior vaginal wall will be beneficial.

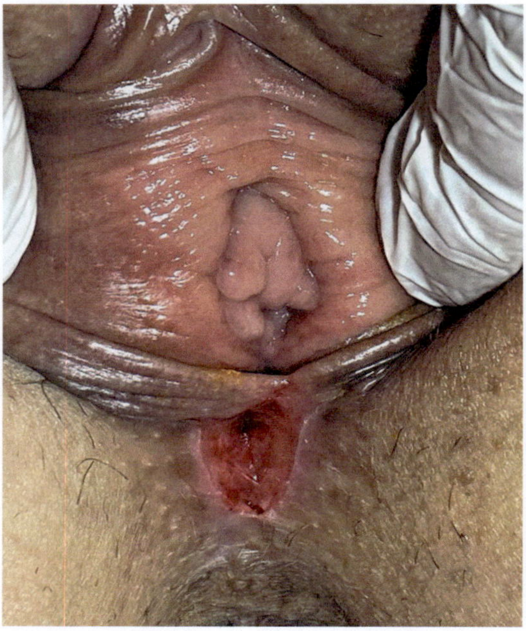

Fig. 12.8 Perineal granuloma fissuratum. The patient complaints of recurrent tears and bleeding after each coitus. This condition is due to decreased tissue elasticity in the perineum after vaginal tightening and perineal reconstructive surgery

12.6 Complications

One of the most common complications in perineoplasty is the perineal entrance being narrowed more than desired. This may cause pain during sexual intercourse or inability to have sexual intercourse. Therefore, as time passes, vaginal muscle hypertonicity ("hypertonic vagina") may also develop. If the narrowness is not so much, relaxation with fingers or dilators exercises can be recommended. If the narrowness is too much and the introital area is fibrotic, lost its elasticity, so does not stretch during penetration, the fibrotic band should simply be removed surgically. Laser cutting is also among the options that can be preferred.

12.7 The Postoperative Term

Postoperative procedures are similar to those in vaginoplasty operations.

12.8 Perianal Aesthetics

Skin tags in the perineum can extend to the perianal area. In some cases, unwanted skin excess or hard fibrotic tissue may occur after previous anal surgery such as for hemorrhoids. This situation can be eliminated primarily in line with general aesthetic genital surgery principles (Fig. 12.9).

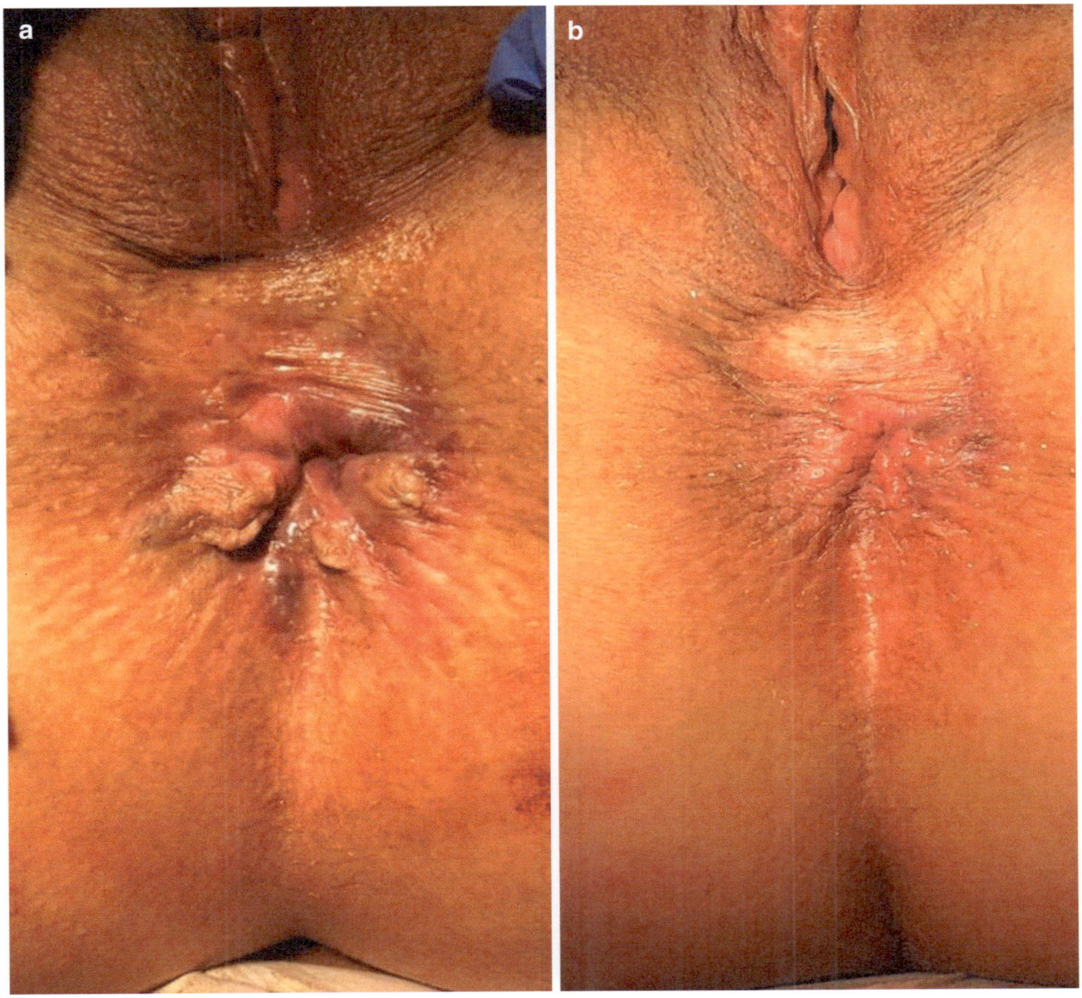

Fig. 12.9 Perianal aesthetics. Removal of hard scar tissue due to previous hemorrhoid surgery. Before (**a**) and 2 months after surgery (**b**)

Appendix

With the purchase of this book, you can use our "SN Flashcards" app to access questions free of charge in order to test your learning and check your understanding of the contents of the book.

To use the app, please follow the instructions below:

1. Go to https://flashcards.springernature.com/login
2. Create a user account by entering your e-mail address and assigning a password.
3. Use the following link to access your SN Flashcards set: ▶ https://sn.pub/tvlq7Q

If the link is missing or does not work, please send an e-mail with the subject "SN Flashcards" and the book title to customerservice@springernature.com.

References

1. Fernando RJ, Sultan AH, Kettle C, Thakar R. Methods of repair for obstetric anal sphincter injury. Cochrane Database Syst Rev 2013;(12):CD002866.
2. Kwon H, Park HS, Shim JY, Lee KW, Choi SJ, Choi GY. Randomized, double-blind, placebo-controlled trial on the efficacy of hyaluronidase in preventing perineal trauma in nulliparous women. Yonsei Med J. 2020;61(1):79–84.

13 Labia Majoraplasty

Ars longa, vita brevis, occasio praeceps, experimentum periculosum, iudicium difficile. (Art is long, life is short, opportunity fleeting, experience misleading, judgment difficult).

Hippocrates

Female external genital cosmetic surgery procedures are viewed by many plastic surgeons and gynecologists as being technically simple operations. They often are. However, they involve many tips and tricks to get the optimum results.

Ptotic, deflated labia majora, is best treated by reduction rather than augmentation. Surgical excision of redundant majora yields consistently excellent results and high patient satisfaction [1].

13.1 Vulvar Laxity

Vulvar laxity, ptosis, and sagging that can occur for different reasons may cause aged and unwanted aesthetic appearance. Vaginal childbirth, natural process of aging, congenital factors, and surgical interventions are considered the main causes of vulvovaginal laxity driven by changes in collagen and elastin fibers. This causes a loss of strength and flexibility within the vaginal wall. As a result, women may experience lack of sensation. Moreover, rapid weight gain, chronic irritation, and vulvar dystrophies may also cause vulvar laxity. Factors such as menopause, during which time collagen destruction accelerates, smoking, malnutrition, and stress may also increase laxity [2]. In some cases, labia majora may be hypertrophic or asymmetrical. The aesthetic operation performed to make sagging, loose, hypertrophic, or asymmetrical labia majora into a smaller, tenser, and symmetrical structure is called "labia majoraplasty." If the goal is to reduce the bulky labia majora, the name "labia majora reduction" is also used.

Labia majoraplasty surgery is also a kind of labiaplasty. However, since labia minoraplasty is performed much more frequently, the term labiaplasty is mostly reserved for internal labial aesthetics.

13.2 Primary Hypertrophy

The condition of excessive volume in the labia majora due to excess adipose tissue is called *"primary hypertrophy,"* and this problem can be solved by liposuction methods. Liposuction can be done with methods such as laser, radiofrequency, or VASER. The fat pad reduction can also be performed.

S. Eserdağ, *Aesthetic and Functional Female Genital Surgery*,
https://doi.org/10.1007/978-3-031-16019-6_13

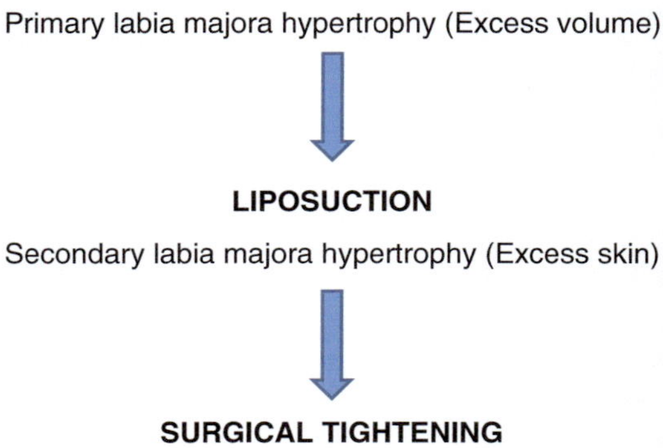

Fig. 13.1 Labia majora hypertrophy and management

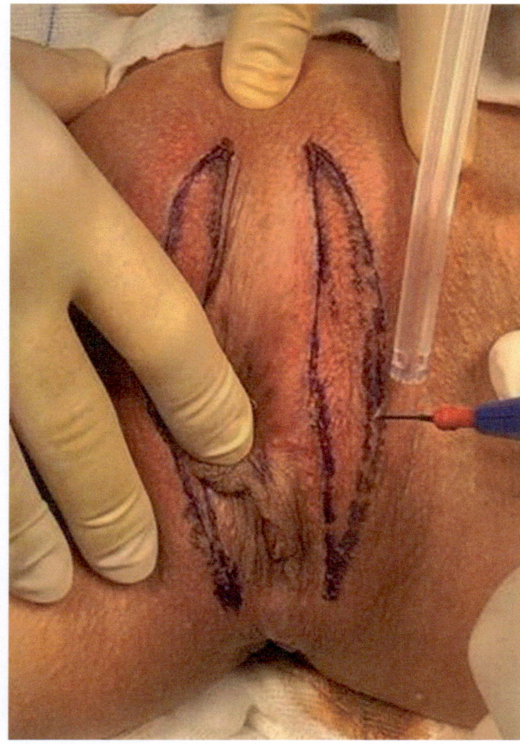

Fig. 13.2 Labia majoraplasty by elliptical excision. RF cutting after elliptical marking. Smoke extractors or aspirators can be used during the incision

13.3 Secondary Hypertrophy

The condition in which excessive skin tissue has been formed due to the decrease in subcutaneous fat and collagen, and therefore wrinkling and loosening occur, is called *"secondary hypertrophy."* In this case, vulvar tightening can be performed by removing the skin tissue with labia majoraplasty. In some cases, adipose tissue can be removed along with the skin using a wedge incision and labia majora reduction can be performed (Fig. 13.1).

13.4 Labia Majoraplasty Surgical Techniques

Majoraplasty operation can be performed using different techniques depending on the degree and extent of the laxity. Some surgery techniques include:

- *Elliptical excision,*
- *Horseshoe excision, and*
- *Teardrop incision (Eserdag).*

Depending on the desired depth, the removal of the tissue can include only the skin, or both layers of skin and subcutaneous tissue, or also involving the fat tissue by opening the fibrous tunic.

13.4.1 Elliptical Excision

First, a vertical elliptical area is marked along the interlabial sulcus from the clitoral hood level to the fourchette lateral below. The more tissue to be removed, the wider the ellipse should be drawn. If the amount of tissue to be removed from both labia is the same (unless asymmetry exists), marking with metric measurement for equal amounts of resection is recommended. Then, the incision is made along the marked line with laser, scalpel, needle-tipped unipolar cautery, or Ellman RF. Care should be taken so that the incision made with needle-tipped cautery or RF does not go too deep (Fig. 13.2).

To the best of our experience, if the incision is made by the scalpel, there is less risk of scarring compared to energy-based devices. It provides safety to use the body of the scalpel instead of its tip. After the incision, the skin and subcutaneous tissues are removed by fine dissection with a no.11 scalpel or fine-tipped metzenbaum scissors. After tissue excision, hemostasis is provided and subcutaneous tissue is closed with continuous or single sutures. For subcutaneous tissue, rapid absorbable sutures with 4/0 round needles are suitable. If the tissue is thick, the closure should be done in two layers. After subcutaneous tissue, skin tissue can be closed with 4/0 sharp needle delayed absorbable suture materials.

If there is labia majora asymmetry, both sides can be equalized by removing more tissue from one side.

13.4.2 Horseshoe Excision

Labia majoraplasty operations can also be performed as a "horseshoe incision" with wide excision. The excision line is extended to the anterior commissure (Fig. 13.3).

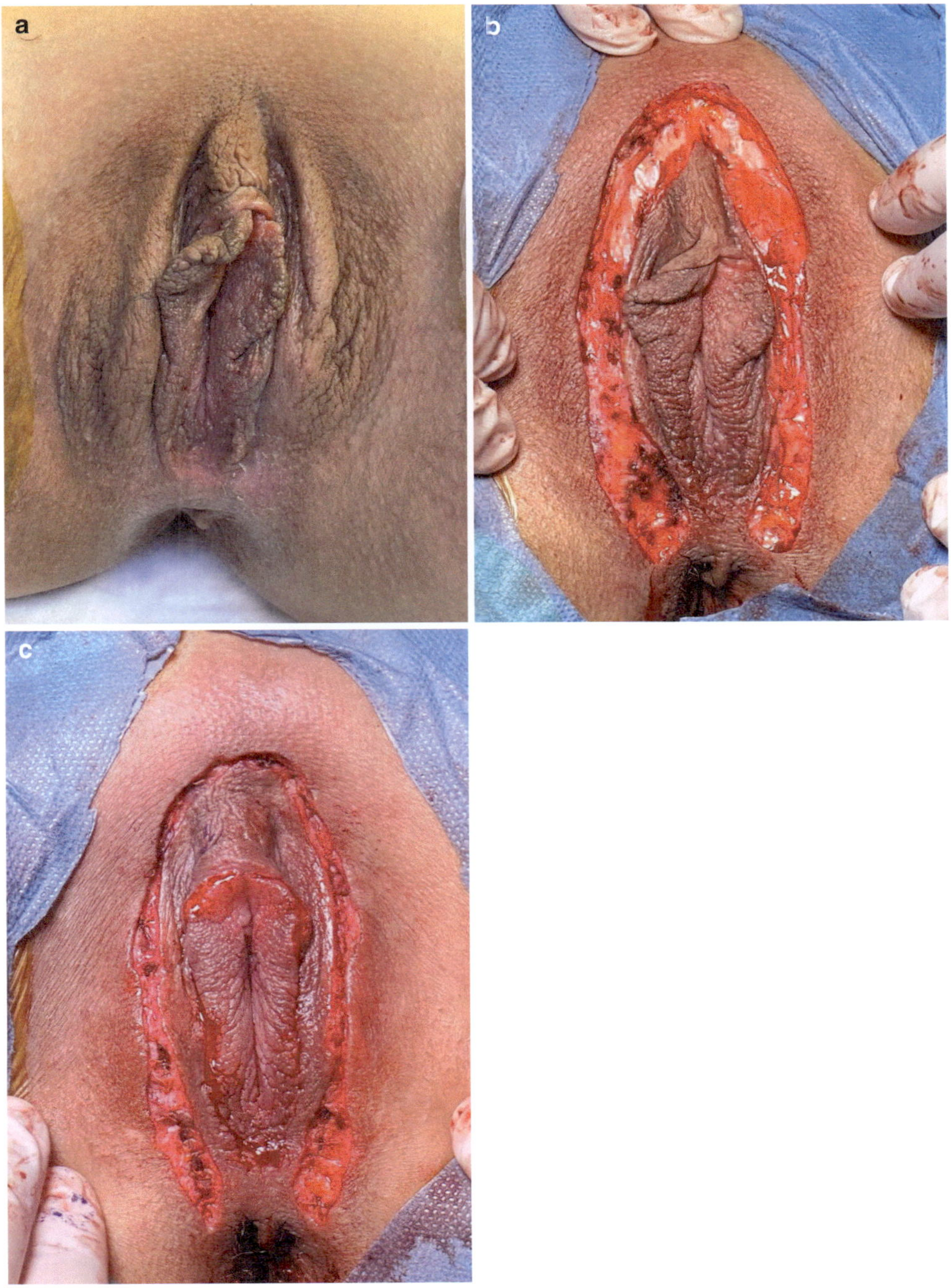

Fig. 13.3 Horseshoe majoraplasty and minoraplasty combined operations. In combined surgery, priority should be in the labia majora. Before (**a**), horseshoe excision in labia majora (**b**), trimming in labia minora (**c**)

13.4.3 Teardrop Incision (Eserdag)

In patients with excessive laxity problems, the labia majora incisions can be extended and brought together on both anterior and posterior commissures. The posterior incision line can be extended to the perineum. So, the maximum amount of correction can be obtained. Due to its shape we named *"teardrop incision"* (Fig. 13.4).

I can say that labia majoraplasty is an easier surgical procedure than labia minoraplasty. However, physician experience in this area is very low due to the fact that it is performed far less frequently.

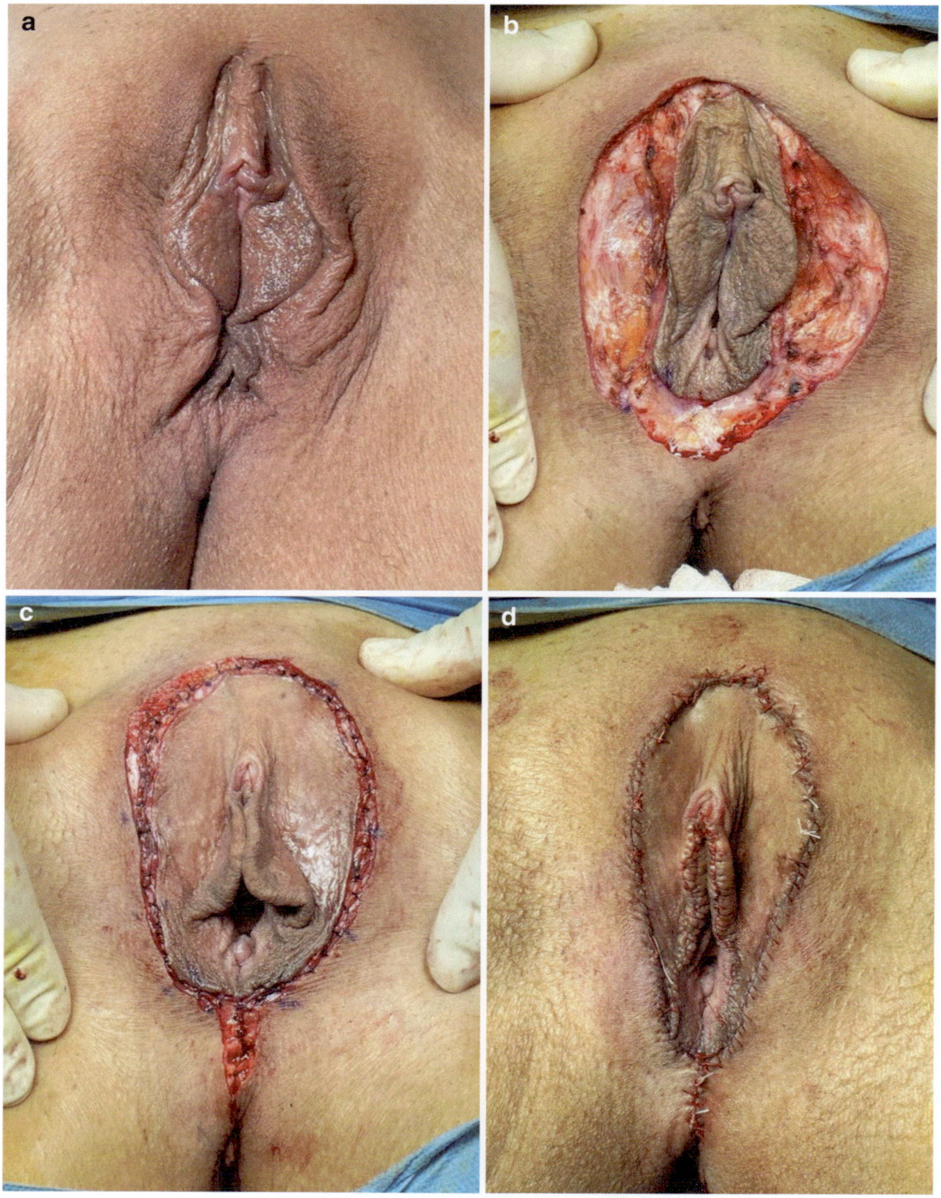

Fig. 13.4 Teardrop incision (*Eserdag*) in majoraplasty. The majoraplasty incision line is extended from the anterior commissure to the posterior commissure and from there to the perineum. This patient also underwent labia minoraplasty operation. Before (**a**), teardrop excision in labia majora (**b**), subcutaneous closure (**c**), labia minora trimming and skin closure (**d**)

Some of the patients with vulvar laxity problems also need a series of combined procedures.

13.5 Majoraplasty with Adipose Tissue Excision (Fat Pad Debulking)

A more invasive surgical excision may be required in primary labia majora hypertrophy cases, which manifest itself not only with excess skin but also with excess subcutaneous and adipose tissue. In this case, the skin, subcutaneous, and adipose tissues can be removed by wedge excision (Fig. 13.5).

In majoraplasty operations involving adipose tissue reduction, attention should be paid to the risks of bleeding and hematoma. Also, the elastic sac and dartos support layers must be properly sutured end-to-end in the closure of the tissues after reduction. Otherwise, there is a risk of perineal hernia, which manifests itself with bulging in the labia majora postoperatively.

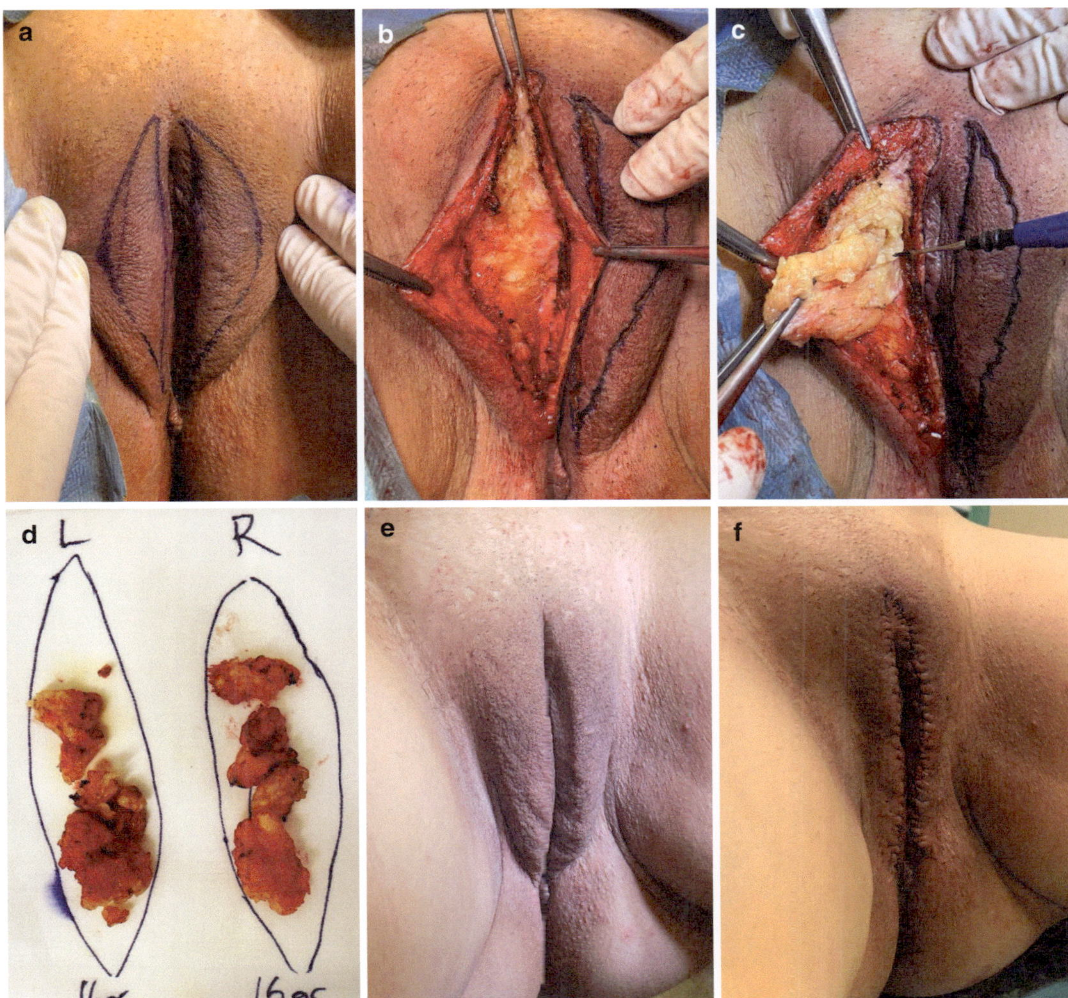

Fig. 13.5 Fat pad debulking. Reduction of the labia majora in a primary labial hypertrophy case. Marking (**a**), elliptical incisions were made and fibrous tunic (elastic sac) was opened (**b**), equal proportions (16 g) of fat were excised from both labia majora (**c**, **d**). The skin and subcutaneous tissues were also reduced along with the adipose tissue. Before (**e**), just after (**f**)

13.6 Combined Procedures

Labia minoraplasty and clitoral hoodoplasty can be performed simultaneously with majoraplasty (Figs. 13.6 and 13.7). Thus, a total vulvoplasty operation will be performed. Similarly, majoraplasty can be performed simultaneously with vaginoplasty and perineoplasty operations (Fig. 13.8). The excised skin area can be extended to the mons pubis border above and to the perineum below ("major majoraplasty" in our own terminology). Sometimes the excised part is much more limited ("minor majoraplasty").

Vaginal tightening operation, laser tightening, genital PRP, or genital RF can be performed simultaneously with majoraplasty. However, if the patient requests fat transfer of the labia majora, it is recommended to wait at least 3 months. Some physicians state that postoperative recovery might be accelerated by injecting PRP to the wound area.

Combined operations of labia majoraplasty and minoraplasty are also frequently demanded by patients. It is recommended to perform majoraplasty first and then minoraplasty in such combined surgeries.

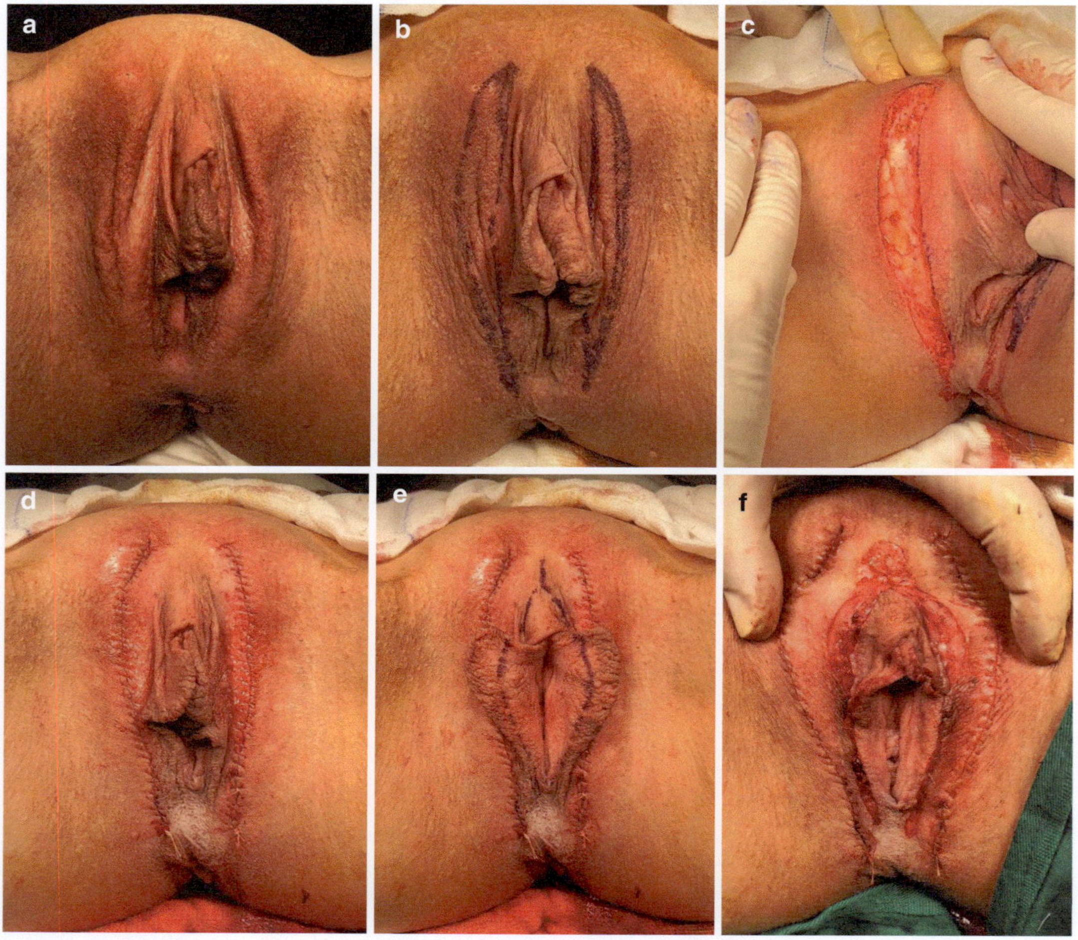

Fig. 13.6 Labia majoraplasty, labia minoraplasty, and inverted-Y clitorohoodoplasty combined operations for severe vulvar laxity. Before (**a**), elliptical marking (**b**), resection (**c**), closure of subcutaneous and skin layers (**d**), marking of labia minora and hood areas (**e**), resection (**f**), closure of subcutaneous and skin layers (**g**), postop view (**h**), before (lateral view) (**i**), just after (lateral view) (**j**)

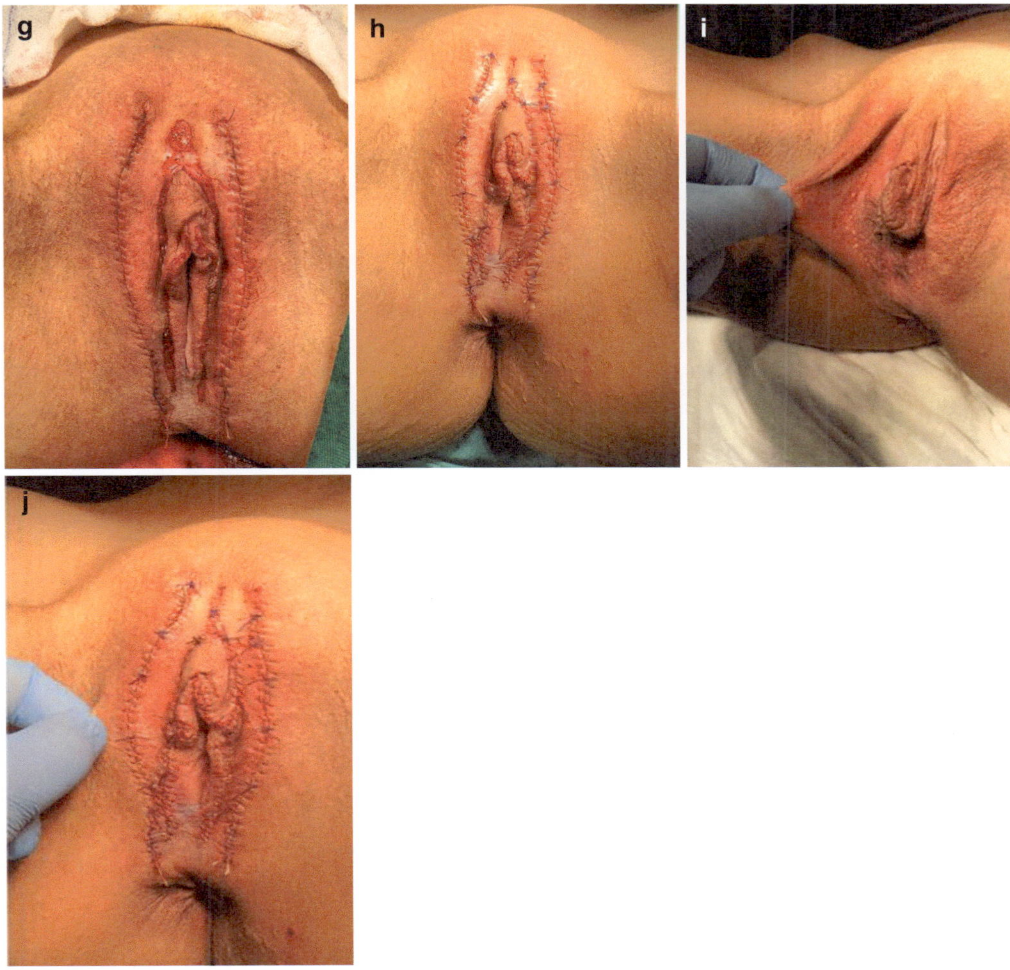

Fig. 13.6 (continued)

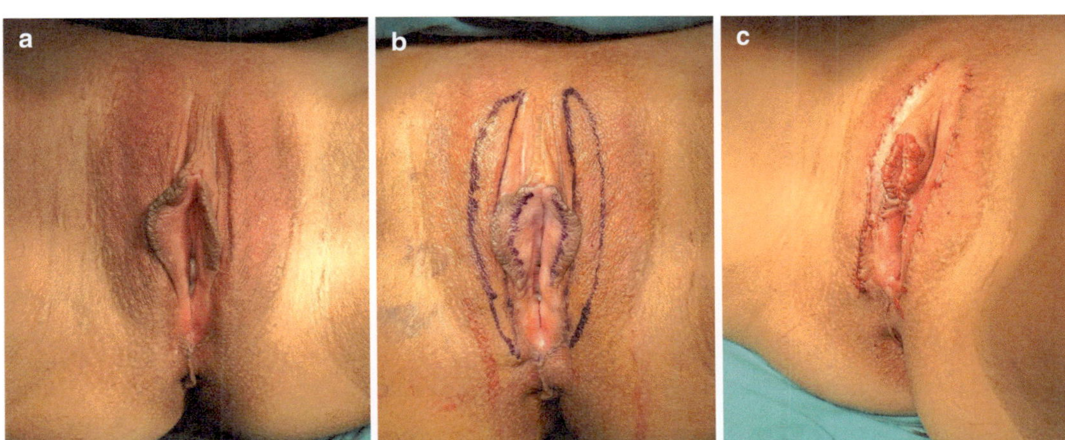

Fig. 13.7 Combination of major labia majoraplasty and minoraplasty. Before (**a**), elliptical marking (**b**), excision and skin closure (**c**, **d**), 2 months after the surgery (**e**, **f**)

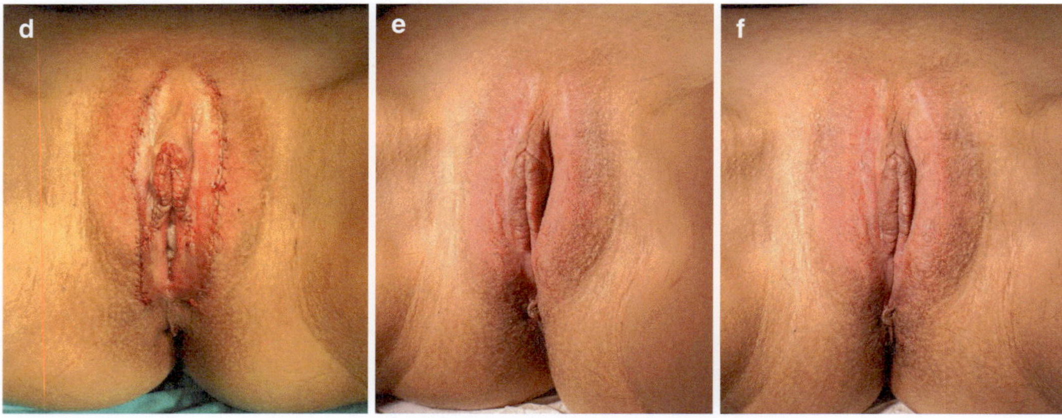

Fig. 13.7 (continued)

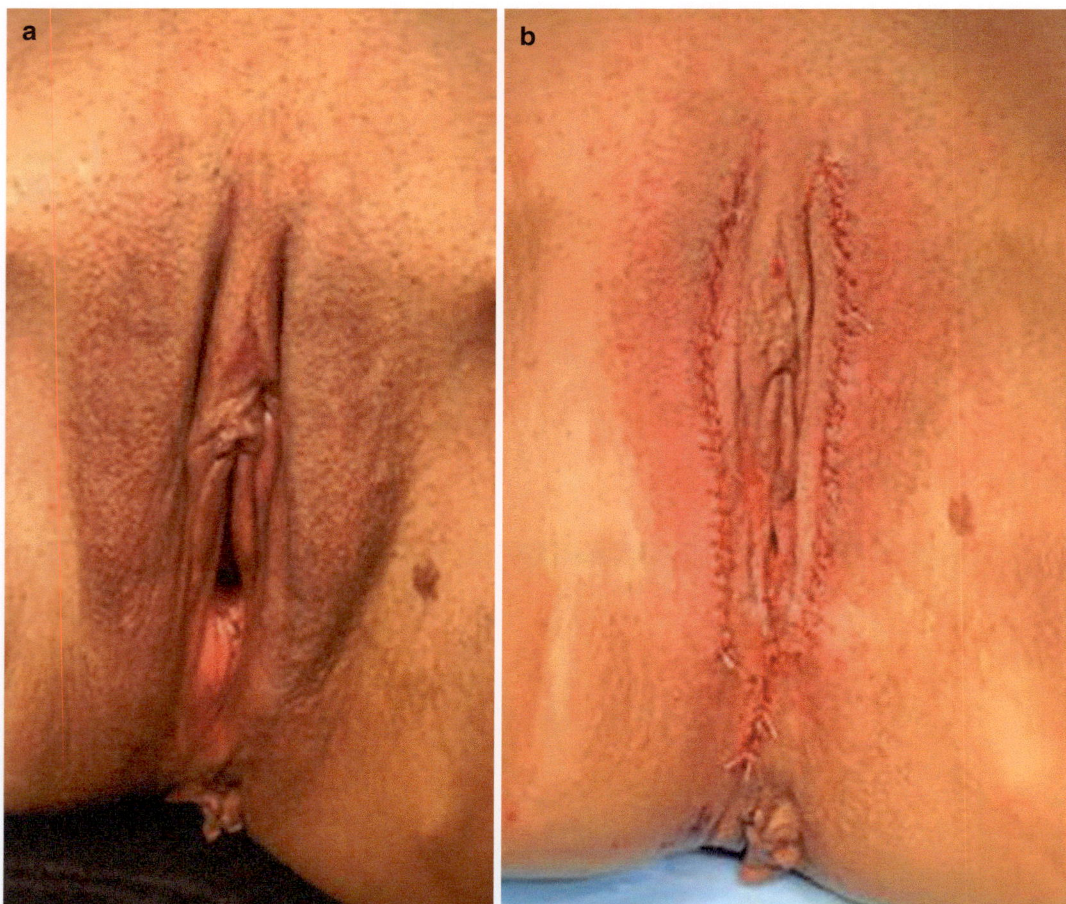

Fig. 13.8 Major majoraplasty, vaginoplasty, and perineoplasty combined surgery. Before (**a**), after (**b**)

13.7 Complications

13.7.1 Acute Term

In majoraplasty operations, complications such as bleeding, hematoma, and allergic reactions can be seen in the acute period. Compared to labia minora operations, the bleeding is less. If the procedure is performed in the office condition and under local anesthesia, hypotension and temporary loss of consciousness due to vasovagal reflex may occur.

13.7.2 Subacute Term

Complications such as excessive edema, infection, and wound dehiscence may occur in the subacute period (usually on the third to fifth postoperative days). Sometimes, Eau de Goulard solution, which has an anti-inflammatory effect and accelerates the healing of the wound, can be used in patients with long-lasting edema. In case of wound dehiscence, some patients may require revision surgery. It is recommended to wait at least 3 months before revision.

13.7.3 Chronic Term

In the chronic period, abscess, hypertrophic scar, inclusion cyst formation, and asymmetry can be observed. Inclusion cysts occur when skin tissue is accidentally buried under the skin. Preoperative metric measurement is important to avoid asymmetry problems.

Since the labia majoraplasty operation results in much more bleeding than minoraplasty, care should be taken for hemostasis. The scar formation that can occur in the postoperative period is generally associated with the incision line being too lateral. Therefore, the operation area must remain in the medial of the vertical line passing through the middle of the labia majora.

Asymmetry is one of the most common problems after majoraplasty. Therefore, the surgery should be designed well from the beginning. In addition, care should be taken to prevent deformations in the form of tissue bulging known as "dog ear," which may occur at the beginning and end of the incision.

Excessive stretching of the tissue in majoraplasty operations adversely affects circulation and wound healing as well as increasing the risk of suture opening.

If revision is required for any problems, wait at least 3 months.

13.8 The Postoperative Term

After labia majoraplasty, patients can be discharged home on the same day. Postoperative care and follow-up are the same as in labia minoraplasty operations.

Appendix

With the purchase of this book, you can use our "SN Flashcards" app to access questions free of charge in order to test your learning and check your understanding of the contents of the book.

To use the app, please follow the instructions below:

1. Go to https://flashcards.springernature.com/login
2. Create a user account by entering your e-mail address and assigning a password.
3. Use the following link to access your SN Flashcards set: ▶ https://sn.pub/tvlq7Q

If the link is missing or does not work, please send an e-mail with the subject "SN Flashcards" and the book title to customerservice@springernature.com.

References

1. Hunter JG. Labia minora, labia majora, and clitoral Hood alteration: experience-based recommendations. Aesthet Surg J. 2016;36(1):71–9.
2. Lalji S, Lozanova P. Evaluation of the safety and efficacy of a monopolar nonablative radiofrequency device for the improvement of vulvo-vaginal laxity and urinary incontinence. J Cosmet Dermatol. 2017;16(2):230–4.

14 Labia Majora Augmentation Via Fat Transfer and Monsplasty

Art is the signature of civilization.

Bernard Shaw

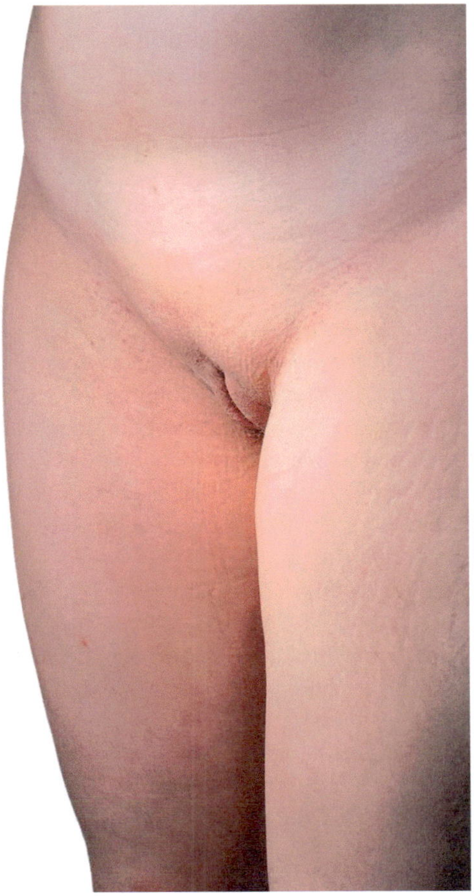

The common desires of many women who prefer aesthetic genital surgery are that the inner lips do not protrude outside the outer lips while standing and with their legs closed and that the labia majora have a flat, plump, and tight structure. One of the annoying situations for women who care about aesthetics is sagging and large outer lips.

In cases with excessive collapse and increased laxity in the labia majora, stretching (tightening) and reduction operations are performed with majoraplasty. The term "surgical majora tightening" can be used for these patients. Some patients who do not have much collapse in the labia majora but have slight depressions and wrinkles prefer to enlarge this area with fat grafting instead of labial reduction. "Labia majora augmentation" will be more appropriate for this group of patients.

14.1 Historical Background

The first fat grafting procedure in history was performed in 1893 by the German physician Dr. Franz Neuber by grafting the fat harvested from the upper arm of a patient into the chin. Two years later, in 1895, another German physician,

S. Eserdağ, *Aesthetic and Functional Female Genital Surgery*,
https://doi.org/10.1007/978-3-031-16019-6_14

Dr. Karl Czerny, repaired his patient's breast defect with the fat graft he received from the lumbar region [1].

Sydney R. Coleman first performed tissue augmentation with autologous fat in 1987, after which this technique spread rapidly. Labia majora augmentation is obtained frequently via fat transfer, hyaluronic acid, and collagen injection.

Autologous fat grafting procedures are most frequently used for breast reconstruction followed by gluteal augmentation, facial augmentation and aesthetics, hand rejuvenation, lip enhancement, penis enlargement, and aesthetic correction. The results obtained depend on the surgeon's experience and technique applied. Evidence-based data on this issue are very limited, so safety and efficacy issues must be specified in the consent forms received from patients [1].

Labia majora augmentation can be performed by autologous fat transfer, hyaluronic acid fillers, or collagen injections.

14.2 Labia Majora Fat Graft Indications

Labial collapse is usually due to poor collagen structure or rapid weight loss. Collapse and wrinkles occur in this area, which is full when overweight, with the reduction in adipose tissue due to rapid weight loss. One of the reasons for the sagging and surface irregularities in the majora is that the adipose tissue protrudes outward as a result of the deterioration of the subcutaneous fascia structures in this area.

Fat graft transfers can be performed for the following medical and cosmetic indications (Table 14.1).

In a case report by Aguilar et al., fat injection was applied to the posterior vaginal wall of a patient, and PRP and HA injections were applied to the subcutaneous area in the perineum. Modified Sabbatsberg scale and improvement in vaginal trophism were detected after the procedure [2].

Table 14.1 Different applications of fat transfer in cosmetic and functional gynecology

• Correcting collapses and wrinkles in the majora
• Hiding the labia minora inside the labia majora instead of surgically reducing the inner labia (labiaplasty)
Covering defects that occurred after previous labia minoraplasty operation that cannot be repaired well surgically
• Providing rejuvenation in the majora by means of mesenchymal stem cells in adipose tissue
• Correcting atrophic episiotomy scars
• Eliminating vulvar atrophy due to lichen sclerosus and menopause to improve symptoms
• Treating stress incontinence
• G-spot augmentation

14.3 Methods

The fat grafting procedure includes fat harvesting, fat processing, and lipofilling. During the application, some special cannulas and auxiliary apparatus are used (Fig. 14.1).

14.3.1 Fat Harvesting (Lipoaspiration)

The most preferred donor site for autologous fat grafting is the abdomen. However, in patients who do not have enough abdominal fat, who are weak, or who have undergone abdominoplasty, it is often impossible to remove abdominal fat. For this reason, lipoaspiration can also be done from the side abdomen (flank), inner thigh, outer thigh, or mons pubis areas.

Fat harvesting is typically performed under general or mild sedation anesthesia. If the patient is comfortable and compatible, the donor area can be marked with a skin pen, and local anesthesia can be performed around the marked area. The local anesthetic agent should be diluted at a rate of 50–60% and should be applied to both the donor and recipient areas, not into the surrounding areas. Lipoaspiration is

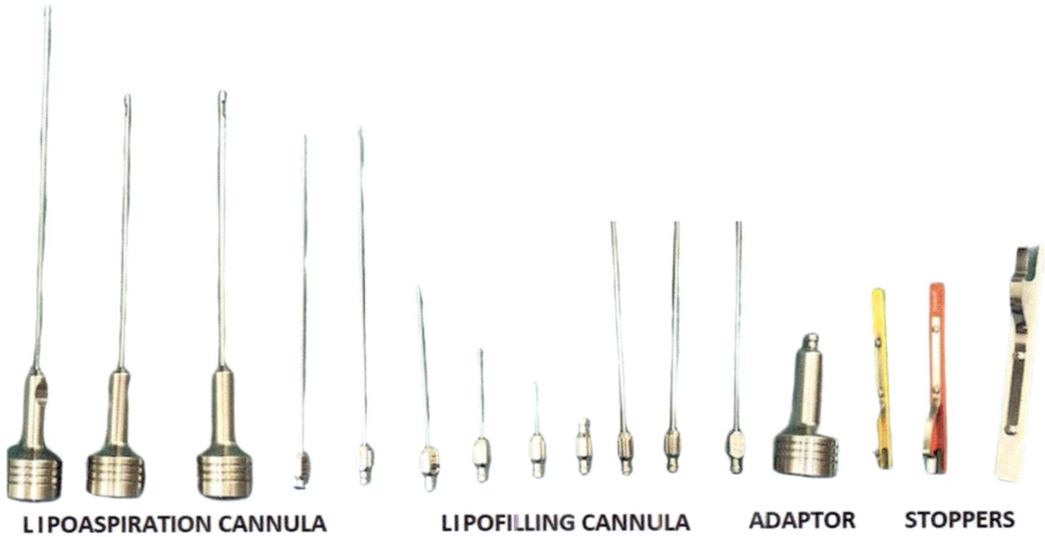

Fig. 14.1 Fat harvesting, fat delivery cannulas, and auxiliary equipment. The adapter is for transferring the extracted fat to small injectors. Stoppers (snapper, injector, locker) serve as safeties to prevent the pistol of the degreasing injector from coming out

performed manually with the help of 3 mm diameter lipoaspiration cannulas attached to a 20 or 60 mL injector, usually through a small incision made into the umbilical region. In line with the needs of the tissue, 20–100 cc of fat is usually aspirated.

It is beneficial to use tumescent anesthesia to reduce bleeding in the donor tissue and to ensure postoperative comfort. Tumescent anesthesia preparation is described in Chap. 8.

14.3.2 Fat Processing

The fat harvested can be processed in different ways according to the experience and preference of the surgeon. These include:

- Centrifuge only,
- Washing + Centrifuge, and
- Dry (no-touch) techniques.

The dry technique may be preferred because, in this technique, the fat harvested from the donor area is prepared to be given after thinning with a simple 3-way stop cock or filters (Fig. 14.2).

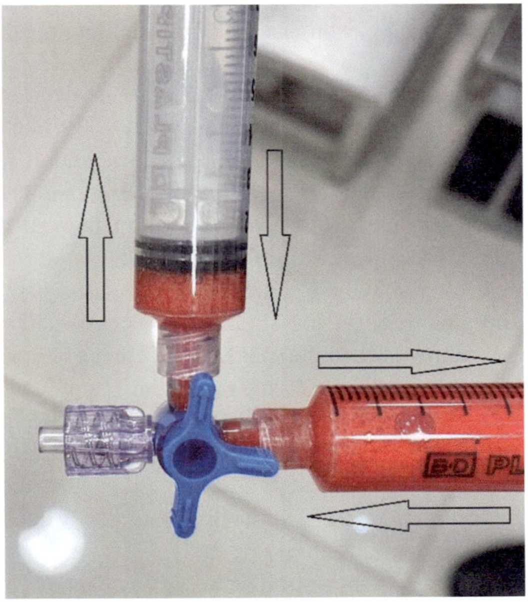

Fig. 14.2 Simple thinning of autologous fat by 3-way stop cock

In the case of tumescent anesthesia, it is more correct to apply centrifuge or washing + centrifuge techniques. In the centrifuge technique, the adipose tissue drawn into the injector is centrifuged at 3000 rpm × 3 min (1 min according to some). As a result of this centrifugation, the fat is separated into the crushed liquid lipocytes in the upper layer, the quality fat tissue to be injected in the middle layer, and the infranatant (blood, water, and aqueous solution) at the bottom. Quality adipose tissue drawn with an injector is given to the majora subcutaneous tissue with the help of a cannula.

In the washing and centrifuge technique, the material taken from the donor area is first washed with sterile water and then centrifuged at 6000 rpm × 2 min. There are discussions about whether the fat graft prepared by this procedure increases the survival rate. Indeed, excessive force applied during the centrifugation can damage the intact adipocytes.

14.3.3 Lipofilling

The lipofilling process is performed through a 1–1.5 mm lipofilling cannula inserted into small holes opened in both laterals of the hood area. The fat that is harvested and thinned is given in equal amounts to the different layers of both labia majora. In order not to confuse the orientation, it is recommended that the fat graft be given in the subcutaneous layers first deeply and then in a superficial plane. Before lipofilling, it should be confirmed that there is no intravascular access by applying negative pressure with the injector. The procedure should be performed by retrograde injection after the blunt-tipped thin cannula is fully inserted into the tissue and by giving a light curvature suitable for the majora structure (Fig. 14.3). Immediately after the procedure, the fat is homogeneously spread in the tissue by hand massage without squeezing.

Majora augmentation with fat can also be performed as a retrograde injection, but with the help of a cannula inserted from the inferior, right, and left sides of the fourchette.

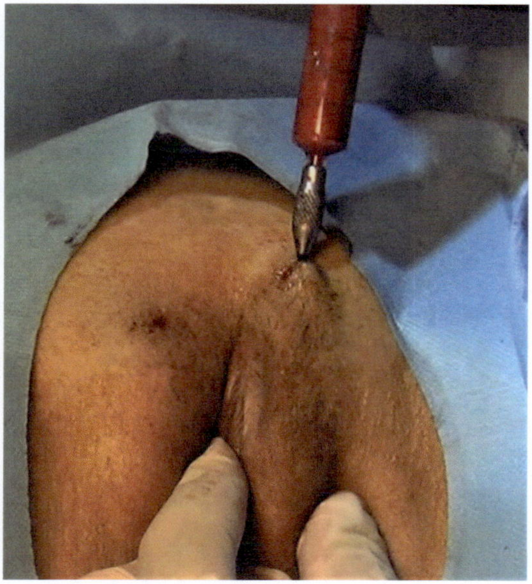

Fig. 14.3 Majora fat transfer from superior to inferior by blunt tip cannula. The lower passages are filled first, and the upper passages are last. The procedure should be done by drawing a slight ellipse in accordance with the curvature of the labia majora

Some authors claim that the prepared fat should be given after being mixed with PRP, thereby increasing the fat cell survival. Tissue necrosis due to devascularization may occur when fat is given without thinning (in particles of 3 mm and above) or when more tissue is transferred to an area. Conversely, not losing much time between fat harvesting and lipofilling processes and low oxygen contact are also important factors for the survival.

Using small cannulas as much as possible in fat harvesting, avoiding fast centrifugation, opening multiple tunnels in lipofilling, and injecting as soon as possible after harvesting are factors that positively affect the success of fat transplantation. The survival rate of the transferred fat six months after the operation varies between 30% and 40%. For this reason, it is beneficial if the amount of fat given in the transfer is a little more.

14.4 Combined Procedures

Labiaplasty, vaginoplasty, and perineoplasty procedures can be performed simultaneously with labia majora augmentation in line with the condition of the patient's tissue and the patient's preference (Figs. 14.4 and 14.5).

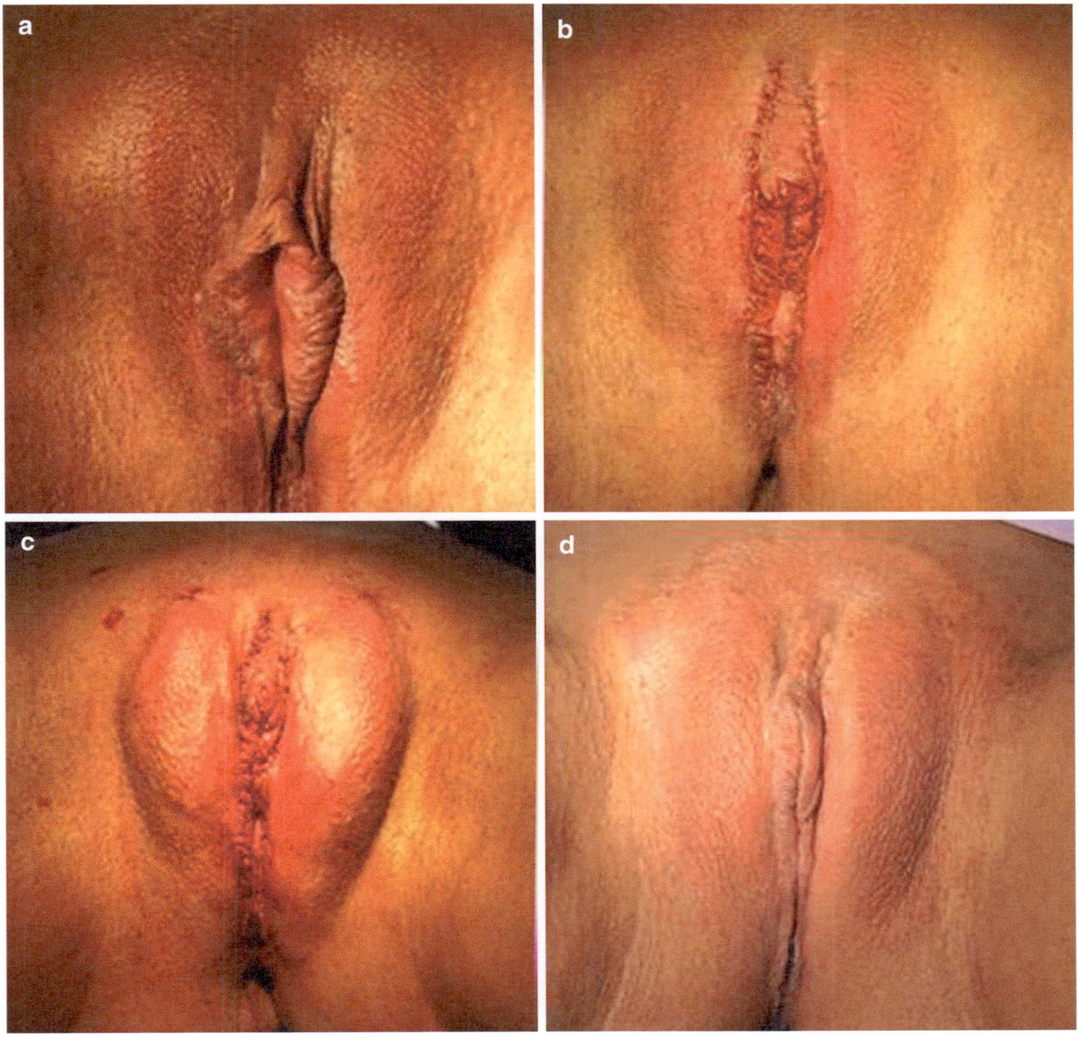

Fig. 14.4 Combined surgery. Labiaplasty, clitorohoodoplasty, and fat injection in the same session. Before (**a**), after labiaplasty and hoodoplasty (**b**), after fat injection (**c**), postoperative 12th month (**d**)

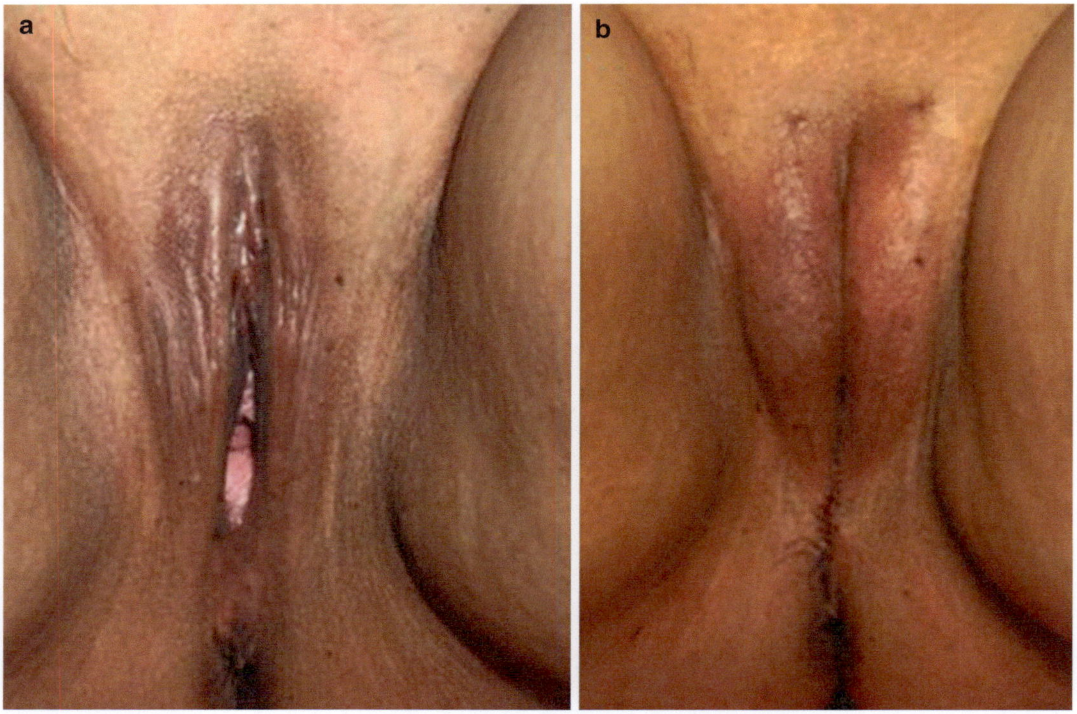

Fig. 14.5 Combined surgery. Vaginal tightening, perineoplasty, and majora fat transfers. Before (**a**), after (**b**)

14.5 Fat Transfer to Different Regions

Fat harvested from the donor area can also be used for the treatment of atrophic cesarean scar (Fig. 14.6), G-spot enlargement (Fig. 14.7), or even the treatment of deep skin grooves on the face. There are also different opinions regarding the use of fat in stress urinary incontinence treatment.

It is common practice to thin the harvested adipose tissue and mix it with PRP and then inject it into the genital or non-genital areas. As in other areas, a cannula should be used in fat transfer for G-spot augmentation.

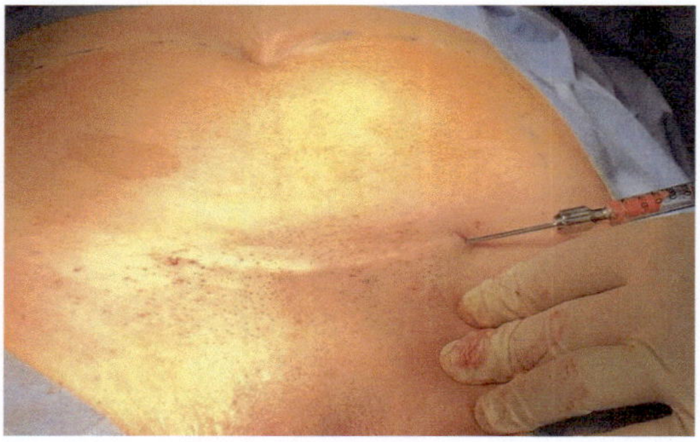

Fig. 14.6 Injection of the prepared fat from the abdomen under the scar tissue for the treatment of cesarean scar

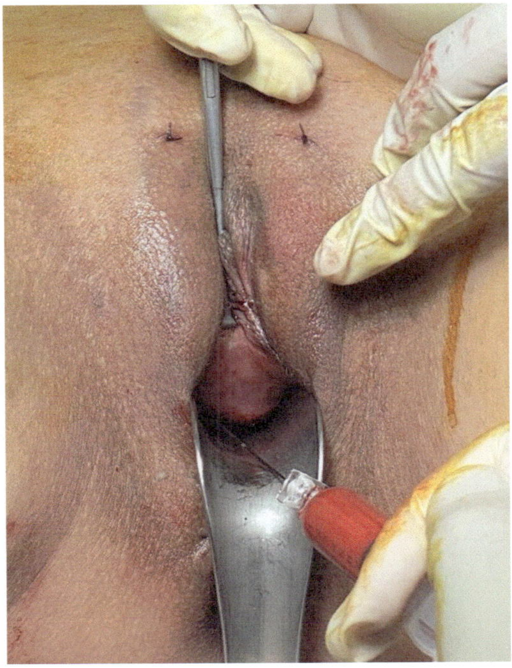

Fig. 14.7 Anterior wall augmentation with autologous fat transfer. After some of the fat harvested from the abdomen was used for labia majora augmentation, the remaining part was transferred to the anterior wall by a thin cannula

14.6 Operation Success

It is expected that 30–40% of the adipose tissue transferred will survive. Therefore, the volume of the fat transferred may be a little more than needed. In the lipofilling process, an average of 20–50 cc of fat can be given to each labia depending on the need. This amount can be increased a little more in patients with severe collapse. Fat survival depends on the following factors:

- Blood circulation of the donor area
- Blood circulation of the recipient area
- Fat preparation technique
- Transfer type
- Duration time between harvesting and lipofilling
- Air exposure of the harvested fat that will be used for lipofilling
- Postoperative care of the patient

In order for adipose tissue to remain alive, oxygen and nutrients must reach that area via blood vessels. After the transfer, while the adipose tissue is fed by diffusion for the first few days, vitality will continue with the development of capillary blood circulation in the following periods. Capillary circulation provides vascular nutrition up to a maximum 3 mm distance. However, if sufficient blood circulation is not provided, fat cells die and are resorbed by the body. In cases where sufficient volume cannot be obtained or the volume decreases rapidly over time, the procedure can be repeated.

14.7 Complications

The fat transfer procedure must be performed by physicians who have experience in this field. The procedure is contraindicated in very weak patients and those who have problems with bleeding and coagulation.

Fat transfer for majora augmentation has some complications and risks in both the donor area and the recipient area.

Depressions in the form of bleeding, hematoma, infection, and local dimpling may occur in the donor area. Fat removal should be done in the donor area in the form of a fan and in equal volume from all regions. In order to avoid dimpling, the surface should not be worked more than 0.5 cm under the skin.

Bleeding, tissue infection (cellulitis), fat embolism, fat necrosis, calcification, cystic encapsulated mass formation (fat cyst), tissue irregularities, asymmetry, and hypersensitivity are among the complications that can be seen in recipient areas. Cellulites are generally responsive to antibiotics.

Another infrequent, but crucial risk is fat embolism that can reach the retinal and cerebral vessels.

14.8 The Postoperative Term

It is important to apply ice to the majora area in the early postoperative period. Patients who are operated and rested can be discharged with prescriptions for antibiotics and painkillers after bleeding and hematoma control. To prevent bleeding, provide compression with a bandage applied to the donor area immediately after the procedure. The bandage can be removed after 48 h.

It is also important for patients to avoid hot showers, rubbing the genital areas, and avoid brunts for a week. Thermal springs, hot baths, hot pools, wearing tight pants, horse riding, and cycling should be avoided for 1 month. The patient should wait 1 month before sexual intercourse, heavy sports, fitness, and yoga practices. Smoking after the procedure will also negatively affect both collagen formation and oxygenation of replaced adipose tissue. Under normal conditions, the permanence of fat transfer will persist, decreasing gradually over 5 years.

After the procedure, the fat tissue injected into the majora in those who lose weight quickly also diminishes. The application can be repeated at intervals of several years in patients who so desire.

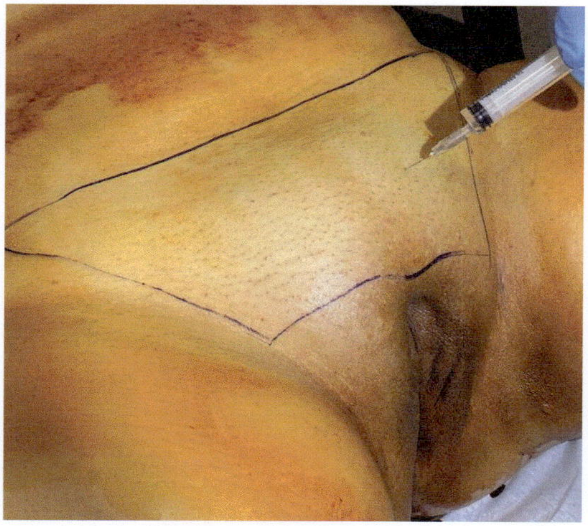

Fig. 14.8 Marking the place where fat will be harvested before the procedure and local anesthetic injection

14.9 Monsplasty

In the mons pubis area, skin excesses or protrusions due to excess fat (mons hypertrophy) can be aesthetically disturbing. Reduction operations for hypertrophy of the mons pubis are called "Mons Reduction" or "Monsplasty." In addition, scars due to cesarean or gynecological operations in the lower abdomen can also become a problem. In these patients, both scar tissue and excess tissue can be removed by wedge excision with surgical procedures in the form of a mini-tummy tuck. In some patients, the mons pubis can be reducted during abdominoplasty operations.

The mons pubis continues anatomically below as the labia majora, and both use the same fascial plane. The excessive sling of the mons pubis during the surgical operation may cause the labia majora, and even the labia minora and clitoral region associated with it to pull upwards. This situation can be observed even in abdominoplasty operations. Excessive suspension causes anatomical dislocation of the genitalia.

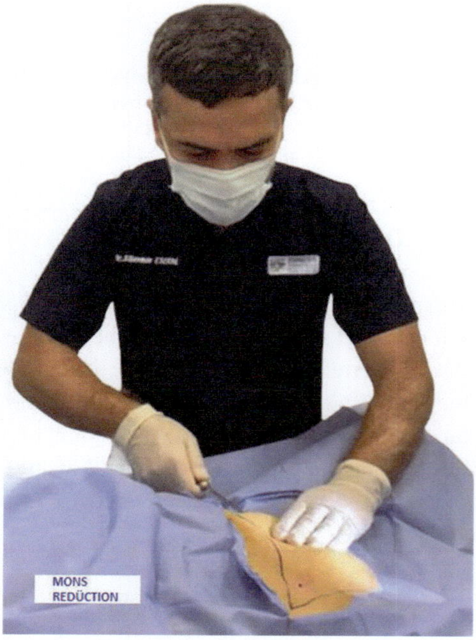

Fig. 14.9 Mons pubis reduction procedure

14.10 Mons Reduction Methods

Mons pubis hypertrophy can usually be resolved by conventional manual lipoaspiration or energy-based liposuction methods. Before the procedure, the patient is asked to go to the toilet and empty her bladder. After the marking (Fig. 14.8), and the injection of local or tumescent anesthesia, bilateral 3 mm incisions are made in the pubis area, fitting the ends of the pfannenstiel incision line. These incisions should not be larger in order not to vitiate negative pressure. The cannula is placed in the incision sites sequentially. While the tissue is pressed and squeezed by the passive hand, the fat tissue is aspirated into the injector with the active hand (Fig. 14.9). Generally between 50 and 200 cc of fat can be aspirated from the mons region (Figs. 14.10 and 14.11).

A secondary benefit can also be obtained by transferring adipose tissue taken with mons reduction to the labia majora, atrophic scar tissue, or anterior vaginal wall. After the adipose tissue is reducted, it can be mixed with PRP if necessary and transferred to the required areas via a thin cannula.

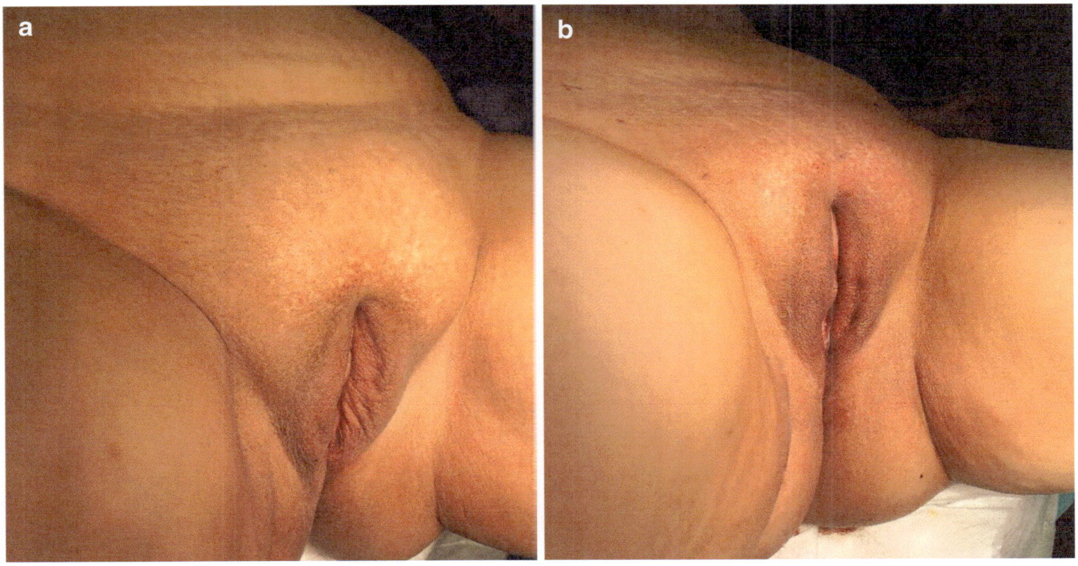

Fig. 14.10 Mons pubis reduction. The large and fatty appearance of the mons pubis can affect the social life. In this case, mons reduction can be done, thanks to manual lipoaspiration methods. Before (**a**) and after (**b**)

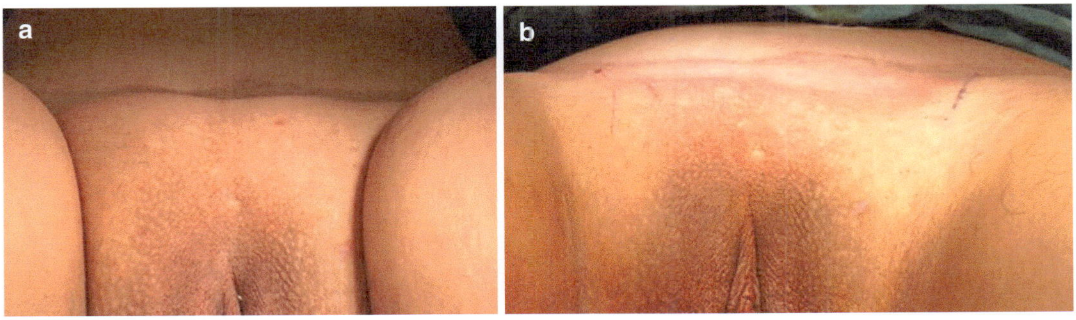

Fig. 14.11 Mons reduction via classical lipoaspiration technique. A total of 120 cc fat was harvested. Before (**a**), just after (**b**)

14.11 Surgical Methods

Mons reduction can also be performed surgically, similar to mini-tummy tuck, especially in cases that have excessive skin sagging or scar revision was also required (Fig. 14.12).

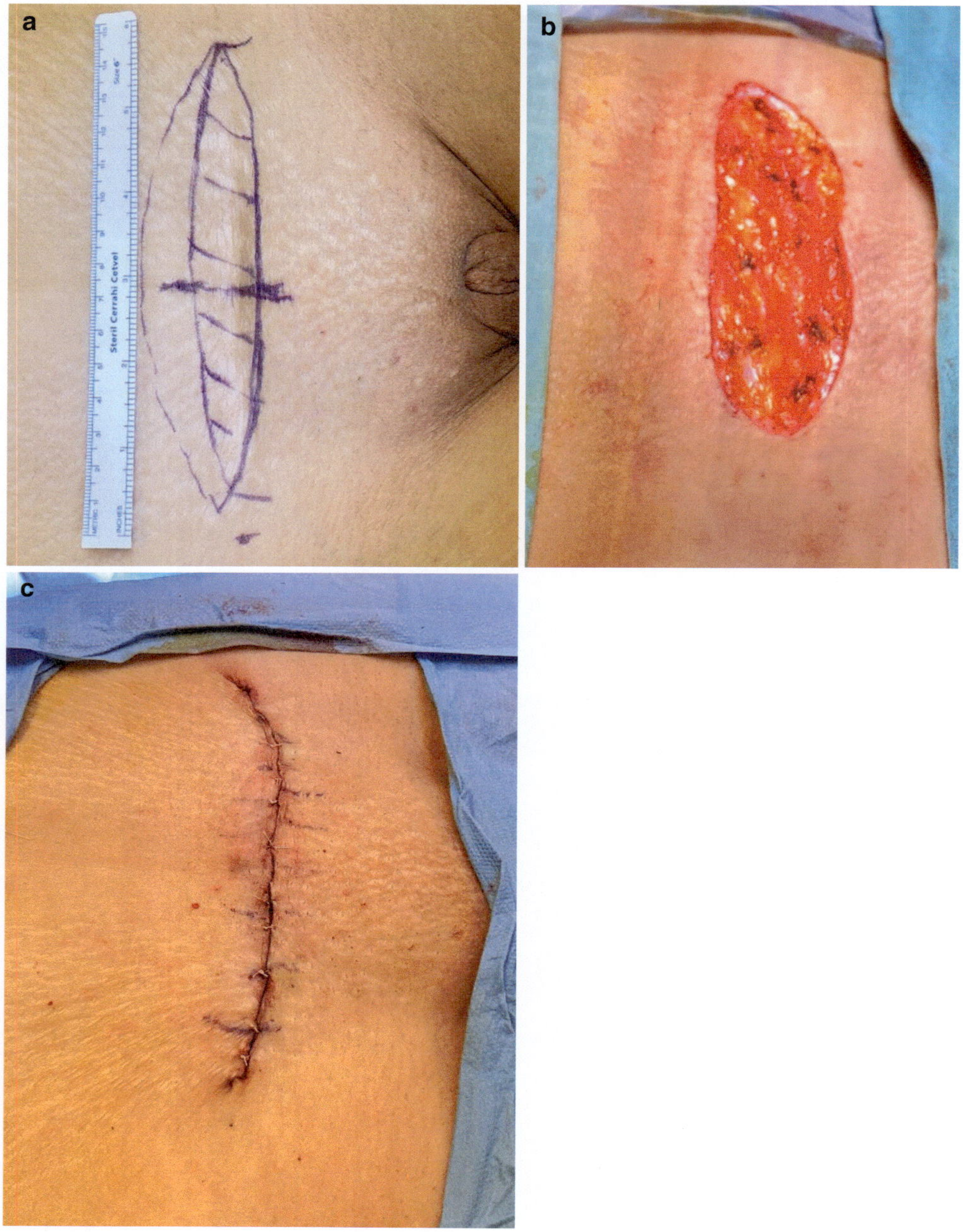

Fig. 14.12 Elliptical removal of excess saggy skin tissue in mons pubis. Cesarean scar revision was also performed at the same time. Marking (**a**), excision of skin and subskin tissue (**b**), suturing (**c**)

14.12 The Postoperative Term

The procedure can be performed as an outpatient procedure under local or sedation anesthesia in the office or hospital. It is beneficial to use anti-pain drugs and antibiotics for five days. Bleeding control is important in the first day. The patient should be informed about being cautious. It is beneficial to keep the bandage applied to the procedure area for 48 h.

If too much fat is removed in patients who have undergone mons reduction with lipoaspiration, sagging in skin may occur. In these cases, surgical correction may be required.

Appendix

With the purchase of this book, you can use our "SN Flashcards" app to access questions free of charge in order to test your learning and check your understanding of the contents of the book.

To use the app, please follow the instructions below:

1. Go to https://flashcards.springernature.com/login
2. Create a user account by entering your e-mail address and assigning a password.
3. Use the following link to access your SN Flashcards set: ▶ https://sn.pub/tvlq7Q

If the link is missing or does not work, please send an e-mail with the subject "SN Flashcards" and the book title to customerservice@springernature.com.

References

1. Fat transfer/fat graft and fat injection ASPS guiding principles, approved by the ASPS Executive Committee, 2009. https://www.plasticsurgery.org/documents/medical-professionals/health-policy/guiding-principles/asps-fat-transfer-graft-guiding-principles.pdf.
2. Aguilar P, Hersant B, SidAhmed-Mezi M, Bosc R, Vidal L, Meningaud JP. Novel technique of vulvo-vaginal rejuvenation by lipofilling and injection of combined platelet-rich-plasma and hyaluronic acid: a case-report. SpringerPlus. 2016;5(1):1184.

15 Hymenoplasty

Nothing is more intolerable than to have admit to yourself your own errors.

Ludwig van Beethoven

As a border between internal and external female genitalia, the hymen is a mucous fold that is located 2–3 cm beyond the vulvar entrance and has different anatomical variations. It has sociological role rather than functional. Hymenoplasty, which is considered to be an AGS operation, is a reconstructive surgery known with terms such as "hymenorrhaphy" and "revirgination" (revirginity). Ethical issues regarding whether this procedure should be done or not are still a matter of debate [1].

The purpose of hymenoplasty is to return the perforated hymen to its original form and to provide bleeding that imitates the first night during sexual intercourse. Hymenoplasty can be done for a short or long term.

15.1 Hymenoplasty Techniques

Hymenoplasty operations can be done with different techniques. These include:

- *Long-term operations*
  - *Vestibulo-introital tightening technique (VITT, Eserdag)*
  - *Luminal reduction hymenoplasty*
  - *Flap operation*
  - *Septum repair*
- *Short-term operations*

15.1.1 Long-term Operations

These include reconstructive operations performed to maintain the hymen for a long time. For this reason, these are also known as "permanent hymen repair."

15.1.1.1 Vestibulo-Introital Tightening Technique (VITT, Eserdag)

The hymenoplasty technique recommended by us (Fig. 15.1), which has the largest series in the literature so far, is in the form of posterior repair, which includes a slight vaginal and vestibular tightening at the same time [2]. In this operation, which we can describe as minor perineoplasty, first the vagina, then the hymen, and finally the perineum are repaired. Sutures of the hymen are laid one by one dorsal, apical, and ventral. To become successful in this technique, tension should not be exerted on the sutures of perforated hymen edges. In the vestibulo-introital tightening

S. Eserdağ, *Aesthetic and Functional Female Genital Surgery*,
https://doi.org/10.1007/978-3-031-16019-6_15

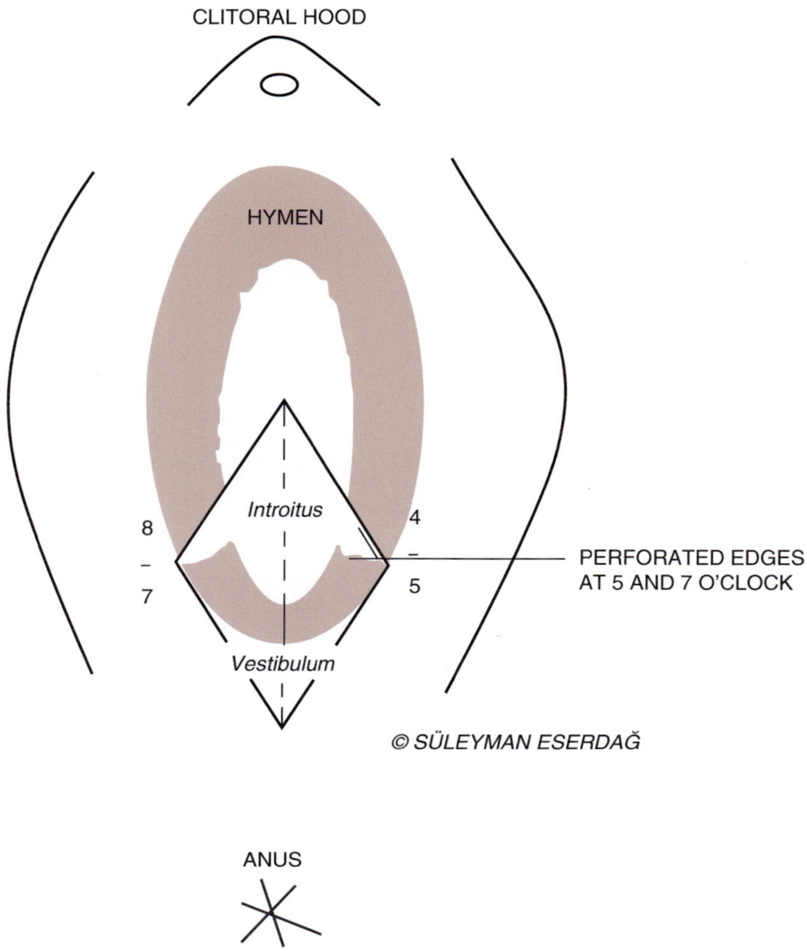

Fig. 15.1 Primary hymen repair (*Eserdag*) performed with the vestibulo-introital tightening technique (VITT) [2]

technique (VITT), the perforated ends of the hymen are repaired, a slight tightening is provided at the vaginal entrance, and the possibility of bleeding during sexual intercourse is increased by the vestibular tightening and the delicate granulation tissue formed in the vestibulum (Fig. 15.2). The operation, performed under local anesthesia, takes approximately 15 minutes. In the operation, 2/0 or 3/0, round needle, long-lasting suture materials are generally used.

In patients with multiple perforation, low-edged hymen, or thin structure, primary repairs by cutting the two sides of the hymen caruncles and suturing them together will not yield results. For these patients, the VITT technique or flap lift operations including vestibular tightening may be more appropriate options.

15.1.1.2 Luminal Reduction Hymenoplasty

In this technique, the epithelialized free edges of each hymen fragment are gently excised along the clefts with scissors or a scalpel, leaving only the tip of the fragments intact. The free margin close to the tips of the remnants is sutured first using a simple interrupted 4-0 rapid sutures, ensuring accurate approximation without step-off at the edge of the hymenal ring. This is followed by a simple interrupted 4-0 rapid sutures on the internal surface and another suture on the external surface of the remnants. This is completed in a sequential fashion for clefts around the lateral and posterior aspects of the vaginal canal until the luminal reduction is accomplished by closure across all clefts. Sutures are not placed at the

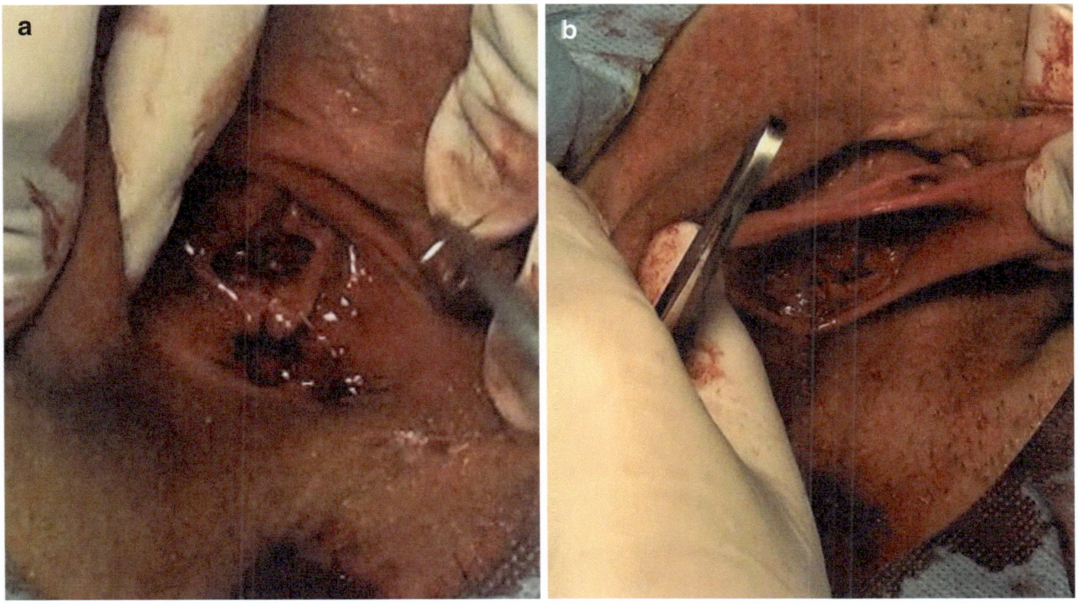

Fig. 15.2 Hymenoplasty with VITT. Approximation of the hymen edges after introital constriction (**a**), just after the operation (**b**)

anterior aspect of the vaginal canal where the hymen remnants can arise from adjacent to the urethra [3].

15.1.1.3 Flap Operation

Another method recommended for long-term hymenoplasty is the flap operation. For this procedure, a large piece of tissue is removed from the posterior vaginal wall. Between 9 and 11 o'clock, the tissue tip is perforated as 1 cm with a sharp clamp behind the hymen and involving the skin-subcutaneous layers. Then the removed flap tissue is hung on this area and sutured. The area where the flap is removed is also repaired. Delayed absorbable sutures (2/0-3/0) are used as suture material. In order for the procedure to be successful, the flap tissue should be removed as thick as possible. After a few months, an appearance resembling a septal hymen occurs.

15.1.1.4 Septum Repair

In some women with septated hymen, the septum and sometimes the edges of the hymen may be perforated during coitus. In these cases, the septal ends hanging in the form of a flap can be cut and re-anastomosed. Or, the septum drooping as a flap and the caruncle of the hymen underneath can be cut and re-anastomosed. For this, it is important that the septum structure should be thick. Also, excessive tension should not be placed on the reconstructed edges.

15.1.2 Short-term Operations

This procedure is applied to women who are planning the coitus within a week at the latest. No incision is needed in this procedure. The vaginal introitus (just behind the hymen) is narrowed as an "introital cerclage" with 4/0 rapid or delayed absorbable sutures (Fig. 15.3). The aim is not to regain the integrity of the hymen but to ensure that bleeding occurs during the first sexual intercourse. During sexual penetration, the tissue will be damaged and more or less bleed. The chance of success is close to 100%. The procedure, performed with local anesthetics, takes only a few minutes.

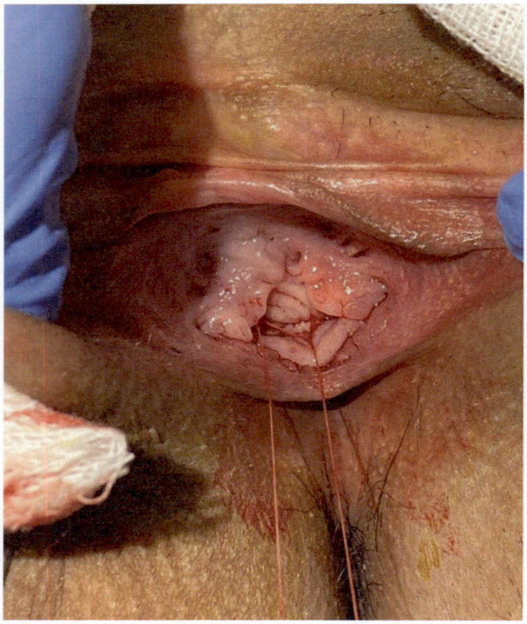

Fig. 15.3 Short-term procedure. Circular subcutaneous sutures are placed just behind the hymen as "purse-string" closure. The aim is to provide bleeding at the first penetration

15.2 Psychological Influences

Many young girls are forced to have sexual intercourse by their boyfriends, relatives, or strangers, involuntarily losing their virginity and apply to gynecologists under intense stress. Some of them accidentally damage their hymen themselves while masturbating unconsciously during childhood. The number of people who feel depressed and even have suicidal thoughts, carrying the regret of their incident inside them, is considerable. Therefore, psychological support should also be provided to these patients. Some patients are referred to physicians who perform hymenoplasty by mental health professionals. Especially in religious or traditional family structure, there are many women who have it done to erase the bad memories of the past, to relax psychologically by "*opening a new page*" in their life, and to regain their self-confidence, even though they do not yet have any candidate with whom to unite their life.

15.3 Combined Procedures

Vaginal tightening can be performed simultaneously with the long-term hymenoplasty operations. It can be performed surgically or by laser, depending on the patient's request and the condition of the tissue. In addition, labiaplasty can be performed together with vaginoplasty. Young girls who were subjected to sexual abuse in childhood and who face the anxiety over this at later ages especially prefer combined hymenoplasty, labiaplasty, and vaginoplasty procedures.

15.4 Complications

Bleeding and infection are among the most common complications. Postoperative abnormal bleeding is usually observed in the first 24 h. Although rare, bleeding can be seen up to the fifth day. Any infections are usually due to missed vaginitis during the operation. Especially in bacterial vaginosis existence, the procedure may fail due to separation of the sutures. In case of failure of the operation, a second operation can be performed. It is recommended that patients be examined again before sexual intercourse in long-term procedures. In cases where the procedure is considered to be unsuccessful or insufficient, a short-term procedure can be performed before marriage.

After hymenoplasty operations, the excessively raised perineum may overly narrow the introitus, making sexual penetration impossible or very painful. In such cases, the perineal entrance should be enlarged (Fig. 15.4).

Combining both sides of the vulvar vestibulum (Fig. 15.5) or labia majora (Fig. 15.6) is also malpractice and can cause serious dyspareunia problem in future sexual life.

Another complication that can be seen after hymenoplasty is "iatrogenic vaginismus" that develops due to psychological contractions. To now, we have encountered vaginismus problem in two patients who had hymenoplasty in the past and could not have intercourse due to excessive contractions during sexual intercourse. In the stories of these patients, there was information that

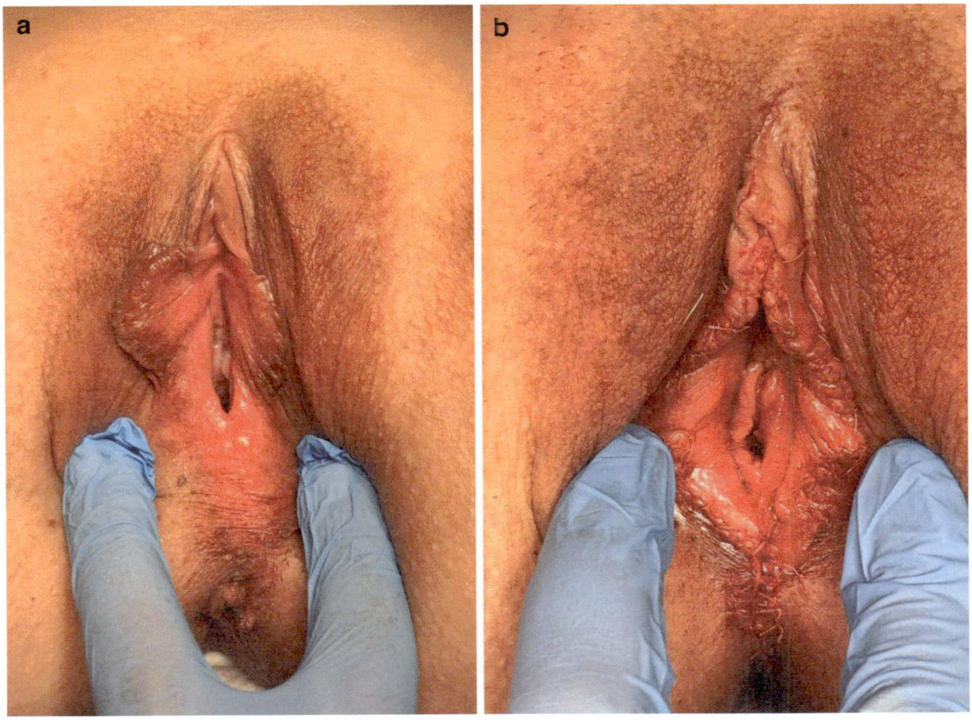

Fig. 15.4 Excessively elevated perineum in hymenoplasty, and inability to have sexual penetration (**a**), after labiaplasty and perineoplasty revision (**b**)

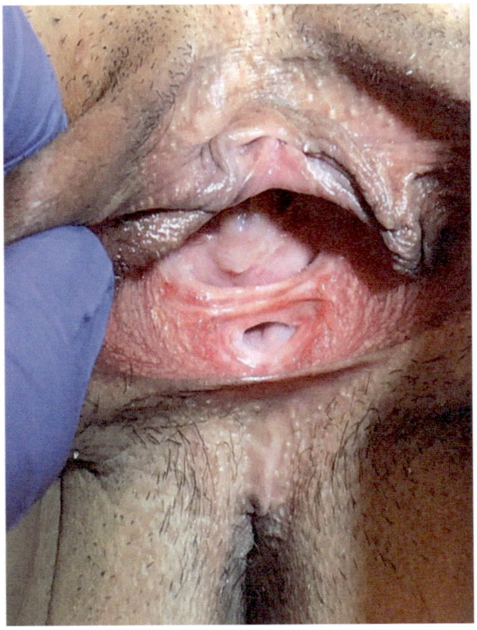

Fig. 15.5 Hymenoplasty malpractice. A horizontal septum was formed by joining both sides of the vestibulum. The vestibulum is a very sensitive area and sexual penetration is not possible after this kind of surgery

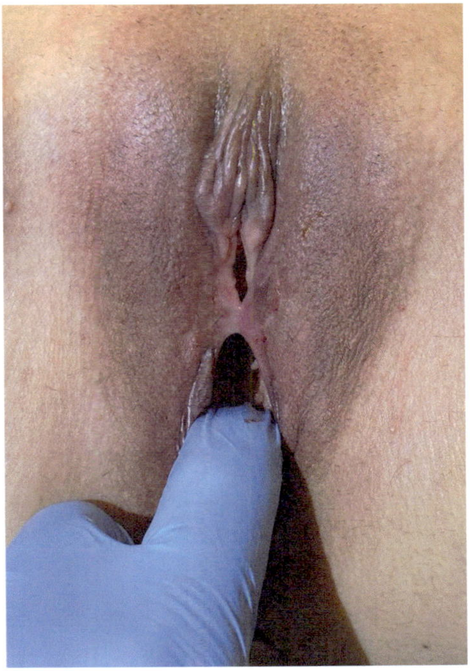

Fig. 15.6 Hymenoplasty malpractice. By combining both labia majora, the vaginal entrance is almost closed

they had been able to have intercourse with their partners before and had a hymenoplasty operation during the marriage process. Their problems were resolved with the cognitive behavioral sexual therapies.

15.5 The Postoperative Term

After long-term hymenoplasty, oral antibiotics and painkillers can be prescribed at a therapeutic dose. Adherence to hygiene rules and dressing if necessary are among the recommendations given. Heavy sports and exercises that involve opening or spreading the legs should be avoided for one month postoperatively. In long-term hymen repair, patients are called for a check-up one month after the operation and within one week before attempting sexual intercourse.

Appendix

With the purchase of this book, you can use our “SN Flashcards” app to access questions free of charge in order to test your learning and check your understanding of the contents of the book.

To use the app, please follow the instructions below:

1. Go to https://flashcards.springernature.com/login
2. Create a user account by entering your e-mail address and assigning a password.
3. Use the following link to access your SN Flashcards set: ▶ https://sn.pub/tvlq7Q

If the link is missing or does not work, please send an e-mail with the subject “SN Flashcards” and the book title to customerservice@springernature.com.

References

1. Bawany MH, Padela AI. Hymenoplasty and Muslim patients: Islamic ethico-legal perspectives. J Sex Med. 2017;14(8):1003–10.
2. Eserdağ S, Kurban D, Kiseli M, Alan Y, Alan M. A new practical surgical technique for hymenoplasty: primary repair of hymen with vestibulo-introital tightening technique. Aesthet Surg J. 2021;41(3):333–7.
3. Vojvodic M, Lista F, Vastis PG, Ahmad J. Luminal reduction hymenoplasty: a Canadian experience with hymen restoration. Aesthet Surg J. 2018;38(7):802–6.

Part III

Non-surgical Operations in the Art of Aesthetic Genital Surgery

16 Vaginal Laser Applications

Imagination is more important than knowledge. Knowledge is limited. Imagination encircles the world.

Albert Einstein

With aging, there are important changes in vaginal histology as in the whole body. These changes affect all layers of the vaginal epithelium. Extracellular matrix components, fibroblast number, vascularization, and water retention capacity decrease. As a result, collagen and elastic fibers decrease, elasticity is lost, the rugae are flattened, the vagina becomes shorter, the epithelium becomes thinner and accordingly, sensitivity to pain occurs. All these changes are accelerated by the decrease in the hormone estrogen experienced during menopause. All treatments prescribed for vaginal rejuvenation are to reduce the speed of these histological changes and relieve symptoms.

There are five different features specified for the ideal vagina: tightness, presence of rugae, mucosal integrity, elasticity, and axis. Genital rejuvenation (GR) covers all procedures performed to improve these five features and rejuvenate the vulva and vaginal tissues. Laser, radiofrequency (RF), PRP, and mesotherapy are the most common non-surgical procedures for GR. Regenerative procedures such as stromal vascular fraction (SVF) and mesenchymal and amniotic fluid stem cell applications have also started in recent years.

16.1 Laser Physics

It will be beneficial to know some laser concepts, parameters, physics, and light-tissue interactions in order to perform medical interventions related to laser correctly and on-site.

A laser is a device that emits light through a process of optical amplification based on the stimulated emission of electromagnetic radiation. The word "LASER" is an acronym for "Light Amplification by Stimulated Emission of Radiation." The basis of laser technology goes back to Einstein's quantum theory in 1917. The first laser use in practice begins with the 694 nm wavelength Ruby crystal laser developed by Theodore H. Maiman in 1960. The use of laser, which increased in the following years, has gained a place in many medical and cosmetic fields.

Laser energy is produced within the laser cavity. The following are present inside the laser cavity:

1. Power supply (flashlamp, direct current electrical energy)
2. Medium: Laser medium can be solid, liquid, or gas

S. Eserdağ, *Aesthetic and Functional Female Genital Surgery*,
https://doi.org/10.1007/978-3-031-16019-6_16

3. Optical cavity or tube (resonator)
4. Distribution systems. They are flexible or flat fiber optic systems that carry the rays partially reflected from the tube to the target tissue.

Thanks to these parts, laser systems can direct the rays coming from the light source to a certain point by amplifying them by collecting them in a certain tube [1].

The name of the laser is based on its medium and the wavelength it creates, such as Er:YAG 2940-nm laser, or Argon laser, Nd:YAG laser, CO_2 laser, krypton laser.

16.2 Laser Parameters

The effect of laser light on tissue is determined by

- Wavelength,
- Spot size,
- Density,
- Features such as application time and intervals are important. In addition, the optical properties of the tissue are also important.

16.2.1 Wavelength

The wavelength is the distance between two successive peaks. Every source of light has a different wavelength in space as shown in Fig. 16.1 and Table 16.1. Each laser has its own wavelength as well. Waves obtained by laser systems are divided into three types: continuous, pseudocontinuous, and pulsed. Although continuous lasers have continuous pulses, their peak power is low. Peak power is higher in pulsed lasers. Since the pseudocontinuous pulsed laser frequency is high, they always appear to be pulsating. Carbon dioxide (CO_2) lasers frequently used in AGS are continuously pulsed.

The pulse duration of all lasers with a short pulse width is below 1 microsecond (μs). Long wavelength lasers produce light above 590 nm. The pulse frequency is expressed in the number of beats generated per second and is indicated with hertz (Hz). When the structure of light is examined, there are energetic particles in it that move at high speed. These particles are called photons. Short wavelength = high energy = high-energy photons.

16.2.2 Distance

Fractional laser expresses that the application is in the form of light beams moving parallel to each other. The interval between light beams passes as "distance." In some lasers, the "density" parameter is used instead of distance. Density and distance are inversely related; as one increases, the other decreases.

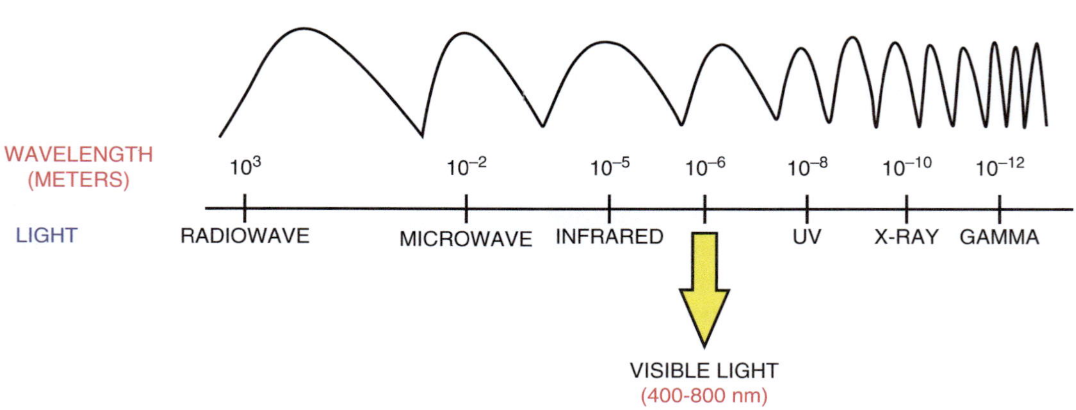

Fig. 16.1 Wavelengths of light (electromagnetic spectrum)

Table 16.1 Wavelengths of light

Ultraviolet (157–400 nm)
Visible light (400–800 nm)
Near-infrared (800–3000 nm)
Mid-infrared (Intermediate infrared) (3000–30,000 nm)
Far infrared (>30,000 nm)

16.2.3 Overlap (Stack)

The effect and penetration depth can be increased by applying the laser on the same spot again. For easier understanding, let us imagine *a nail hammering into the wood*. Each hammer blow will increase the penetration of the nail into the wood a little more. The same is true for laser. Overlapping (or stack mode from one to five) can be increased to stimulate collagen synthesis in deeper tissue. Conversely, there is no need to increase the overlap in genital bleaching treatments, as laser beam should stay more superficial.

16.2.4 Moving Time

This is the time between every two pulses. Time can be gained by reducing moving time as you gain experience.

16.2.5 Energy

In physics, energy is defined as the capacity to do work. The energy unit of the laser is mjoule. Since Energy = Power × Time, laser energy is calculated by the formula Joules (joules) = watt × seconds. So 1 watt of power in 1 s is equivalent to 1 J (1000 mJ) of energy.

16.2.6 Power

Power is the amount of work done per unit time. Power expresses the speed at which the energy required to complete a job is spent. Hence, it shows how fast the work is done. How much energy is used per unit time while operating the laser is measured with the concept of power. The unit of power is the watt. It is calculated as watt = J/s. Although the energy applied to the tissue in the laser is the same, the effect obtained may be different. For example, the 10-Watt application that lasts 9 s and the 90-Watt application that lasts for 1-second produce the same energy as 90 J. However, the effects on the tissue are quite different from each other.

16.2.7 Energy Current (Fluence)

This is the amount of energy given per unit area. It is expressed as fluence = J/cm^2. Most laser systems measure a unit area of cm^2. Therefore, energy flow is also called power or energy density.

16.2.8 Energy Density (Irradiance)

This is the amount of power given per unit area. The units of irradiance are W/cm^2. Energy density indicates the capacity to cut, vaporize, and/or coagulate tissue. For example, cutting can be done with high energy density and coagulation can be done with low density for hemostasis.

16.2.9 Spot Size (Beam diameter)

Laser spot size is the cross-section of the laser light beam. It is usually expressed in mm. Spot size also affects fluence and irradiance directly. Energy flow and energy density are inversely proportional to the square of the radius of the spot size. When the spot size is halved, fluence and irradiance are quadrupled. Spot size is also important in terms of laser light penetration. Smaller spot size allows more light diffusion through the skin. Spot size between 7 and 10 mm provides maximum penetration to the mid-dermis or deeper targets. Penetration decreases if the spot size is over 10–12 mm.

16.2.10 Pulse Duration

Laser light can create continuous waves or pulse waves. Pulse duration is expressed in μs or ms. Continuous waves can emit constant beams of light, causing non-selective tissue damage. The exposure time to laser light beams determines the rate of laser energy generated. Pulsed laser, however, causes selective tissue damage. With much shorter pulses in new laser systems, increased selectivity and specificity are possible.

Millisecond (10^{-3}) duration pulses are considered long, nanosecond pulses are considered short. Q-switched lasers take 3–7 ns to pulse. Therefore, their damage to the surrounding tissues is also minimal.

16.2.11 Thermal Relaxation Time

After the laser light is absorbed by the target tissue, heat loss occurs by spreading to neighboring tissues. The time taken to transfer 50% of the heat generated in the tissue after laser to the surrounding tissue is called the thermal relaxation time and varies in relation to the size of the target structure [2]. Laser devices work on the basis of sending monochromatic fixed wavelength high-energy light to the tissue. Specific wavelengths affect the tissue they penetrate. Each laser has its own chromophore substance in the tissue to which it shows affinity. Chromophores are a group of atoms that give color to the skin and absorb light of a certain wavelength. The most important chromophores of skin tissue are hemoglobin, melanin, water, and carotene.

After the laser light is absorbed by the chromophore, a thermal effect occurs. By changing the wavelength, energy amount, and pulse duration of the light, it can be ensured that it acts selectively on target molecules such as melanin, hemoglobin, water, or carotene. If there is not enough absorption in the tissue, the laser-related effect will not occur [3]. Cytokines that occur as a result of thermal damage trigger the tissue remodeling process. Thus, a “rejuvenation” process begins.

In the effect of laser light on tissue, wavelength, the diameter of the light, density, and properties such as application time and intervals are important. In addition, the optical properties of the tissue are also important.

16.3 Properties of Laser Light

Laser light is monochromatic, bright, coherent, and unidirectional. The features related to laser light are listed below.

16.3.1 Collimation (Alignment in One Direction)

While conventional light can be scattered everywhere, laser light has light beams that travel parallel to each other. This feature is called collimation.

16.3.2 Coherence

This is the movement of laser light beams in the same phase with each other. Laser light is high energy and intense; it has the ability to focus on a very small point.

16.3.3 Reflection, Transmission, and Absorption Properties

Laser light also has the ability to pass through the tissue (transmission), reflect, and absorb. Transmission refers to laser light that passes through tissue without any effect. Reflection is when light hits the tissue and travels to different places. It has been shown that laser light is reflected at a rate of 4–7% [4]. Absorption is the absorption of laser light by the tissue. Only the absorption feature of the laser provides the effect we desire.

As the tissue selectively absorbs the laser light, thermal damage occurs due to the heat generated. If the energy absorption rate is low, thermal energy is produced; if this ratio is high, explosive shock waves are produced that cause mechanical deterioration. If exposure to light is continued after thermal energy is generated, the generated heat will spread to neighboring tissues. Therefore, the most appropriate wavelength, current, and pulse duration should be selected for an effective and selective treatment.

16.4 Which Laser Should Be Used in Which Indication?

The target chromophore in vascular lesions is hemoglobin. The absorption peaks of hemoglobin are 418, 542, and 577 nm. The most effective lasers on this chromophore are 488–514 nm argon laser, pulsed dye laser (PDL), Nd:YAG laser, and 568 nm krypton laser.

To give another example, the target chromophore in epilation is melanin. Short wavelength lasers such as Ruby 694 nm or Alexandrite 755 nm are preferred to affect melanin. However, due to the burns and hyperpigmentation risks of these lasers, especially in people with dark skin color, Diode 800 and Nd:YAG 1064 lasers are used, which have lower affinity for melanin and therefore can go deeper.

Laser treatments by different devices have taken part in many medical and cosmetic fields (Table 16.2).

Table 16.2 Some of the lasers used in medicine

Ruby 694 nm Q-switched laser
Alexandrite 755 nm LP laser
KTP 532 nm Q-switched laser
Nd:YAG 1064 nm Q-switched laser
IPL 540–950 nm light source
IPL 570–950 nm light source
Diode 800 laser
Er:YAG 2940 nm laser
CO_2 10,600 nm laser
Krypton 530–647 nm laser
Helium-Neon (He/Ne) 632 nm laser
Argon 488–514 laser

16.5 Lasers in Gynecology

The first use of laser in gynecology started with cervical condyloma treatments in the 1970s. Later, they were used in laparoscopy for the treatment of pelvic pathologies, hysteroscopy for submucosal myoma and polyp treatment, PGD with very small spot size (1–5 μm), hatching of zona pellucida, and assisted reproductive methods for blastomere biopsy.

The use of lasers for vaginal tightening, SUI treatment, vulvar bleaching, and vulvovaginal rejuvenation purposes started in the 2010s. CO_2 and Erbium:YAG lasers are most commonly used in these treatments. Both have H_2O (water) as their chromophore, and their wavelengths are different from each other. Both lasers can be used in different dermatological problems. None of these lasers has FDA approval for non-surgical vaginal rejuvenation and tightening, genitourinary syndrome of menopause, sexual dysfunctions, or SUI treatment. FDA has approved applications such as treatment of abnormal or precancerous cervical lesions and condyloma, and also for incision, excision, ablation, vaporization, and coagulation of body soft tissues in medical specialties, including aesthetic and gynecology.

16.5.1 Carbon Dioxide Lasers

Carbon dioxide lasers, which have been used in facial rejuvenation for years due to their fractional properties, are ablative (capable of destruction) gas-mediated lasers with an infrared beam at 10,600 nm wavelength. They are the most powerful continuous-wave lasers to date. Tissue penetration is high, and they can reach the "lamina propria" layer of the dermis, which is an important region for collagen production. The laser beam can penetrate the tissue up to 20–30 μm with a shot in less than 1 millisecond. Thermal damage can reach up to 100–150 μm in the thick layer of the tissue. It has even been reported that it causes thermal coagulation up to 1 mm.

With the photothermal effects of CO_2 lasers, the temperature inside the tissue can rise above 60 °C. Because of these properties, these lasers are also used for tissue cutting in labiaplasty. In addition, ablative effects are used in hypertrophic scar treatments and in the treatment of dermatological problems such as condyloma, moles, actinic keratosis, sebaceous adenoma, and angiokeratoma.

16.5.2 Er:YAG (Erbium:YAG) Lasers

These are lasers with a wavelength of 2940 nm, infrared beam, short pulse duration (0.1–3 ms), high power (2.5 J/cm^2), and 1–6 mm diameter [5]. Er:YAG lasers have two different forms. The standard form is ablative and short pulse, while the SMOOTH form operates in a non-ablative and special pulsed mode. The non-ablative intraurethral probe developed is intended for frequent recurrent urinary infections, incontinence treatments, and menopausal genitourinary syndrome treatments. Er:YAG lasers are used in the same range of indications as CO_2 lasers in cosmetic and functional gynecology.

The name Er:YAG comes from the initials of the Erbium-doped Yttrium Aluminum Garnet material in solid mediums (Er:$Y_3Al_5O_{12}$). Their affinity for water is 10 times higher than CO_2 lasers. Therefore, heat penetration in water-rich vaginal tissue is limited. They are suitable for epidermal applications and used in the treatment of acne scars, burn scars, melasma, hyperpigmentation, and wrinkles in the skin as well as being very effective in the treatment of small tumors, condyloma, and actinic keratosis [6]. Complaints such as erythema, edema, and pain after treatment are less frequent compared to ablative CO_2 lasers. But the amount of bleeding in surgical incision procedures is higher than CO_2 lasers.

16.6 Laser Indications: Use in Gynecology and Dermatology

CO_2 and Er:YAG lasers can be used in the genitals and different areas of the body for various functional and aesthetic indications. They can be used in surgical applications such as soft tissue excision, incision, ablation, vaporization, and coagulation. For this purpose, they have a place in dermatology, plastic surgery, gynecology, ENT, invasive, and endoscopic general surgery branches.

Functional indications of laser:

- Stress urinary incontinence (SUI) treatment in patients without prolapse
- Vaginal tightening and rejuvenation treatments
- Increasing sexual pleasure
- Symptomatic treatment of menopausal genitourinary syndrome
- Treatment of vaginal dryness (especially in patients whose use of estrogen is contraindicated during menopause)
- Treatment of recurrent vaginitis and vaginal yeast infections
- Treatment of vulvar vestibulitis syndrome
- Symptomatic treatment of genital lichen sclerosus disease

Cosmetic indications of laser:

- Labia majora, perineal, and perianal area bleaching
- Labia majora and perineal area tightening, resurfacing
- Cutting tissue in operations such as labiaplasty, vaginal tightening, and hymen removal (Fig. 16.2)

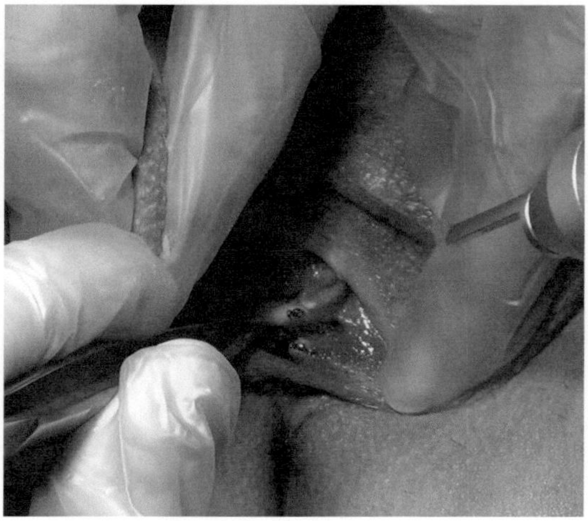

Fig. 16.2 Laser cutting and removal of the hymen (laser hymenectomy)

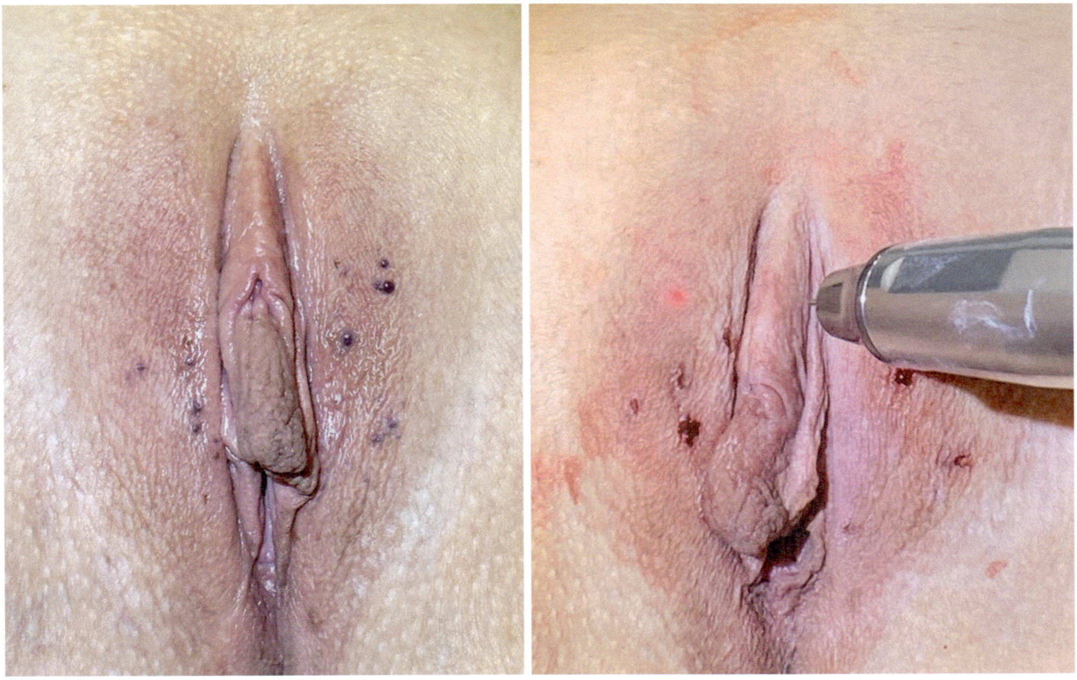

Fig. 16.3 Hemangiomata and laser coagulation in the vulva. Dermal hemangiomas, which are benign vascular lesions, can be treated with laser

- Acrochordon, nevus, hemangioma, and hemangiomata treatments (Fig. 16.3)
- Genital wart (Fig. 16.4) and molluscum contagiosum treatments
- Scar treatments
- Striae and fissure treatments on the skin
- Facial rejuvenation (antiaging, wrinkle treatment, pore tightening, lifting)

Cutting and coagulation procedures are performed by the surgical probes of the lasers (Fig. 16.5).

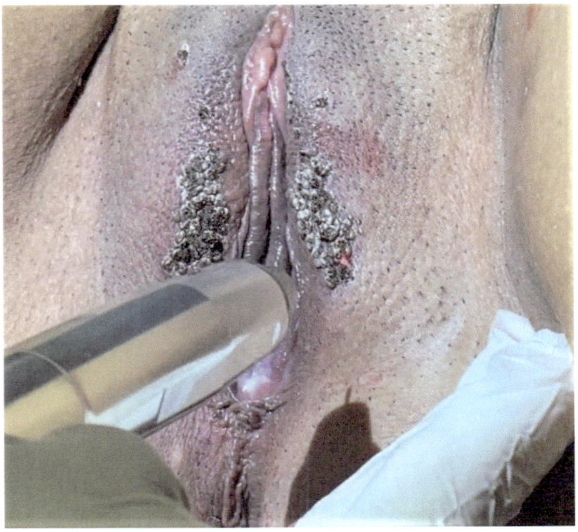

Fig. 16.4 Condyloma ablation by laser

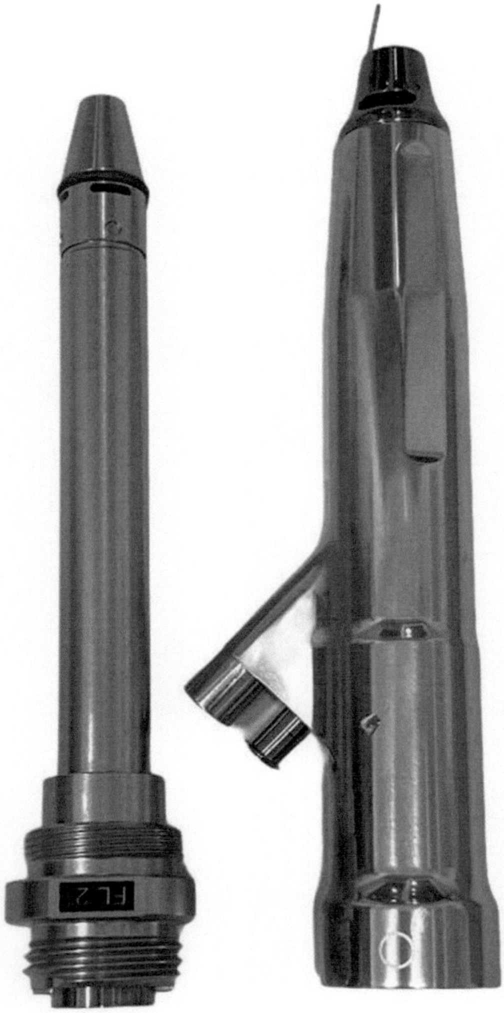

Fig. 16.5 The surgical probe (left) and its cover (right), which are the cutting and coagulation components of the SmartXide™ laser

16.7 Vaginal Laser Contraindications

Vaginal laser is not recommended in the following cases:

- Moderate and severe POP cases

Laser application is not recommended in moderate to severe POP cases with or without stress incontinence. Muscle and fascia defects can only be corrected by surgical operations.

- Pregnancy

All elective aesthetic, reconstructive, and laser procedures should be avoided during pregnancy.

- Puerperium

Vaginal laser can be applied in the puerperium from the third month after birth. There is no harm in applying it during breastfeeding.

- Menstruation period

Vaginal laser should be avoided due to vaginal wetness and susceptibility to infections during the menstrual period.

- Active HPV or HSV presence

Vaginal laser is not applied in the presence of active HPV or HSV, as it may increase the spread of the infection. Laser should not be used in other active genital infections.

- Uncontrolled diabetes mellitus (DM)

In uncontrolled DM patients, blood glucose regulation should be achieved first; otherwise, the inflammation period can be extended after the laser treatment.

- Immune system problems

Laser is contraindicated in acquired and congenital immune system problems and those using immunosuppressant drugs.

- Body dysmorphic disorder (BDD)

As stated in the ACOG bulletin, these patients may have different emotional changes after surgery. In addition, as the expectations of patients with BDD about the procedure to be performed can be very high, dissatisfaction rates after the procedure are also high.

- Psychiatric or serious psychological disturbances

Laser is not recommended for situations such as depression, anxiety, OCD (obsessive-compulsive disorder), or psychosis.

- Mentally disabled

All aesthetic operations are contraindicated for people with mental disabilities.

- Abnormal Pap smear test

The procedure is also contraindicated in patients with abnormal cellular pathology in the cervix or vagina.

- Cancer or suspected cancer

Laser application is also contraindicated in undiagnosed genital cancer or precancerous conditions.

- Photosensitivity

Photosensitive persons should be excluded from laser applications.

- Patients with overly high expectations

Patients with high expectations and those who are insecure overly detailed, indecisive, and having dilemmas in their minds should not be persuaded to undergo laser treatment. This group of patients may present different psychopathologies after the procedure.

There is no need to remove the contraceptive intrauterine device (IUD) before the vaginal rejuvenation procedures.

16.8 Preparation

It is important to evaluate by pelvic examination and ultrasound before vaginal laser. There should be no suspicion of malignancy in the ultrasound evaluations of the patients to be treated. Patients with intense vaginal or cervical infections during vaginal examination should have these infections treated first. In addition, there should not be any pathology in the smear tests performed in the previous year. In those who do not have a smear test within a year, a smear test should be done before the procedure. In patients with a low pain threshold, a mild anesthetic effect can be achieved by applying topical anesthetic cream into the vagina 10–15 min before the procedure. In very rare cases, the procedure can be performed under sedation anesthesia in line with the patient's demands. It is important for the patient to be informed in detail by the physician before the procedure and for the patient to sign the consent form afterward.

Goggles, mask, and operation garment must be used during all laser treatments on the internal and external genitalia. It will even be beneficial to give goggles to the patient. In a possible HPV infection, the mask prevents contamination of the practitioner by the viruses suspended in the air by particulates due to the ablative effect of the laser. If you are treating genital warts with laser or cautery, it is recommended to use double masks and goggles. The goggles both protect you from the contaminated air and prevent the emitted laser light from reaching your eyes by reflection from the application area. Garment also prevents possible contamination to your clothes and other parts of your skin. The room should be ventilated and disinfected after each procedure.

Many laser companies have produced special probe covers for their own devices for vaginal applications. Sterile packaged laser probe covers should be used exclusively for each patient.

In some countries, the rooms where the laser applications are applied have to meet some special conditions by regulations.

16.9 Laser Applications for Vaginal Rejuvenation

The patient is first examined by inserting a speculum in the lithotomy position on the gynecological examination table. During the examination, the vulva, vagina, and cervix are inspected. If there is no contraindication for the procedure, vaginal discharge and vaginal fluids are cleaned with a dry gauze. Afterward, the speculum is removed and the laser probe is inserted into the vagina, pushing it to the deepest part (until cervix). In order for the laser probe to move easily in the vagina, some vaseline can be applied on the probe, but not on the tip. Water-based gels should be avoided.

After the laser parameters are set, laser scanning is started from 12 o'clock, preferably clockwise. The probe is rotated a total of two complete turns (360°) so that there is a pulse at 45°. After the second round, the probe is withdrawn 1 cm and the same process is repeated (two turns). The laser probes already have metric dimensions to guide. In this way, the entire vaginal canal is scanned until the laser reaches the hymen (by making two full turns and withdrawing 1 cm). Afterward, the probe is pushed back in, to the bottom, this time one round in one area and again one cm after each round, scanning is provided up to the hymen level. Thus, the intravaginal laser will be scanned three times in total. Although three scans are sufficient most of the time, four or even five scans can be performed in some cases.

Vaginal laser application takes an average of 20 min, and thanks to the robotic arms produced by some companies, this duration can be reduced to 3 min. The energy used according to the patient's age, tolerance, and tissue conditions is between 80 and 120 mJ/pixel in young patients. It can be reduced to 50–60 mJ/pixel during menopause.

Table 16.3 Vaginal rejuvenation steps with CO_2 laser. This is the recommended protocol for CO_2 lasers such as FemiLift and Beladona

• Inform the patient and obtain her consent. Make sure she has had a smear test in the past year and the result is negative and that the patient is not pregnant
• Increase comfort by topical creams into the vagina 10–15 min before the procedure
• Switch on the device and set parameters
• In the lithotomy position, first inspect the external genital area, then the vagina and cervix by inserting a speculum
• After the inspection and drying of vaginal and cervical secretions with gauze, remove the speculum
• After applying vaseline on the probe or probe cover of the laser, insert the probe by pushing it up to the fornix
• Start scanning with a laser at 12 o'clock. Rotate the probe twice 360° in the same place, with a pulse every 45°
• Complete the 360-degree rotational treatment twice with 45-degree rotations by withdrawing the probe 1 cm
• Continue the process in this manner until the back of the hymen (introitus)
• Then push the probe back to the fornix, this time make a 360-degree turn
• Again, withdraw one cm each to the introitus (a total of three scans have been completed). If there is a lot of pain in the introitus, reduce the energy to a tolerable level
• Re-inspect the inside of the vagina by inserting the speculum, locally scan the missing areas
• Finish the procedure by cleaning the serous discharge and ablated mucosa in the vaginal canal with gauze

16.10 Steps of Laser Vaginal Rejuvenation (LVR) Procedure

The steps of laser vaginal rejuvenation are summarized in Table 16.3.

In the MonaLisa Touch™ technique made with Smart Xide™, another CO_2 laser brand, the application method is different. With the 60 W Smart Xide laser, it is possible to shoot 360° homogeneously at the same time, thanks to the movable mirror placed inside the scanner head. Therefore, there is no need to rotate the probe 360° (Fig. 16.6). Moreover, Smart Xide™ is the only laser device combined with RF today.

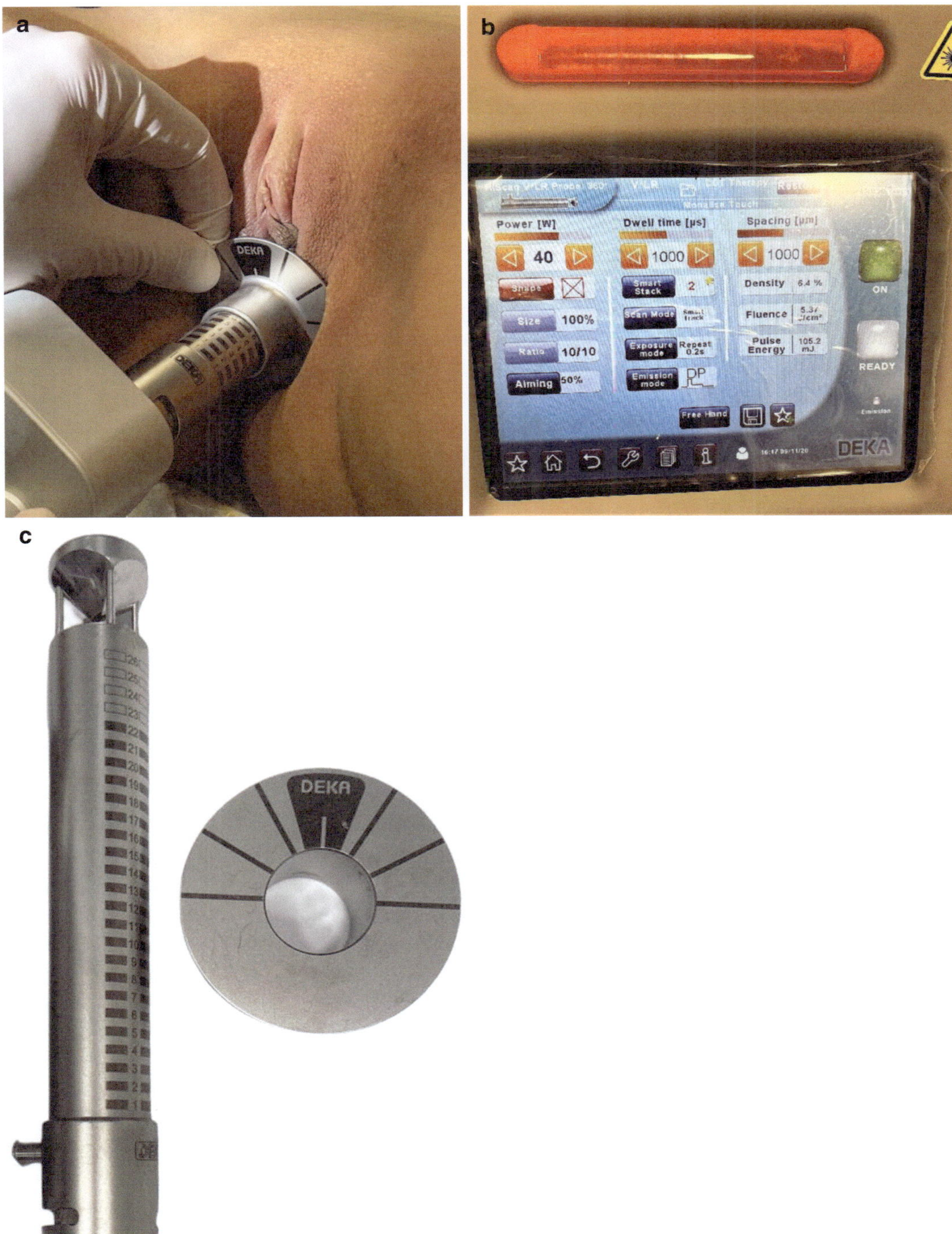

Fig. 16.6 Vaginal rejuvenation with MonaLisa Touch Technique. Application (**a**), device screen (**b**), and vaginal probe and its ring (**c**)

16.11 Application Protocol

The classical protocol for vaginal tightening and SUI treatments is three sessions in total, with an average interval of 1–1.5 months. Afterward, a single touch-up session is performed in the 12th month. The same procedure can be repeated every 2–3 years in line with the demands and complaints of the patient. In our own practice, we do the applications in two sessions with 1.5–3 months intervals. If necessary, the number of sessions can be increased up to 3–5. The frequency of application in lichen treatment is 2–4 sessions every 3–4 months, depending on the response of the patient's tissue.

16.12 Some Laser Devices on the Market

Especially in recent years, many laser companies have entered the field of genital rejuvenation. The table contains some laser devices and treatment protocols (Table 16.4).

The ring leaning against the labia allows and guides the easy insertion of the probe. After the entire vaginal probe is placed in the vagina, the scanning process is started. After each shot, one step is withdrawn based on the marked nails on the probe, so that the entire vagina can be scanned within a few minutes.

Table 16.4 Some laser devices in the market and their treatment protocols

Device name/ company	Type	Treatment protocol
SmartXide™ (DEKA)	Fractional CO_2 laser	3 treatments every 4–6 weeks
FemiLift™ (ALMA)	Fractional CO_2 laser	3 treatments every 4–6 weeks
Beladona™ (WONTECH)	Fractional CO_2 laser	3 treatments every 4–6 weeks
Youlaser MT™ (QUANTA)	10,600 nm ablative CO_2 and 1540 nm non-ablative GaAs (gallium arsenide) dual laser	3 treatments every 4–6 weeks
FotonaSmooth™ (FOTONA)	2940 nm non-ablative Er:YAG	3 treatments every 4 weeks
Petit Lady™ (LUTRONIC)	2940 nm Er:YAG	3 treatments every 2 weeks

How many pulses are made to the vagina in a single session? How much energy is emitted in total?

With a simple mathematical calculation, we can calculate how many shots will be made. Since a pulse is thrown at 45°, 8 pulses occur in a 360-degree cycle (round). Since the size of the vagina varies between 8 and 10 cm, 64–80 pulses are taken in an average vaginal canal scan. When the entire vaginal canal is scanned three times, the total number of pulses will be between 192 and 240. This roughly corresponds to a total energy of 20–25 J.

In order to perform the vaginal scanning process completely, it is recommended to check the inside of the canal with a speculum after three scans and re-scan the areas that have not been scanned sufficiently.

FemiLift™ lasers from Alma Company are based on scanner and patented pixel technology (Fig. 16.7). Laser energy is transmitted to the tissue with DOE (Diffractive Optical Element). DOE divides the beam into 81 microscopic pixels in a 9 × 9 shape. The advanced robotic arm technology (FemiLift Smart) provides convenience to the practitioner. FemiLift lasers used for cosmetic gynecology have a power of 30 W and a base value of 100 mJ/pixel (100 mJ = 0.1 J). If we remember the formula Joule = Watt × Seconds, the ablation time in the scanner technology is 30 W × T (Time) = 0.1 J, T (Time) = 0.1/30 W = 3.3 ms (milliseconds). Since a pixel consists of 9 × 9 = 81 points, the power of a point is 30 W/81 points = 0.37 W. Since it will be 0.37 W × T = 0.1 mJ, the time required for thermal effect is T = 0.1/0.37 W = 270 ms.

The FotonaSmooth™ laser system is a laser that produces light at a wavelength of 2940 nm in the mid-infrared spectrum and can operate in both fractional ablative and non-ablative modes. It has two different dual models, FotonaSmooth SP and SP Plus, with 2940 nm Er:YAG and 1064 nm Nd:YAG lasers. In addition, there is a non-ablative intraurethral probe developed for stress incontinence treatment (Fig. 16.8) and a robotic arm called "G-Runner."

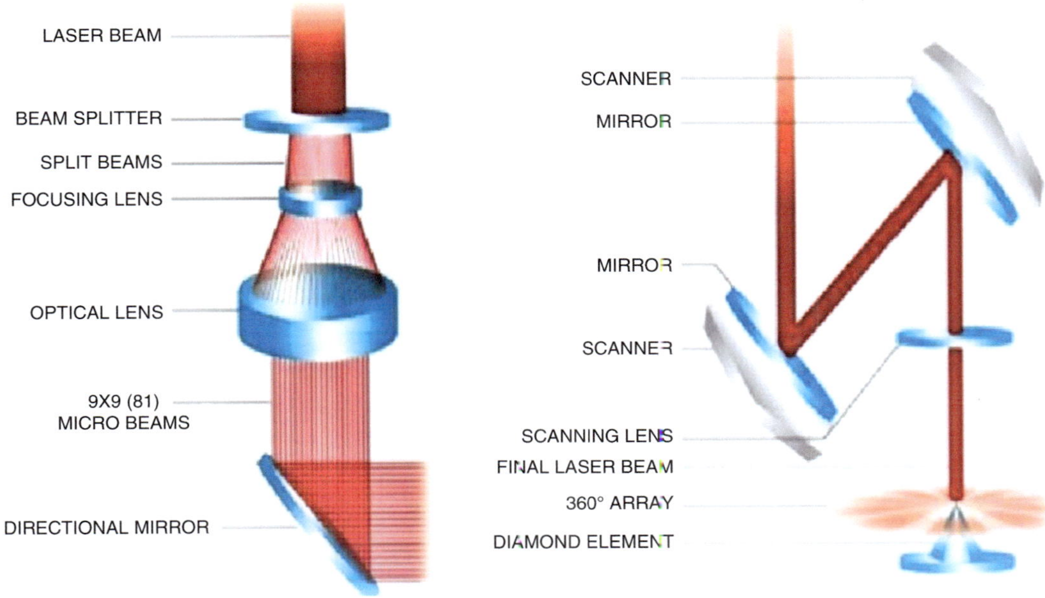

Fig. 16.7 Laser pixel technology that belongs to Alma Company

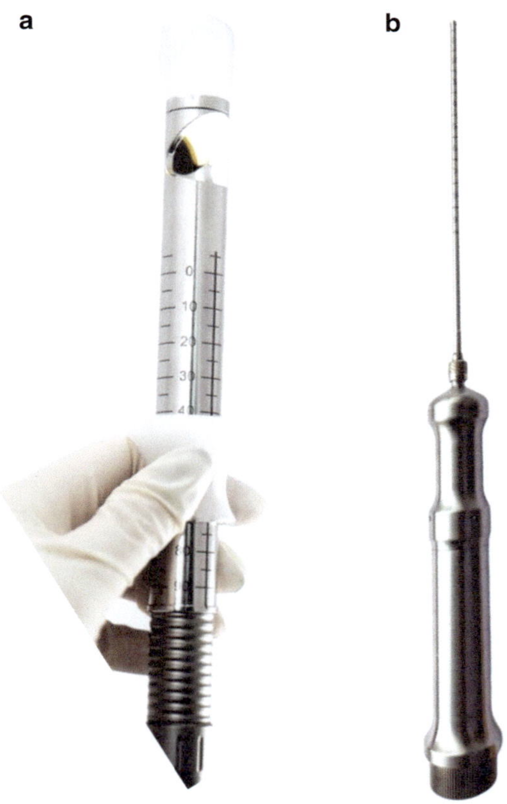

Fig. 16.8 FotonaSmooth™ non-ablative vaginal laser probe (**a**) and intraurethral probe (**b**)

16.13 Laser Applications for Stress Urinary Incontinence (SUI) Treatment

Laser is a good indication for those who have mild POP or who have stress incontinence without POP. The patient is first prepared for the procedure as for the vaginal tightening procedure. The probe tip is then pushed against the cervix. The 11-12-1 o'clock alignments are scanned twice. Then, the same application is repeated on the entire anterior wall until the probe reaches the hymen level by withdrawing one cm each time. After reaching the hymen boundary, the laser probe is pushed to the first starting point (deep) again, and the 11-12-1 o'clock alignments are scanned until the hymen is reached once again. As a result, the entire front wall is scanned three times. If necessary, four to five scans can be made on the anterior wall.

To summarize, while four quadrants of the vagina are scanned three times in total for vaginal tightening, only the anterior vaginal wall (at 11-12-1 o'clock) is scanned three times in total in SUI treatment. The energy used according to the patient's age, tolerability, and tissue condition is between 80 and 120 mJ/pixel in young patients.

16.14 Laser Applications in Menopausal Genitourinary Syndrome (GSM)

Menopausal genitourinary syndrome (GSM) is a new concept that includes all symptoms resulting from changes in the entire vulvovaginal region, urethra, and urinary bladder due to the decrease in estrogen and other sex steroids (Table 16.5). It is formerly known as "vulvovaginal atrophy (VVA)," "urogenital atrophy," and "atrophic vaginitis." Postmenopausal women may experience all of these symptoms or just some. The vaginal and urethral epithelia develop from the same estrogen-dependent tissue origin embryologically. Therefore, the decrease in estrogen during menopause affects both regions. Vulva, vagina, urethra, and bladder are the most affected organs in GSM, which is experienced by 50% of women during menopause. The diagnosis can be made by characteristic symptoms, physical examination, and laboratory tests. On examination, the vagina is pale, dry, and sensitive, and the ruga structures are also reduced. Vaginal pH is generally above 5. Vaginal Maturation Index (VMI), which shows the proportion of mature parabasal, intermediate, and superficial squamous cells, is helpful in diagnosis. Serum estrogen levels are not diagnostic.

Table 16.5 Symptoms of GSM

Genital symptoms
– Vaginal dryness
– Itching, burning, and irritation in the genital area
Sexual symptoms
– Dyspareunia due to reduced lubrication and sensitivity
– Decreased sexual intimacy
– Lack of sexual desire, arousal, and difficulty of having orgasm
Urinary symptoms
– Frequent urinary tract infections
– Stress incontinence
– Pollakiuria, urgency, and dysuria
Quality of life
– Decreased confidence
– Sleep problems
– Disruption of social functions

The first-line treatment in GSM is the use of nonhormonal vaginal lubricants and moisturizers and the continuation of sexual intercourse. At moderate and severe levels, local estrogen treatments are very effective and well-tolerated, especially in patients with pain, burning complaints in the genital area, dyspareunia, and complaints about urinary retention or voiding. In this way, the vaginal epithelium thickens, secretions increase, vaginal flora improves, and vaginal pH decreases. In general, the complaints of vaginal dryness and urogenital symptoms decrease. However, fractional lasers may be a good option, especially since estrogen therapy is contraindicated for patients who have received breast cancer treatment or who are being followed up due to suspicious lesion(s) in the breast. Even in these patients, laser and PRP can be combined. The aim is again to increase the synthesis of collagen connective tissue.

For those who are not contraindicated to use estrogen and have symptoms of vulvovaginitis due to menopause, it would be a more correct approach to treat the vaginal mucosa with local estrogen treatments for at least one month and then to perform laser or RF treatment. The amount of energy used in vaginal laser treatment during menopause is between 50 and 80 mJ/pixel depending on the condition and tolerance of the patient's tissue. The lower energy applied is due to the decrease in both the thickness of the mucosa and the amount of water within the tissue.

Conversely, in patients whose GSM symptoms continue to cause severe discomfort despite the estrogen treatments they receive, laser and PRP sessions applied from time to time along with estrogen therapy can be relieving. In these patients, especially for the symptoms of vaginal dryness and vulvovaginal atrophy, hyaluronic acid injections, stromal vascular fracture (SVF) injections, and some mesotherapy products for regeneration may also be preferred.

Laser can also be applied to the external genital areas in menopausal vulvar atrophies.

I applied vaginal CO_2 laser therapy to two patients who had previously been diagnosed with interstitial cystitis and had tried many medications and treatment methods. After the first application, I observed a significant reduction in the symptoms of dysuria and pollakiuria in both of them.

16.15 Laser for Symptomatic Treatment of Lichen Sclerosus

Lichen sclerosus et atrophicus is a chronic benign inflammatory skin disease that can frequently involve the genital area and is thought to be autoimmune, causing mucocutaneous atrophy and many related symptoms. It can involve the genital area, perineum, and perianal area. Vaginal involvement is extremely rare. Its true prevalence is unknown but is thought to occur in one in 59 women. Although the exact cause is not known, it is thought to be a multifactorial disease that includes genetic, hormonal, autoimmune, and inflammatory factors. The definitive diagnosis can be made by clinical findings and biopsy. Vulvar lichen sclerosus is discussed in detail in Chap. 5.

Lichen sclerosus et atrophicus frequently causes skin atrophy and many related symptoms in the genitalia. Pain, burning, stinging sensation in the genital area, itching, inability to wear tight pants, dyspareunia, sexual desire problems, orgasmic dysfunctions, and dysuria are the most common patient complaints. When these patients are not treated, the vulvar architecture progressively deteriorates; the inner and outer labia become pale or even disappear (resorption) over time, the clitoris becomes embedded, and the introitus narrows. It is stated that the risk of vulvar squamous cell carcinoma is between 2–6%. For this reason, it is essential to take a biopsy before treatment and to follow the progress with serial biopsies.

Ultra-potent steroids such as clobetasol propionate, which are administered topically for LS treatment, suppress tissue inflammation on the one hand and increase skin atrophy in long-term use on the other. Therefore, use for more than 2 months should be avoided. It is generally recommended to reduce the dose to 2–3 times per week after 6–8 weeks of daily use.

Fractional lasers can be used in the symptomatic treatment of lichen sclerosus disease. Increasing the inflammation in the inflammatory skin tissue with laser and PRP can be compared to the "*firefighters putting out the fire with a fire*." The healing period will follow the inflammation process.

In laser treatment, the application energy is higher and the density is kept lower compared to bleaching treatments. A treatment with 20 W of power, 4 density, 1.0 irradiation time (dwell time), and 2 passes is recommended. The dose can be adjusted according to the response of the tissue. Depending on the response of the tissue, it can be applied as 2–4 applications every 3–4 months. It is also recommended as 3–4 applications with FemiLift laser once a month, with light-medium energy of 10–20 mJ/pixel.

In addition, the injection of freshly prepared PRP into the subcutaneous tissue immediately after laser application will further increase the effectiveness of the treatment (Fig. 16.9). However, laser therapy for active lichen patients with excessive inflammatory, watery lesions is not recommended.

Performing the treatment with mild sedation anesthesia and local anesthesia infiltration will increase patient comfort. Also, if there are functional complaints due to buried clitoris, perineal scarring, or vaginal stenosis, reconstruction can be performed with simple surgical procedures in the same session. The healing process may take a few weeks.

Successful results are also obtained with radiofrequency (RF) treatments. All these applications can also be supported by topical estrogen and liposomal testosterone treatments. Fat grafting or stromal vascular fraction (SVF) treatments may also be recommended in resistant patients.

In patients with excessive adhesions and difficulty in urination or coitus, the vaginal entrance should be opened by surgical interventions.

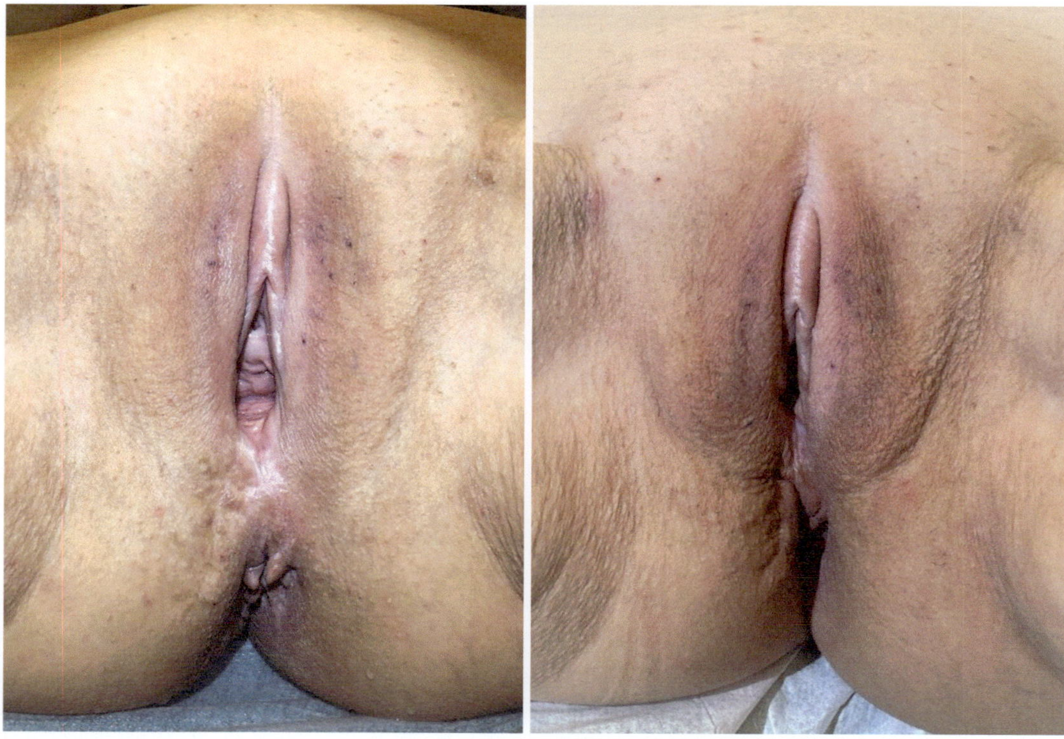

Fig. 16.9 Appearances after one-session laser and PRP application to a lichen patient. Left, before; right, after 2.5 months. An obvious improvement in the patient's symptoms was also observed

16.16 Post-Laser Histological Changes

The technical characteristics of the energy-based technology and the physiological properties of the target tissue are factors that directly affect cellular activation that causes tissue restoration. These include many factors such as the wavelength of the laser, energy density, pulse duration, spot diameter, absorption by tissue, tissue hydration, oxygenation, blood circulation, keratinization if the application area is the skin area, and surrounding tissue properties. For example, since the vagina is drier, more sensitive, and its epithelial tissue is thinner during the menopausal period, the amount of energy applied should be kept lower than in the premenopausal period.

After the laser treatment, wound healing initiates with the inflammatory response and continues with the proliferation and remodeling phases (Note: Recommended to read "Physiology of Wound Healing" first in Chap. 6).

16.16.1 Inflammation Phase

Immediately after laser treatment, tissue changes characterized by edema, hyperemia, and release of chemical mediators occur (Fig. 16.10). This stage, which occurs in the first 72 h, is the inflammatory process due to acute thermal damage. During this period, collagen tissue shrinks and decreases due to high temperature. Vaginal mucosa will have desquamation due to ablation in a few days (Fig. 16.11).

The inflammation process begins with the cytokines released as a result of thermomechanical tissue destruction (ablation) by the laser beam. The supraphysiological heat zone (Heat Zone) causes the HSP 70 (Heat Shock Protein 70) mediator to be released by creating the "Heat

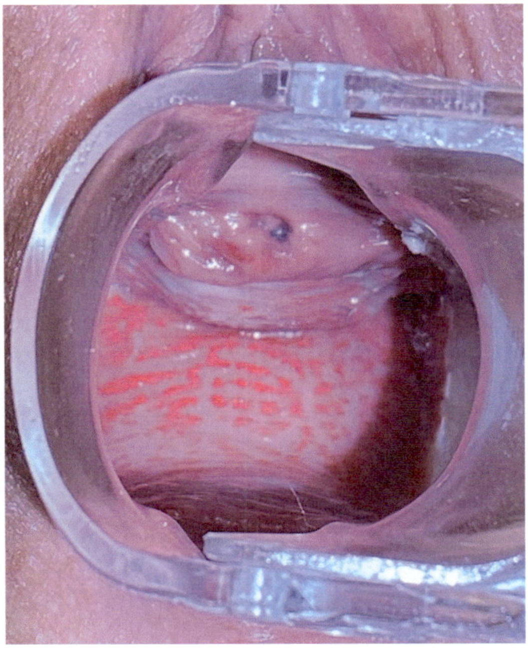

Fig. 16.10 Vaginal mucosa appearance just after fractional carbon dioxide laser application. Pay attention for hyperemia and edema

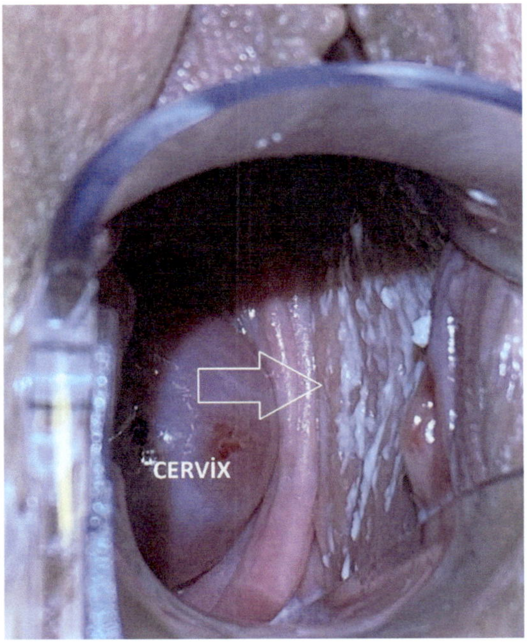

Fig. 16.11 Desquamation of vaginal mucosa after CO_2 laser (three days after the procedure)

Shock Response" in the tissue. This mediator also induces the release of TGF- β, which is a *key element in the inflammatory response*, fibrogenic process, and new collagen and extracellular matrix production. Also, basic fibroblast growth factor (bFGF) that stimulates angiogenic activity with endothelial cell migration and proliferation, epidermal growth factor (EGF) that stimulates re-epithelialization, platelet-derived growth factor (PDGF) that stimulates fibroblasts for the production of extracellular matrix components, a local increase of different cytokines such as vascular endothelial growth factor (VEGF), which regulates vasculogenesis and angiogenesis, have been demonstrated histochemically.

16.16.2 Proliferation Phase

The process after inflammation is the proliferation phase, and in this phase, the fibroblasts gathered in the damaged area begin new collagen synthesis and start the healing process. During this period, the synthesis of dermal matrix material also increases.

16.16.3 Maturation Phase

After 30 days, the inflammation has ended, mature collagen and elastic fibers have been formed, and the tissue regeneration process has taken place. This period, also known as the "remodeling period," will continue for a few more months, increasing its effect.

The purposes of energy-based therapies such as laser or RF are to provide collagen contraction, new collagen formation, vascularization, and infiltration of growth factors into the tissue, thereby increasing the moisture, tightening, and elasticity of the vaginal mucosa. The same devices have been used by dermatologists for years in areas such as the face, neck, and décolleté, and their effectiveness in these areas has been shown in many studies. Scientific studies on the genital area are still limited.

Table 16.6 Histological changes in vaginal tissue after laser treatment

I. Inflammation (acute thermal damage) phase (48–72 h)
• Edema
• Release of chemical mediators
• Collagen shrinkage
II. Proliferation phase (next 30 days)
• Collection of fibroblasts
• Formation of new dermal matrix molecules
• Formation of new collagen fibers
III. Remodeling phase (following 30–40 days)
• End of inflammatory infiltration
• Formation of mature collagen fibers
• Increasing the tension of collagen fibers
• Neovascularization
• Formation of new elastic fibers

Histological changes during wound healing period have been summarized in Table 16.6.

16.17 Collagen Structure and Types

Collagen is a type of protein that gives the tissue its shape; it consists of fibers that are not stretchy, is resistant to stretching and tension, and is the main material of skin and other tissues. Collagen makes up about 30% of all protein found in mammals. Collagens are synthesized by fibroblasts and stored in the extracellular matrix. They have structural roles, are important in organization, and provide intra-tissue shape. Their general structure is in the form of a triple helix, and they consist of amino acids that come together to form the triple helix of the extended fibril. Thirty different types of collagen have been identified so far, and their names are designated in Roman numerals [7].

16.17.1 Collagen Types

Type I is found in skin, bone, vessels, tendon, ligament, fascia, and organ capsules. Type I collagen is 90% of the collagen in the body. It is the main component of the organic part of the bone. For example, some diseases with autosomal dominant inheritance such as osteogenesis imperfecta occur as a result of Type I collagen mutation.

Type II is found in cartilage. It is the main collagenous component of cartilage. For example, chondrodysplasias are caused by Type II collagen mutations.

Type III consists of reticulum-forming fibers. It is found in the stroma (within loose connective tissue) of organs. For example, there is a Type III collagen defect in the vascular type in Ehlers-Danlos syndrome.

Type IV is found in basal lamina structure.

Type V is found on cell surfaces, hair, and placenta.

Energy-based therapies stimulate fibroblasts and increase Type I collagen production in the extracellular matrix. The mechanism takes place as follows: collagen fibrils have a triple helix structure consisting of protein chains linked to each other by interchain bonds. Intramolecular hydrogen bonds are broken and contracted with the heat generated during energy-based treatments. As a result of this contraction, the long, triple helix structure of collagen folds and turns into a thicker and shorter form. Thus, tissue tightening occurs. Partially denatured collagen may also signal for neocollagenesis.

Collagen can be used in dentistry, orthopedics, cardiac surgery, cardiac support, bone grafting, burn treatment, wound healing, and tissue regeneration as well as being widely used in the field of cosmetics. It can also be used orally to support bone, joint, heart, and skin health.

Elastin fibers synthesized by fibroblasts have a shorter and branched structure. By wrapping around collagen bundles, they increase resistance to stretching with their stretching properties.

16.18 Comparison of Laser and Surgical Tightening Operations

Procedures performed with laser and surgical vaginal tightening have advantages and disadvantages compared to each other. Since laser procedures are carried out in an office condition, they are easy, extremely low-risk, and easily tolerable. Vaginoplasty operations, however, offer advantages such as repairing fascia defects, permanent reconstruction of the vagina, and obtaining optimal results when performed together with perineoplasty (Table 16.7).

Table 16.7 Comparison of laser vaginal rejuvenation (LVR) and surgical vaginal rejuvenations (SVR)

Comparison	LVR	SVR
Technique	Non-surgical/easy	Surgical/difficult
Anesthesia	(−)	(+)
Topical cream	(−) Perineum only (+)	(+) If local anesthesia is planned
Aesthetic repair	(−)	(+), if perineoplasty is done
Tightening	The entire vaginal canal (four walls)	Posterior vaginal wall, about 6–8 cm
Mechanism	Increasing collagen and elastic fibers	Fascia repair and approximation of muscle layers
Duration	3–20 min (depending on the device)	60 min
Repetition	(+)	(−)
Antibiotic and analgesic	(−)	(+)
Downtime	No	7 days
Activities	The same day	1 month later
Sexual abstinence	7 days	1.5 months; sometimes 2 months

16.19 Survey Studies and Scientific Data

Although clinical results of laser and RF procedures in terms of safety and efficacy have been evaluated in some peer-reviewed journals, objective, validated measurements and scales are still insufficient. Commonly used indexes include:

1. Female Sexual Function Index (FSFI) [8],
2. Millheiser Vaginal Laxity Scale [9],
3. Millheiser Sexual Satisfaction Scale [10],
4. Visual Analogue Scale [11],
5. Incontinence Survey International Research [12],
6. Satisfaction Scores (Likert Scale) [13],
7. Vaginal Health Index [14].

Some publications on vaginal rejuvenation by carbon dioxide lasers (Table 16.8) and Erbium:YAG lasers (Table 16.9) are summarized below.

16.20 Scientific Data

Table 16.8 Some publications on vaginal rejuvenation by carbon dioxide lasers

Study	Result
Salvatore et al. [15] 77 postmenopausal patients	Significant increase in FSFI scores (14.8–27.2) 17 patients' inactive sexual life
Gaspar et al. [16] CO_2 + PRP + PFE	Significant reduction in sexual complaints
Filippini [17] 386 postmenopausal patients	Decrease in dyspareunia due to vaginal epithelial atrophy
Perino [18] 48 postmenopausal patients	Safety, efficacy, and satisfaction in reducing vulvovaginal symptoms
Pieralli [19] 50 patients (aged between 41 and 66)	VHI score: 8.9–21.6 (<15 VVA) VAS: improvement in dyspareunia 52% of patients is satisfied at 11 months

Table 16.9 Some publications on vaginal rejuvenation by Erbium:YAG lasers

Study	Results
Adrian [20]	Increased tightening
Gambacciani [21]	Significant reduction in vaginal
Gambacciani [22]	dryness and dyspareunia
45 postmenopausal patients	
Vizintin [23]	Effective and safe to treat vaginal laxity

16.21 Combined Procedures

Laser vaginal tightening can be performed together with procedures such as labiaplasty, vulvar bleaching, or PRP. Even in patients with stress incontinence without vaginal enlargement and POP, posterior vaginal tightening and anterior wall laser application can be combined. If vaginal laser and PRP are to be combined in sexual pleasure treatments, first laser treatment and then PRP should be applied.

Vaginal laser procedure can be combined with magnetic chair application, especially in SUI patients.

16.22 Complications

No major complications have been reported after laser application. If the energy applied in CO_2 lasers is high, the inflammation process may be prolonged. Infections such as previously undetected or subclinical bacterial vaginosis may also become symptomatic after laser treatment. Such patients may experience decreased healing speed, more edema, and pain. If the treatment extends beyond the vaginal border during the procedure, complaints such as redness, pain, and blistering in the vaginal entrance and vestibular area may occur.

Because CO_2 lasers have a more ablative effect when the energy or pulse number is high, the healing process in the tissue due to inflammation may be delayed. Accordingly, pain and bleeding complaints can be seen during intercourse. These complaints may extend up to the second month after the procedure. Therefore, laser parameters and sessions should be adjusted for the patient's tissue conditions, complaints, and age.

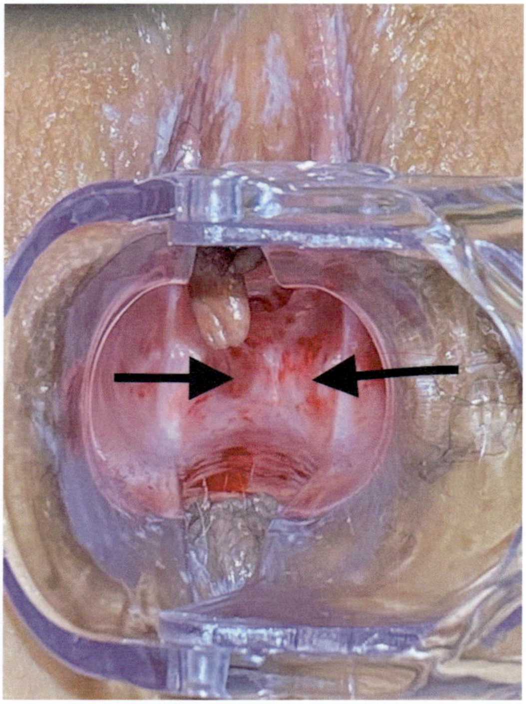

Fig. 16.12 Post-laser vaginal adhesion. The area about one cm wide between both arrows shows the fibrotic adhesion that divides the vagina like a longitudinal septum. The procedure was performed on a 48-year-old patient who had been in menopause for 2 years to eliminate dyspareunia due to vulvovaginal atrophy, with a total of 24 pulses to the entire vaginal canal at 80 mJ/pixel. This adhesion that developed after the procedure was simply cut open with scissors

Surgery should be recommended to patients who are not satisfied with vaginal tightening or improved in SUI complaints after three sessions.

The possibility of vaginal adhesion after laser treatment (Fig. 16.12) is extremely low. I have encountered vaginal adhesion in only three of the more than 9000 applications I have done so far.

16.23 The Post-Procedure Term

The vaginal laser procedure is a non-invasive application. It does not require anesthesia and immediately after the procedure, patients can return to work without needing to rest. Therefore, it is referred to as a *"lunch time management."* There are no other restrictions other than a 7–10 days prohibition on coitus. On the day of the procedure, some patients may experience mild itching, rash, edema, vaginal bleeding, tenderness, dysuria, weakness, nausea, headache, dizziness, hot flashes, and fever, although rare. Some patients state that they feel like *"flu-like syndrome."* Muscle and joint pains can be seen. Most of these complaints are due to cytokines released by the inflammation that starts in the vagina. Since the main purpose of laser application is to initiate this inflammatory process, it would be a more appropriate approach to recommend 1000 mg paracetamol in one dose instead of NSAI drugs that suppress inflammation for those with such complaints. If there is no evidence of infection, antibiotics are not required. If bacterial vaginosis is undiagnosed or subclinical before the procedure, inflammatory phase may become more severely and the wound healing process may be delayed.

Pinkish discharge is normal for the first few days after the application. The discharge then becomes very watery and gradually decreases and ends spontaneously between 5 and 14 days after the procedure.

Since the collagen production after laser treatment begins in the third week, the tightening effect felt by the patient herself and her partner during sexual intercourse also occurs after the third week. Suggestion to perform Kegel and other pelvic exercises that patients can start immediately after the procedure also increases the tightening effect.

In order to relieve concerns, it is beneficial to give the patients a written paper stating the expected situations and what to do after the procedure.

Appendix

With the purchase of this book, you can use our "SN Flashcards" app to access questions free of charge in order to test your learning and check your understanding of the contents of the book.

To use the app, please follow the instructions below:

1. Go to https://flashcards.springernature.com/login
2. Create a user account by entering your e-mail address and assigning a password.
3. Use the following link to access your SN Flashcards set: ▶ https://sn.pub/tvlq7Q

If the link is missing or does not work, please send an e-mail with the subject "SN Flashcards" and the book title to customerservice@springernature.com.

References

1. Ergenekon G, Aybey B. Lazer Fiziği ve Lazerlerin Dermatoloji'de Kullanımı. Turkiye Klinikleri J Int Med Sci. 2005;1(52):1–13.
2. Koç E, Dicem. Lazere Giriş ve Genel Bilgiler. Türk Derm. 2012;1:2–6.
3. Anderson RR, Parrish JA. Selective photothermolysis: precise microsurgery by selective absorption of pulsed radiation. Science. 1983;220(4596):524–7.
4. Carroll L, Humphreys TR. LASER-tissue interactions. Clin Dermatol. 2006;24(1):2–7.
5. Öztürkcan SBC. Dermatolojide Lazer ve Işık Sistemi. Turk Klinikleri J Cosm Dermatol. 2009;2:1–8.
6. Lee WR, Shen SC, Al-Suwayeh SA, Li YC, Fang JY. Erbium:YAG laser resurfacing increases skin permeability and the risk of excessive absorption of antibiotics and sunscreens: the influence of skin recovery on drug absorption. Toxicol Lett. 2012;211(2):150–8.
7. Ricard-Blum S. The collagen family. Cold Spring Harb Perspect Biol. 2011;3(1):a004978.
8. Rosen R, Brown C, Heiman J, Leiblum S, Meston C, Shabsigh R, Ferguson D, D'Agostino R Jr. The female sexual function index (FSFI): a multidimensional self-report instrument for the assessment of female sexual function. J Sex Marital Ther. 2000;26(2):191–208.
9. Millheiser LS, Pauls RN, Herbst SJ, Chen BH. Radiofrequency treatment of vaginal laxity after vaginal delivery: nonsurgical vaginal tightening. J Sex Med. 2010;7(9):3088–95.
10. Davis D, Shaver PR, Widaman KF, Vernon ML, Follette WC, Beitz K. I can't get no satisfaction: insecure attachment, inhibited sexual communication, and sexual dissatisfaction. Pers Relat. 2006;13:465–83.
11. Lukacz ES, Lawrence JM, Burchette RJ, Luber KM, Nager CW, Buckwalter JG. The use of visual analog scale in urogynecologic research: a psychometric evaluation. Am J Obstet Gynecol. 2004;191(1):165–70.

12. Avery K, Donovan J, Peters TJ, Shaw C, Gotoh M, Abrams P. ICIQ: a brief and robust measure for evaluating the symptoms and impact of urinary incontinence. Neurourol Urodyn. 2004;23(4):322–30.
13. Sullivan GM, Artino AR Jr. Analyzing and interpreting data from Likert-type scales. J Grad Med Educ. 2013;5(4):541–2.
14. Bachmann G. Urogenital ageing: an old problem newly recognized. Maturitas. 1995;22(Suppl):1–5.
15. Salvatore S, Nappi RE, Parma M, Chionna R, Lagona F, Zerbinati N, Ferrero S, Origoni M, Candiani M, Leone Roberti Maggiore U. Sexual function after fractional microablative CO_2 laser in women with vulvovaginal atrophy. Climacteric. 2015;18(2):219–25.
16. Gaspar A, Addamo G, Brandi H. Vaginal fractional CO_2 laser: a minimally invasive option for vaginal rejuvenation. Am J Cosmet Surg. 2011;28:156–62.
17. Filippini M, Del Duca E, Negosanti F, Bonciani D, Negosanti L, Sannino M, Cannarozzo G, Nisticò SP. Fractional CO_2 laser: from skin rejuvenation to vulvo-vaginal reshaping. Photomed Laser Surg. 2017;35(3):171–5.
18. Perino A, Calligaro A, Forlani F, Tiberio C, Cucinella G, Svelato A, Saitta S, Calagna G. Vulvo-vaginal atrophy: a new treatment modality using thermo-ablative fractional CO_2 laser. Maturitas. 2015;80(3):296–301.
19. Pieralli A, Fallani MG, Becorpi A, Bianchi C, Corioni S, Longinotti M, Tredici Z, Guaschino S. Fractional CO_2 laser for vulvovaginal atrophy (VVA) dyspareunia relief in breast cancer survivors. Arch Gynecol Obstet. 2016;294(4):841–6.
20. Gaspar A. Comparison of two novel laser treatments in aesthetic gynecology. J Laser Health Acad. 1012;1:S10.
21. Gambacciani M, Levancini M, Cervigni M. Vaginal erbium laser: the second-generation thermotherapy for the genitourinary syndrome of menopause. Climacteric. 2015;18(5):757–63.
22. Gambacciani M, Torelli MG, Martella L, Bracco GL, Casagrande AG, Albertin E, Tabanelli S, Viglietta M, D'Ambrogio G, Garone G, Cervigni M. Rationale and design for the Vaginal Erbium Laser Academy Study (VELAS): an international multicenter observational study on genitourinary syndrome of menopause and stress urinary incontinence. Climacteric. 2015;18(Suppl 1):43–8.
23. Vizintin Z, Lukac M, Kazic M, Tettamanti M. Erbium laser in gynecology. Climacteric. 2015;18(Suppl 1):4–8.

17 Genital Bleaching Treatments

An art, which has an aim to achieve the beauty, is called a philosophy or in the absolute sense it is named wisdom.

Al-Farabi

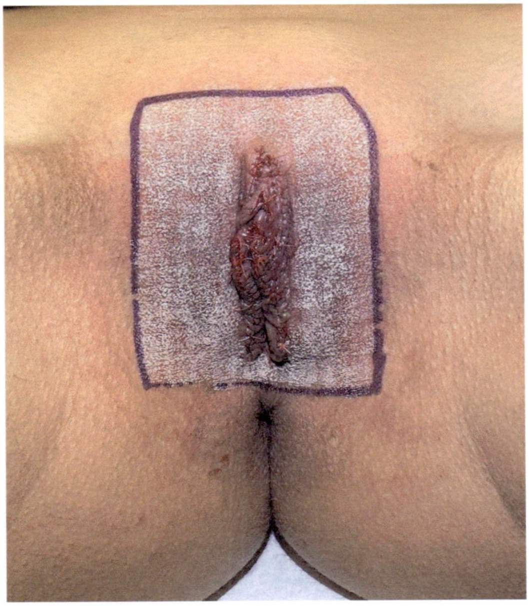

Demands by patients for ano-genital bleaching have rapidly increased, especially in recent years.

Bleaching treatments are also referred to as "vulvar bleaching" or "pudenda bleaching." However, the term "genital whitening" is not correct. As a matter of fact, the process is not whitening but bleaching in the color tone. It will be useful to read the skin (Chap. 4) and wound healing (Chap. 6) sections before entering genital area bleaching treatments.

17.1 Skin Color Types

It is possible to talk about the structural and acquired skin color according to the melanin content in humans. Structural skin color is the color we have at birth and is genetically determined. Acquired skin color develops as a result of ultraviolet light, some hormones, drugs, and diseases. Six different skin types were defined according to the "Fitzpatrick classification" in humans (Table 17.1). These skin types are further detailed with the "Von Luschan scale."

S. Eserdağ, *Aesthetic and Functional Female Genital Surgery*,
https://doi.org/10.1007/978-3-031-16019-6_17

Table 17.1 Fitzpatrick classification used for skin color typing in humans [1]

Skin type	Appearance	Sunburn	Tanning	Von Luschan scale
I	Pale white skin It is very light colored skin Blue, green eye color (celtic type)	Always	Never tans	1–5
II	Fair skin Common in Europeans Blue, gray, green eye color	Usually	Tans with difficulty	6–10
III	Average (Fair) skin color It has a medium light tone Common in Southern Europeans. Brown eyes and brown hair	Sometimes mild burn	Tans medium	11–15
IV	Light-brown skin Common in the Mediterranean. Brown or black eye color	Rarely	Tans easily	16–21
V	Dark-brown skin Black eye color	Very rarely	Tans darkly easily	22–28
VI	Black skin Skin is very dark. Black eye color	Never	Heavily pigmented. Natural skin color is black and skin color does not darken. Tans very easily	29–36

17.2 Causes of Hyperpigmentation

Skin hyperpigmentation may occur due to an excess of pigment localized in the dermal or epidermal layer. Hyperpigmentation may occur due to hereditary or acquired causes such as drug use, chronic diseases, hormonal, and postinflammatory factors.

Among the most common causes of vulvar hyperpigmentation in women are exposure to ultraviolet rays, tanning beds, use of oral contraceptives, PCOS, laser hair removal, waxing, pregnancy, postinflammatory hyperpigmentation (PIH) and smoking. Some systemic diseases like Addison's disease, Cushing's disease, acanthosis nigricans, intertriginous, Peutz–Jeghers syndrome, Coeliac disease, Cronkhite–Canada syndrome, porphyria, haemochromatosis, B12 and folic acid deficiency, atopic dermatitis, Graves' disease, aromatase deficiency, mercury poisoning, Graves' disease and some medications also increase darkening. Darkening of the genital and anal area can cause some social and psychological negativity, especially insecurity during sexual intercourse. Ano-genital area bleaching is a rapidly increasing trend in women, and, interestingly, in recent years, also in men.

17.3 Hyperpigmentation Treatments

CO_2 laser, Er:YAG laser, and Q-switched (switched) lasers are most frequently used for hyperpigmentation treatments. In addition, chemical peel products, spot-removing solutions, some creams, and mesotherapy products are among the other applications. Bleaching in the genital area occurs as a result of the peeling of the epidermis layer of the skin as a result of ablation due to the thermal effect on the tissue with the fractional head of Er:YAG or CO_2 lasers. Q-switched lasers, however, can lighten the color by affecting the melanin secreted by melanocytes in the basal layer. For this purpose, it is also used in the treatment of tattoo removal, Café-au lait macules, birthmarks, melasma, freckle, age spots. The skin takes its color from dermal and epidermal components and subcutaneous blood vessels. Therefore, the target should be directed to the region where the darkening belongs.

Before laser application, the energy and density parameters of the laser are adjusted according to the skin color of the person. In those with dark skin color, energy should be applied in lower doses due to the risks of burns, scar tissue formation, and postinflammatory hyperpigmentation. The dose can be increased a little more for light-skinned people.

17.3.1 Treatment Protocol

The application area should be shaved. The procedure can be performed under sedation or local anesthesia. If it is to be performed under local anesthesia, it will be beneficial to apply topical anesthetic creams containing lidocaine 25mg/g and prilocaine 25 mg/g (5% Emla Cream™), or BLT cream™, or magistral 12% benzocaine, 4% lidocaine, and 8% tetracaine combination 45 min prior. In practice, first the genital area is cleaned with an external chlorhexidine-like disinfectant solution and dried. Preferably a white marking pencil a white is then used to draw a rectangle around the hyperpigmented area. Then, if the patient is hypersensitive to pain, the application area is numbed with a syringe containing 1/2 or 1/3 diluted local anesthetic solution and a long dental needle attached to its tip. The treatment area is checked by touching it with the needle tip (prick test) to ensure that it has become numb. Then, the physician wears protective goggles, and the fractional probe of the laser is brought into full contact with the tissue and the scanning process is started. The entire marked rectangular area is scanned once or twice. Scanning can be done in the square mode of the probe, with 5–7 W and 6–8 density. If the patient's skin color is dark, the power may be lower; if light, it may be slightly higher. Average treatment time is 3–4 min (Fig. 17.1).

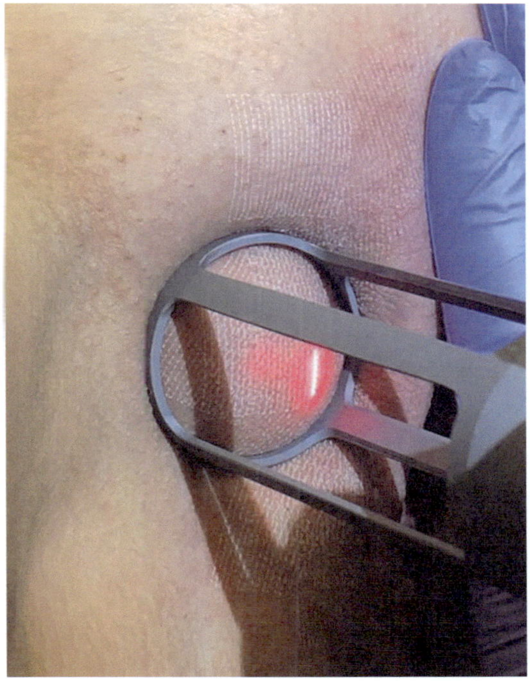

Fig. 17.1 Genital bleaching with fractional carbon dioxide laser

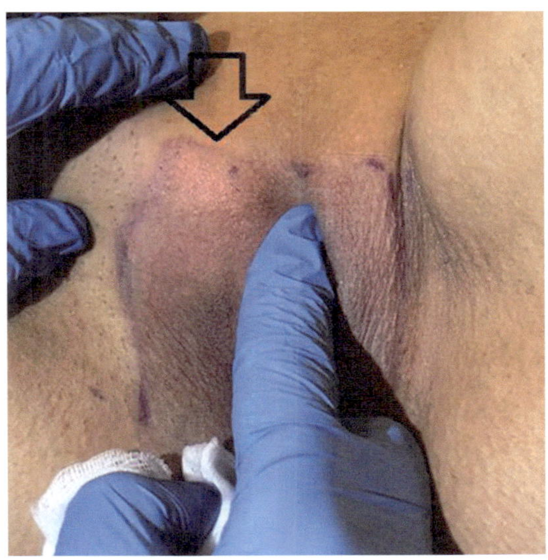

Fig. 17.2 Immediately after the procedure. The area indicated by the arrow shows the epidermis after peeling by wiping with wet gauze

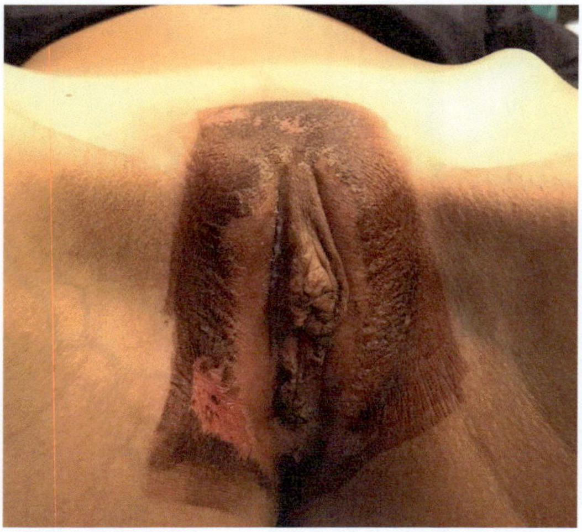

Fig. 17.3 Seven days after bleaching with CO_2 laser. The ablated skin tissue first darkens and then begins to peel off

After the procedure effects of ablation are seen immediately (Fig. 17.2). The ablated epidermal layer of the skin first darkens and then peels off (Fig. 17.3). The sessions can be repeated 2–3 times, once every 4–6 weeks. It is important to avoid breathing the vaporized tissue in air during the laser procedure and to wear a mask during the procedure.

Bleaching procedure can also be combined with surgical operations (Fig. 17.4).

The skin color of the patient is important when laser treatment is performed. Since melanin pigment is greater in those with dark skin color, the absorption rate increases. Consequently, risks such as burns, scar development, and postinflammatory hyperpigmentation increase. Therefore, the amount of energy applied should be kept lower.

In bleaching therapies, when the density is intense (that is, distance of light beams is close to each other), the penetration of the energy to a very deep depth is not desired. Therefore, energy should generally remain low and density remain high. However, if the vulvar surface tightening and vulvar resurfacing are desired by increasing subcutaneous collagen, the opposite is applied; that is, the energy should be slightly higher and the density is lower.

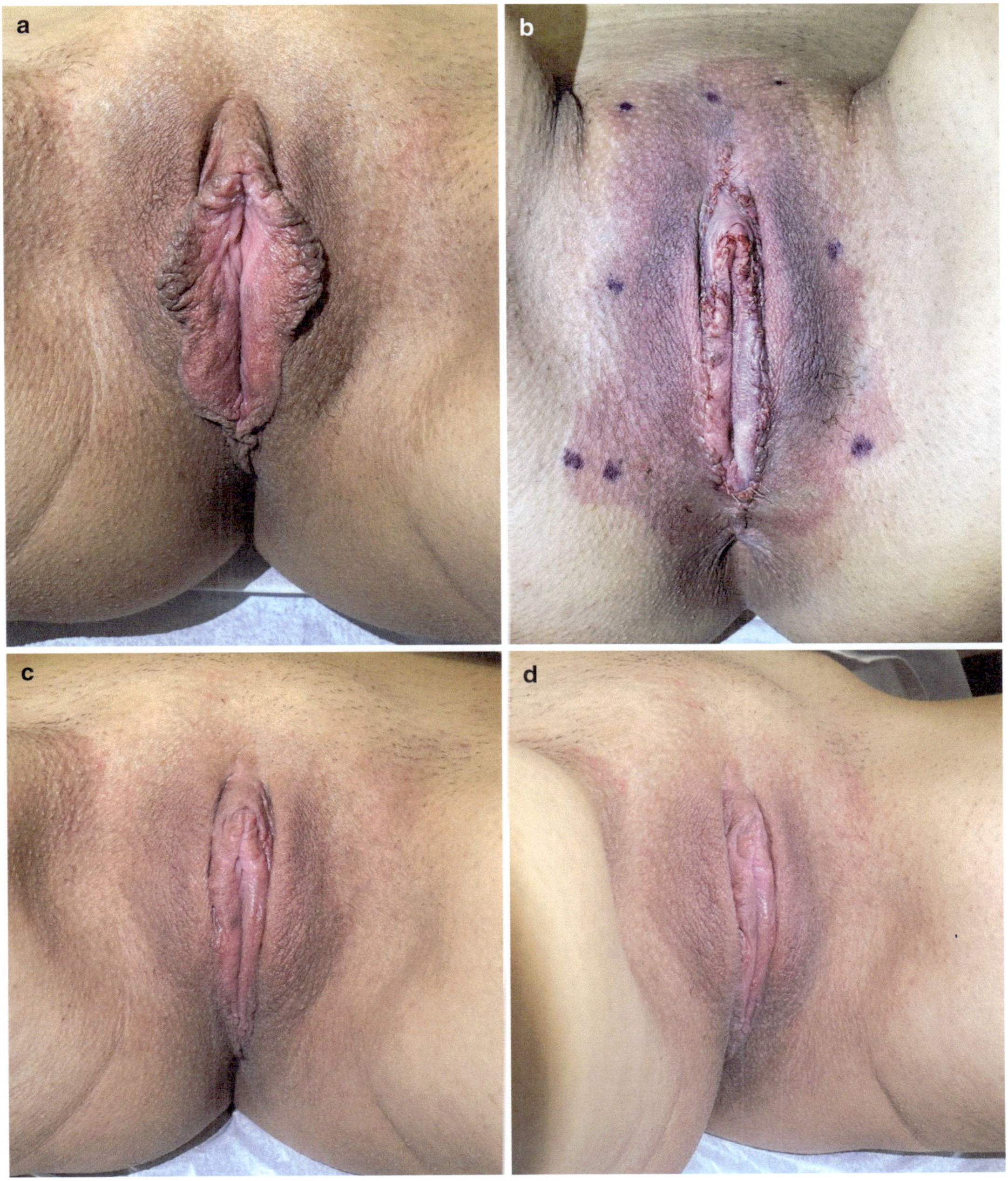

Fig. 17.4 Bleaching with laser and mesotherapy immediately after labiaplasty and hoodoplasty operations. Before (**a**); after labiaplasty, hoodoplasty, laser and mesotherapy bleaching procedures (**b**); two months after the operation (**c**, **d**)

17.4 Lasers with Q-switched Technique

Lasers with wavelengths between 400 and 1100 nm target the melanin chromophore. These wavelengths are visible in the electromagnetic spectrum and are compatible with near-infrared light. Although all lasers in this range are effective on melanin pigment, especially those in the green, red, and infrared bands are more effective. The only important criterion is not the wavelength of the light, but also the pulse duration and sufficient fluency. For example, green and blue light lasers cause more damage to the tissue with the long-pulsed continuous waves they emit. The Q-switched technique has enabled the production of Q-switched alexandrite, Q-switched ruby, and Q-switched Nd:YAG lasers.

Q-switched lasers are lasers that work with the selective photothermolysis principle without damaging the surrounding tissue with very short pulses such as 3–7 ns. In recent years, pico lasers with much shorter pulse duration have also been produced.

17.5 Post-procedure Term

After a few days following the bleaching process with carbon dioxide and erbium lasers, the epidermal skin becomes brown and then peels off spontaneously. The live, bright, and pinkish skin tissue from underneath will show a younger appearance. However, there are dermal pigment components and vascular structures other than those in the epidermis that give the skin its color. Therefore, the results obtained in all patients may not be equally satisfactory. It would be a correct approach to inform the patients that there will be 30–35% bleaching. Some mesotherapy products can also be applied intradermally in the same session to increase effectiveness.

It is normal to have complaints such as burning, itching, stinging, and pricking for a few weeks after the laser procedure. Topical anesthetics and cortisone-containing creams given after the procedure provide a more comfortable passage of this process. Collagen-containing soothing creams and moisturizers may also be recommended. Silver-containing creams used in burn treatment should be avoided. In addition, lightening creams can be started after 2–3 weeks. The final results are seen an average of 1 month after the procedure. A single session may be sufficient, or a total of 2–4 sessions can be performed every 1–2 months if necessary. Usually there is no need for a prohibition on sexual intercourse. The next day, the patient can take a shower with warm water and wash the genital area without rubbing it with soap. When necessary, paracetamol group drugs can be used as pain relief.

It is important to protect the area from the sun for a month after laser bleaching. For this reason, it is more appropriate to avoid performing the procedure in summer.

17.6 Contraindications

Laser treatments should not be applied in the following cases for vulvar bleaching:

- Presence of bacterial or viral genital infections
- Genital malignancy or suspected malignancy
- Pregnancy or breastfeeding period
- Impaired immune system
- Keloid history
- Use of isotretinoin in the last 12 months
- Scleroderma
- History of heavy radiation therapy
- Burns in the treatment area
- Photosensitivity
- Patients with psychiatric or mental problems
- Patients with overly high expectations
- Those with skin type VI

17.7 Complications

If the laser energy is set high during the bleaching procedures, it may cause complications such as permanent hypopigmentation, burns, scar formation, and postinflammatory hyperpigmentation. If the application is not made homogeneously, demarked areas such as "checkerboard" appearance may occur in the genital area (Fig. 17.5).

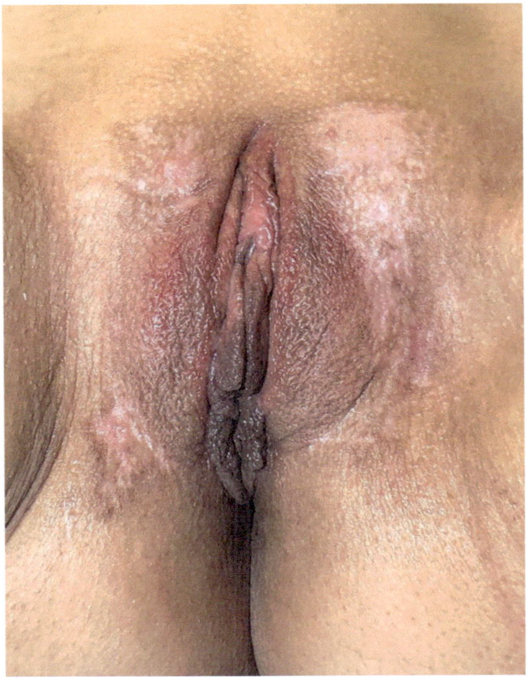

Fig. 17.5 Laser bleaching complication. Color contrasts that develop after application

17.8 Postinflammatory Hyperpigmentation (PIH)

Postinflammatory hyperpigmentation (PIH) is the darkening of the skin seen after all events that cause damage to the skin such as inflammation like infection, acne, eczema, technology-based skin treatments, chemicals, wax, and laser epilation. It may develop due to inflammation of the epidermal, dermal, or both areas. It is evaluated visually and with Wood's lamp, skin biopsy, and color scales.

Postinflammatory hyperpigmentation originating from epidermis can be in different color tones from light to dark brown. For first-line treatments, peeling-effective acidic solutions should be preferred. For this, 2% or 4% hydroquinone, which provides efficiency by inhibiting tyrosinase, Kligman formula (5% hydroxyquinone-0.1% tretinoin, 0.1% dexamethasone mixture), which was first developed in 1975, modified Kligman formula (4% hydroxyquinone-0.05% tretinoin), 0.01% fluocinolone acetonide mixture), and retinoids can be used. Retinoids increase the turnover of keratinocytes, decrease melanosome transfer, and act by inhibiting tyrosinase transcription. Retinoids have three forms: tretinoin, adapalene, and tazarotene. 50% glycolic acid or 20–30% salicylic acid can be applied in the second-step treatment of epidermal postinflammatory hyperpigmentation.

Postinflammatory hyperpigmentations of both epidermal and dermal origin are brown in color mixed with grayish black. In such darkening, first epidermal and then dermal treatment should be applied.

Q-switched 1064 Nd:YAG and 1550 nm erbium-doped lasers should be preferred in the treatment of blue-gray and black dermal-origin postinflammatory hyperpigmentations. Table 17.2 shows the options that can be used in treatment [2].

Table 17.2 Treatment strategies of PIH [2]

Causes of PIH:
Skin damage and prolonged inflammation
Infections, acne, eczema, technology-based skin treatments, chemicals, wax, laser epilation

↓

Diagnosis:
Anamnesis, examination, Wood's lamp, biopsy

TYPE	COLOR	TREATMENT
Epidermal PIH	Brown (from light to dark brown)	Acidic solutions
Both epidermal and dermal PIH	Brown in color mixed with grayish black	First acidic solutions, later laser treatments
Dermal PIH	Blue-gray and black	Q-switched 1064 Nd:YAG and 1550 nm Erbium-doped lasers

17.9 Other Methods Applied in Bleaching Treatment

There are products with different contents for bleaching purposes. Some of these include:

- *Trichloroacetic acid (TCA)*
- *Different chemical agents*
- *Ready-to-use solutions*
- *Injectable mesotherapy preparations*
- *Dermabrasion and microdermabrasion*
- PRP

17.9.1 Trichloroacetic Acid (TCA)

TCA is one of the peeling agents commonly used in dermatology. It provides rejuvenation under the skin by causing necrosis in the epidermis. TCA is especially used in the treatment of wrinkles, actinic keratosis, melasma, lentigo simplex, and acne scars. It also has an antiaging effect. It can be applied at a concentration of 20% in the genital area. Since excess remaining on the tissue will increase the irritation effect, the skin should be washed directly with saline after a short wait. Postinflammatory hyperpigmentation may occur if TCA is left on too long. It can be a suitable treatment alternative, especially for large anogenital hyperpigmentations (Fig. 17.6).

17.9.2 Different Chemical Agents

Lactic acid is an effective chemical agent in hydration, peeling, and bleaching of the skin. Thus, it increases the quality of the skin.

Azelaic acid has antimicrobial and keratolytic properties. It has antioxidant and bactericidal properties.

Mandelic acid has exfoliative, bactericidal, and moisturizing properties. Chemical peel applications can be done in 4–6 sessions every 15 days.

Advantageous aspects of chemical agents are that they can be used on all skin types, they can be applied to larger areas than laser, and there is no need for local anesthetics before the procedure. Patients can easily tolerate the erythema and desquamation that may occur after application.

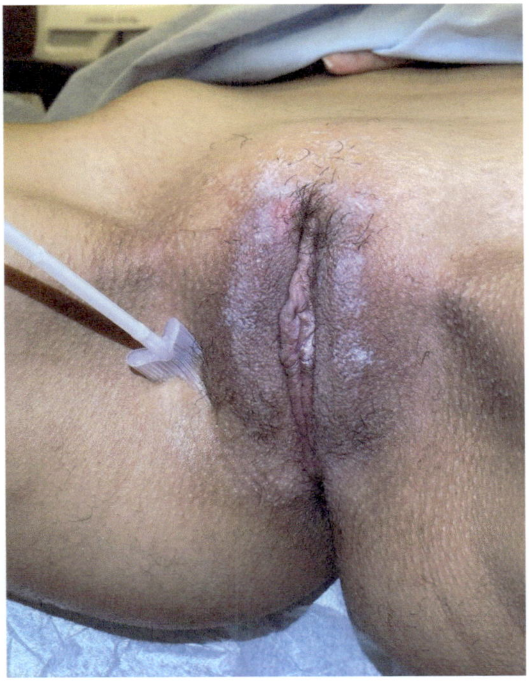

Fig. 17.6 Bleaching process with 20% of TCA. It can be done simply by applying the solution to the genital area with a disposable smear brush. When the burning sensation occurs, the area is washed with isotonic saline

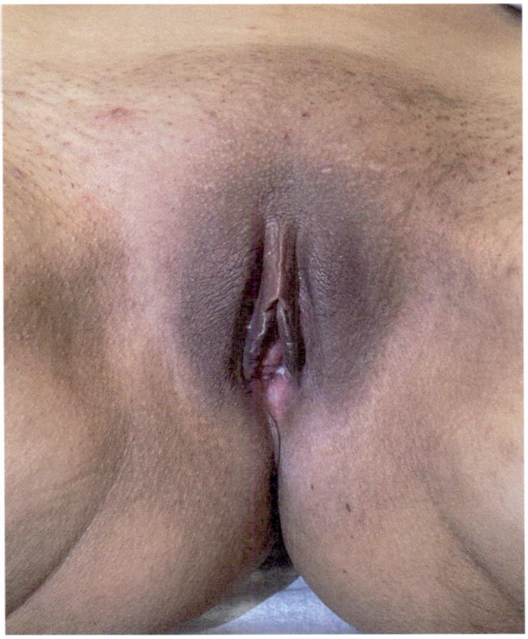

Fig. 17.7 Extensive hyperpigmentation

Chemical peeling applications may be considered in broad hyperpigmentations extending to the pubis and inner thighs (Fig. 17.7).

After the procedure, soap or creams should not be used for the first 24 h. Washing should only be done with water, and drying should be done with light touches without rubbing the area. Activities such as gymnastics and swimming should be delayed for 3–5 days. In addition, comfortable cotton and non-synthetic underwear should be preferred.

Another option for the treatments of wide hyperpigmentations and skin rejuvenation is dermamelan™ intimate (by Mesoestetic company). It is possible to have visible results by a single clinical session in labia majora, perianal area, mons pubis, inner thighs, and groins. The treatment is started at the clinic with the applications of peeling solution, and then mask cream, and after the area is covered with occlusive film the patient is discharged home. As home application regimen, she washes the area with lukewarm water 2 h later, applies crystal fiber intimate mask over the treated area for 10–15 min, and starts to use daily gel cream at nights 48 h after the end of the clinic treatment.

17.9.3 Ready-to-Use Solutions

There are also some products that can be used on the genital area in the clinic or by the patients themselves at home. Chloroacetic acid, kojic acid, rucinol, and glutathione in these products have lifting and bleaching properties. Ingredients such as papain, genistein, retinol (vitamin A), bisabolol, and licorice root extract have regenerating and soothing properties. A total of 4–6 sessions with an interval of 10 days are recommended for the desired results.

Hyperpigmentation treatment agents and mechanisms of actions are summarized in Table 17.3.

Table 17.3 Hyperpigmentation treatment options and mechanism of actions [1]

Treatment	Mechanism of action				
	Tyrosinase inhibition	Melanosome transfer inhibition	Increased epidermal turnover	Antioxidation	Other
Hydroquinone	•				
Mequinol	•				
Retinoic acid	•	•	•		
Azelaic acid	•				
Arbutin/deoxyarbutin	•				• Melanosome maturation inhibition
Licorice	•				
Kojic acid	• Interacts with copper				
Soy		• PAR-2 (Protease-activated receptor 2)			
Ascorbic acid (vitamin C)	• Interacts with copper			•	
Niacinamide		•			
N-acetyl glucosamine	•				
Aloesin	•				
Mulberry				•	
Rucinol	•				
Emblica	•			•	
Pycnogenol				•	
Mulberry	•			•	
Coffeeberry				•	
Green tea	•			•	
Silymarin	•			•	
Grape seed extract				•	
Orchid				•	
Belides		•		•	
Tranexamic acid				• Inhibits UV-induced plasmin activity in keratinocytes	•
Polypodium leucotomos				•	
Glutathione	•			•	
Chemical peel			•		
Dermabrasion			•		
Pigmented-specific laser					• Destroys melanin

17.9.4 Injectable Mesotherapy Preparations

Mesotherapy preparations containing products such as vitamin C, glutathione, and tranexamic acid can be applied intradermally with 30G mesotherapy needles without going too deep. In order to achieve the desired color change, generally 3–5 applications with 10–14 day intervals are required (Fig. 17.8).

17.9.5 Dermabrasion: Microdermabrasion

This is the process of mechanically peeling the damaged or hyperpigmented areas of the skin by means of a fast rotating device. It is also used in acne scars, wrinkles, and melasma treatments.

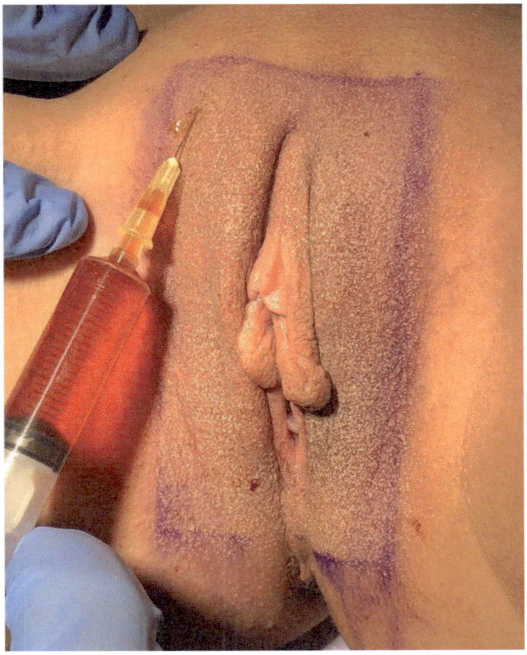

Fig. 17.8 Bleaching with mesotherapy. This is done by creating intradermal papules without going deep into the skin tissue. It can also be applied in the same session with laser treatment

17.9.6 PRP

PRP can be applied for both regeneration and bleaching of the skin due to its growth factor content. However, the bleaching effect is limited.

Appendix

With the purchase of this book, you can use our "SN Flashcards" app to access questions free of charge in order to test your learning and check your understanding of the contents of the book.

To use the app, please follow the instructions below:

1. Go to https://flashcards.springernature.com/login
2. Create a user account by entering your e-mail address and assigning a password.
3. Use the following link to access your SN Flashcards set: ▶ https://sn.pub/tvlq7Q

If the link is missing or does not work, please send an e-mail with the subject "SN Flashcards" and the book title to customerservice@springernature.com.

References

1. Sachdeva S. Fitzpatrick skin typing: applications in dermatology. Indian J Dermatol Venereol Leprol. 2009;75(1):93–6.
2. Chaowattanapanit S, Silpa-Archa N, Kohli I, Lim HW, Hamzavi I. Postinflammatory hyperpigmentation: a comprehensive overview: treatment options and prevention. J Am Acad Dermatol. 2017;77(4):607–21.

18 Genital Radiofrequency Applications

The good physician treats the disease; the great physician treats the patient who has the disease

Sir William Osler

Vaginal rejuvenation (VR) includes all applications that include optimal repair and correction of the vagina and adjacent organs, both aesthetically and functionally. Transferred by Arabic medicine into Western Europe, the concept of VR first defined in the texts "*On Treatments for Women*" written by Trotula (Trota of Salerno) in 12th century as the suturation of postpartum lacerations, restoring virginity and treatment of leaky bladder [1].

18.1 Increasing Trend in Vaginal Rejuvenation

Nowadays, more than 20 million women worldwide are faced with pelvic organ prolapse, birth ruptures, and incontinence problems with the prolongation of life expectancy. Vaginal relaxation syndrome and vulvovaginal laxity usually occur as a result of vaginal delivery, aging, and atrophy. Such problems bring along sexual problems and self-esteem problems as well as functional problems in women. A study conducted by the International Urogynecology Association in 2012 showed that 84% of physicians believed that vaginal laxity was not reported, and 95% thought that the increase in laxity negatively affected sexual function [2]. In the ACOG Bulletin, it was stated that 40% of women experience psychological problems due to their sexual problems, and only 14% of them talked to their physicians [3]. These issues, which women avoided even talking to their physicians about in past and were regarded as taboo, have become more easily shared today. Public awareness programs, physician training, and media played major roles in removing such barriers in communication.

Today, laser, radiofrequency, and HIFU are among the most frequently used non-invasive energy-based treatments for VR as alternatives to surgery. Although these technologies are completely different from each other, their main purpose is the same: to initiate the healing process by creating temporary thermal damage to the tissue. All these technologies are very old. The reliability of these methods, which have been used in the field of cosmetic dermatology for years, has also been proven by many scientific studies in this field. However, it has only been since the early 2010s that the vaginal and vulvar probes of these devices were developed and found a place in the field of cosmetic gynecology. Despite many positive results, evidence-based studies are

S. Eserdağ, *Aesthetic and Functional Female Genital Surgery*,
https://doi.org/10.1007/978-3-031-16019-6_18

still inadequate. For this reason, energy-based device applications such as vaginal laser and radiofrequency, whose use is increasingly common every year, still do not have FDA approval for the genital area.

18.2 Radiofrequency (RF) Technology

Radiofrequency is a technology that creates a thermal effect on tissue, just like laser. The name radiofrequency comes from being in the same wave frequency range as radio and TV. The energy produced is non-ionizing electromagnetic current with a frequency between 3 KHz and 300 GHz. The encounter of current with resistance from the tissue is called impedance. Thus, heat is generated and electric current transforms into thermal energy. The more impedance and electric current in the target tissue, the more energy is generated. Tissues with high impedance, such as subcutaneous adipose tissue, produce more energy and have deeper thermal effects. Unlike laser light, there is neither diffraction nor chromophore absorption in the tissue. Therefore, RF can be applied on all skin types. In cosmetic dermatology, frequencies between 0.5 and 40 MHz are generally preferred for skin rejuvenation [4].

The indications in RF applications often coincide with the laser indications. Unlike laser, RF does not have bleaching effect in the genital area. Genital RF treatments are mostly performed for SUI treatment and vaginal rejuvenation. Studies have shown that non-ablative RF can be used in tightening the vaginal canal [5, 6]. In addition, it has indication areas such as increasing sexual pleasure, facilitating orgasm function, and symptomatic treatment of genitourinary syndrome (GSM) due to menopause. In a study conducted by Red Alinsod, improvement in vaginal laxity, sexual satisfaction, atrophy, orgasm problems, and SUI symptoms were found after RF treatment [7].

RF is also used in the treatment of vaginal dryness and symptomatic treatment of genital lichen sclerosus disease and vulvar vestibulitis, especially in patients whose use of estrogen is contraindicated during menopause.

Different devices have been produced by combining RF technology with many different technologies for skin rejuvenation. Monopolar (unipolar) RF devices are generally used in cosmetic gynecology. However, especially in recent years, bipolar and tripolar devices have also been produced. Deka Company succeeded in producing a device that combines CO_2 laser and bipolar RF technologies.

18.3 Mechanism of Action

After the electric current produced in the device spreads into the tissue through the probe, it encounters water in the dermis and turns into thermal energy, with a warming up to 45 °C occurring in the tissue. The resulting thermal energy initiates a tissue regeneration and repair process, just like laser. Unlike laser, it reaches deeper, i.e., subcutaneous tissue, and does not create ablation.

Genital RF can also be applied to the vulva. By increasing collagen connective tissue synthesis, it can reduce wrinkles and smooth the surface. It is completely non-invasive and non-ablative. Sexual intercourse is not prohibited after the procedure. It does not require anesthesia and there is no need for rest. RF devices can also be used for lipolysis in the vulva and mons pubis due to their deep penetration properties. Since RF does not work based on light like laser devices, the skin color and skin type of the person are not important in dose adjustment. Another advantage is that most of these devices are portable. In addition, the comfortable manipulable probe arms provide convenience to the practitioner. Thin probe structures can also be tolerated more easily by patients (Fig. 18.1).

In monopolar radiofrequencies, the electromagnetic current is between the probe and the ground line, while in bipolar radiofrequency it is between two poles.

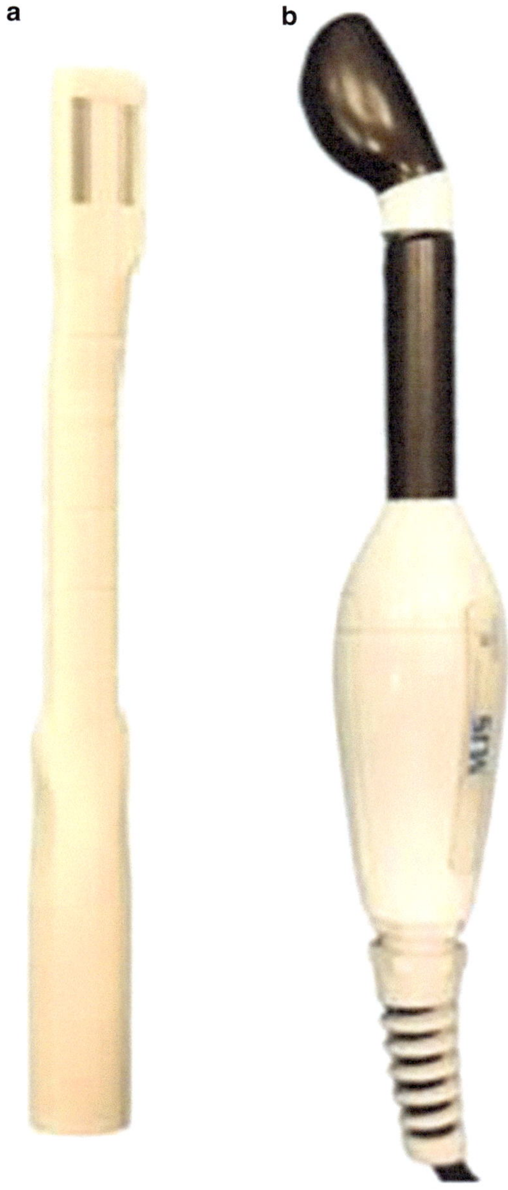

Fig. 18.1 RF probes; bipolar (**a**) and monopolar (**b**)

18.4 Indications for Use in Gynecology and Dermatology

Radiofrequency devices are used in the genital area for different functional and aesthetic indications.

Functional indications:

- Stress urinary incontinence (SUI) treatment in patients without prolapse,
- Vaginal rejuvenation treatments,
- Increasing sexual pleasure,
- Increasing orgasm function,
- Symptomatic treatment of menopausal genito-urinary syndrome,
- Vaginal dryness treatment, and
- Symptomatic treatment of genital lichen sclerosus disease.

Tadir et al. specifically demonstrated that the formation of new elastin after RF treatment helps in the treatment of vaginal laxity [8]. The increase in glycogen content was also shown histologically in the same study.

Aesthetic indications:

- Labia majora and perineal tightening and resurfacing,
- Scar treatments,
- Vascular lesion treatments,
- Acne vulgaris treatment, and
- Facial rejuvenation (antiaging, treatment of wrinkles and pores, lifting)

The RF devices have been used in cosmetic dermatology since the 2000s and in cosmetic gynecology since the early 2010s.

18.5 Some RF Devices on the Market

Genital RF devices have different models just like laser devices (Table 18.1).

There is a thermometer at the probe tip of the ThermiVa™ RF device, and the device adjusts its own temperature (Transcutaneous Temperature Controlled RF) (Fig. 18.2). A temperature of 42–46 °C should generally be reached for the effectiveness of the process. For vaginal rejuvenation, the treatment of each vaginal wall takes an average of five minutes, so that the four vaginal walls and introitus are scanned over a total of 20 min. In the external genitalia, the probe, moving in the style of "*painting with a brush on a canvas*" is circulated over the labia majora, minora, clitoral area, vestibulum, and perineum. Each side is treated for 5 min, so one-session treatment of the entire vulva takes up to ten minutes in total.

Table 18.1 Some RF devices used for genital rejuvenation

Device name/company	Device type	Treatment protocol
ThermiVa™ (Thermiaesthetics)	Temperature-controlled RF	3 treatments every 4–6 weeks
Viveve™ (Viveve Medical)	One-session monopolar RF with surface cooling	1 treatment
Venus Fiore™ (Venus Concept)	Multipolar RF with pulsed electromagnetic field	3 treatments per week
ReVive™ (Viora)	Bipolar RF	4–6 treatments every 2–3 weeks
Protégé Intima™ (BTL Aesthetics)	Focused RF	2–4 treatments every 2–3 weeks
Pellevé™ (Ellman International)	Monopolar RF	3 treatments every 2–3 weeks
Votiva™ (Inmode)	Bipolar RF	3 treatments every 2–4 weeks
C500 Urogyne™ (Capenergy)	Monopolar RF (tecartherapy-diathermy)	4–6 treatments per week

The C500 Urogyne™ device can operate at three different frequencies (0.8, 1.0, and 1.2 MHz) that can be adjusted manually to maximize tissue absorption. The efficiency of RF increases as the absorption of energy by the tissue increases, just like in laser. With the different probe heads for the C500 device, it can be applied both inside the vagina and on the vulva. It is mostly used for stress urinary incontinence, vulvovaginal rejuvenation, and sexual enhancement indications in women. There is also a thin probe developed for anal incontinence treatment. Intracavitary (vaginal and anal) probes have a temperature sensor. It can also be used in incontinence treatments after prostatectomy surgeries in men (Fig. 18.3).

In monopolar radiofrequency devices, as the amount of energy and frequency increases, the tissue penetration depth also increases. While

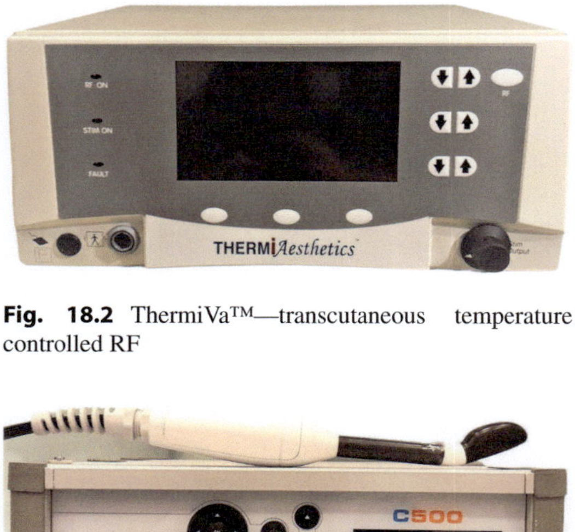

Fig. 18.2 ThermiVa™—transcutaneous temperature controlled RF

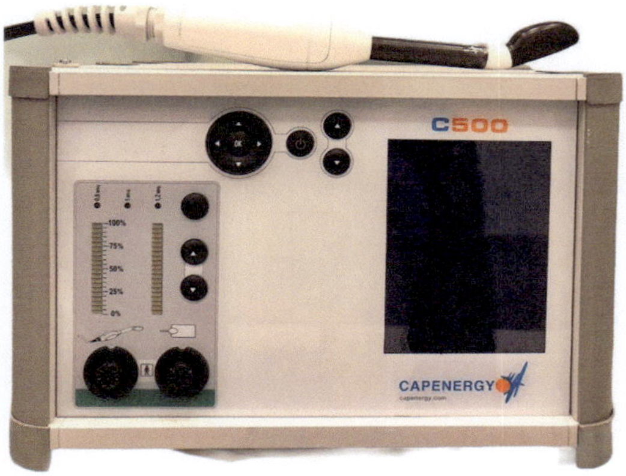

Fig. 18.3 C 500 Urogyne™—monopolar non-ablative RF device

low frequency can only pass through connective tissue, high frequency can emit electromagnetic transmission to all cells of the body. The frequency that penetrates the cell membrane is 1 MHz. As the surface area increases, the amount of energy dispersed also increases.

Surface-cooled, single-session monopolar radiofrequency technology called Viveve™ has also entered the market. Thanks to the cooling system on the probe tip, this technology can provide a high amount of energy such as 90 J/cm^2 to the tissue, and this energy can be reduced to a depth of 3–4 mm, and a high thermal efficiency can be created. It has indications such as increasing sexual pleasure, improving orgasm function, treating vaginal laxity, and SUI. This one-session treatment, which is quite safe, painless, and non-ablative, takes about 30 min on average. The effect continues for 12 months.

The DEKA Company was able to integrate bipolar vaginal RF into the SmartXide™ laser produced for the MonaLisa Touch technique in 2020 (Fig. 18.4).

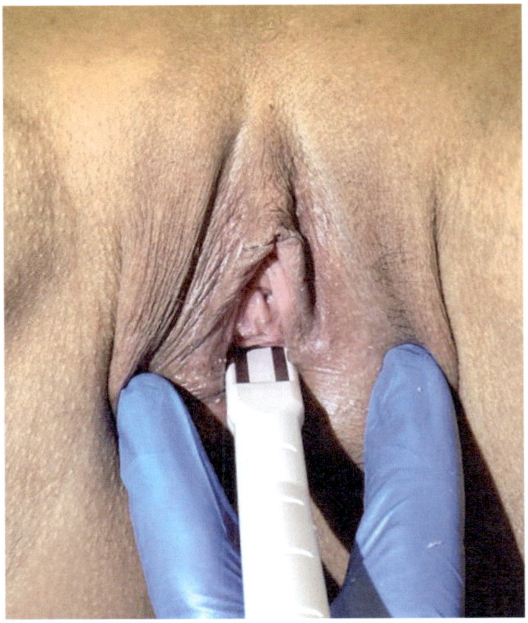

Fig. 18.4 Bipolar vaginal RF application of SmartXide™ laser to anterior vaginal wall for SUI treatment

18.6 Genital RF Contraindications

Genital RF is not recommended in the following situations:

- Moderate and severe POP cases
- Pregnancy
- Puerperium

It can be applied from the third month after birth. It can be applied during breastfeeding.

- Menstruation period

It is not applied during menstruation due to the risk of infections.

- Active HPV or HSV presence

It is not applied in the presence of active HPV or HSV, as it may increase the spread of the infection. It is not applied in other active genital infections.

- Body dysmorphic disorder (BDD)

As stated in the ACOG bulletin, these patients may have different emotional changes after surgery. In addition, as the expectations of patients with BDD about the procedure to be performed can be very high, dissatisfaction rates after the procedure are also high.

- Psychiatric or serious psychological disturbances

It is not recommended for situations such as depression, anxiety, OCD (obsessive-compulsive disorder), or psychosis.

- Mentally disabled

All aesthetic operations are contraindicated for mentally disabled people.

- Abnormal Pap smear

Table 18.2 Comparison of laser and radiofrequency procedures

Comparison	Vaginal laser	Radiofrequency (RF)
Application	Easy	Very easy
Ablation	CO_2 lasers ablative, Er:YAG lasers non-ablative	Non-ablative
Severity of pain	(±)	(−)
Anesthesia	Sometimes anesthetic cream to the introitus	(−)
Penetration	Epidermis	Subcutaneous tissue
Temperature	50–65 °C (higher in CO_2 lasers)	40–45 °C
Mechanism	Amplified light	Electrical current
Vaginal tightening and SUI treatment effectiveness	(+)	(+)
Treatment protocol	3 sessions every 1–2 months	3–6 sessions with 1–4 week intervals
Sexual abstinence	7 days	No restrictions
Return to activities	The same day	The same day
Vulvar bleaching	(+)	(−)
Vulvar rejuvenation	(+)	(+)
Probe	Thick/somewhat laborious to manipulate	Thin/easy to manipulate

It is contraindicated in patients with abnormal cellular pathology in the cervix and vagina.

- Cancer or suspected cancer

It is not applied in genital cancer or in precancerous cases that are not fully diagnosed.

- Pacemaker use
- Patients with overly high expectations

Insecure patients with high expectations can also have a very low satisfaction level.

There is no need to remove the IUD before the procedure for those who use IUD.

Genital radiofrequency devices are similar to vaginal lasers in many ways in terms of usage indications, contraindications, and patient profiles (compared in Table 18.2).

18.7 Preparation

It will be beneficial for all patients who come for vaginal tightening and/or SUI treatment to undergo gynecological examination and transvaginal ultrasound evaluation before the procedure. There should be no suspicion of malignancy in patients to be treated. Patients with signs of vaginitis or cervicitis in their gynecological examination should first be treated for infections. In addition, there should be no cellular abnormality in the smear tests performed in the last year. In those who do not have a smear test within a year, it should be performed before the procedure.

Monopolar devices are generally preferred in RF treatments. Therefore, a grounding plate is placed on an area of the patient's body (usually on pelvic area or below the waist). In order to avoid burns, the grounding plate should have full skin contact.

Many RF companies have produced single-use probe covers for vaginal applications. In some, the probes allow for a certain number of applications. Thus, consumables expenditure affects costs. However, it is possible to cover the probe by a condom in some companies' RF devices.

Physicians, nurses, or physiotherapists trained in this area can perform genital RF procedures. If the treatment is to be carried out by a male physician or health care staff, it is recommended a female assistant to accompany him.

18.8 Performing Genital RF Treatments

Anesthesia is not required as it is a completely painless procedure. First, a speculum is attached and vaginal discharge is cleaned with dry gauze. The probe with its protective cover is inserted into the vagina by applying a little ultrasound gel. By moving the probe continuously posterior and anterior, left and right inside the vagina, each wall of the vagina is scanned equally for five minutes. Thus, the rejuvenation of the whole vagina ends in an average of 20 min. Those with SUI problems should have more scans on the anterior wall. The increase in the intra-tissue temperature during the procedure can be monitored on the temperature gauge of the device. Temperatures of 40 °C and above can be felt by the patient. Since the patient will experience a burning sensation above 44–45 °C, the energy is reduced to a tolerable level. Feedback from the patient is important in temperature adjustment.

For patients who demand vulvar tightening and wrinkle treatment, a total of ten minutes of application, 5 min to each labia, is sufficient with the help of different heads. This application can be done in the same session as vaginal rejuvenation. Thus, the entire vulvovaginal treatment will be completed in 30 min.

In cases of sexual pleasure and orgasm problems, the entire vulva and vagina should be scanned, with emphasis on the clitoral area, vulvar vestibulum, and anterior vagina. Gel should be applied to ensure lubricity in all internal and external genital applications.

18.9 Effects on Orgasmic Function

Orgasmic function is a complex event associated with central, peripheral, and environmental factors. The inability of the person to reach orgasm despite sexual stimulation or having difficulty reaching orgasm is described as "anorgasmia" or "orgasmic dysfunction." This situation can be a source of distress in the person herself or in her relationship with her partner.

Problems that need to be solved in anorgasmia are intertwined just like in other sexual dysfunctions. A holistic approach to all sexual dysfunctions is important, according to the biopsychosocial model defined by Rosen et al. [9]. All of the biological, psychological, sociocultural, and interpersonal factors should be addressed one by one (Fig. 18.5).

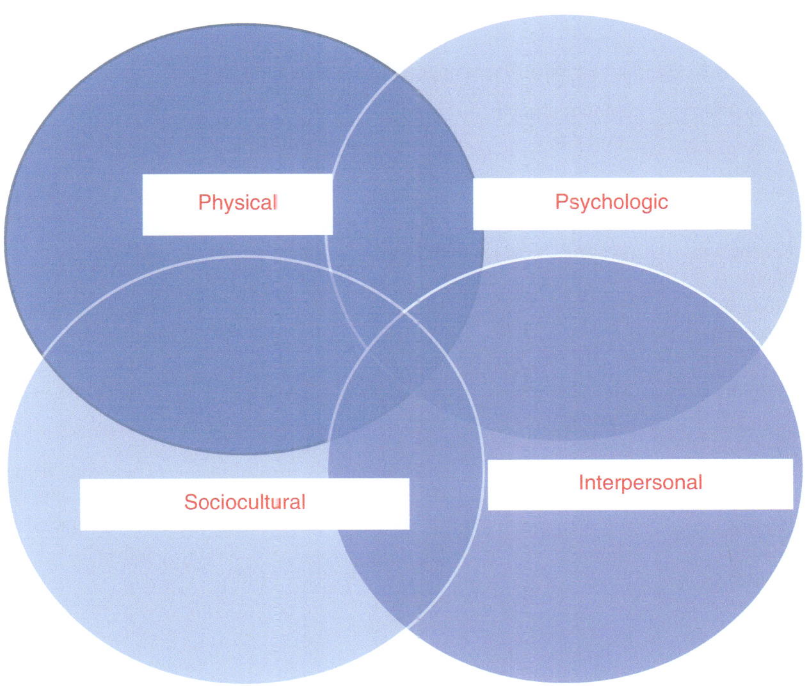

Fig. 18.5 Biopsychosocial model

While some women cannot reach orgasm in any way by sexual intercourse or stimulation of the clitoris by masturbation, some can experience orgasm only by masturbation. Inability to orgasm in any way is usually due to lack of knowledge and experience, not being able to explore the body adequately, and different psychological factors from early childhood. Patients with coital and clitoral anorgasmia can go a long way with the given sexual therapies.

Patients who can orgasm with clitoral stimulation by themselves or with their partner, but who cannot orgasm in any way during sexual intercourse with their partner or who have difficulty are in the group of "coital anorgasmia." In the treatment of these patients, in addition to sexual therapies, stimulation of collagen production with energy-based non-invasive methods, increasing clitoral blood flow, and increasing neural sensitivity of the genital area may also be beneficial. The aim is to treat primarily the biological component in the biopsychosocial model. Energy-based or regenerative treatments such as laser, radiofrequency, HIFU, and stem cell applications are still waiting to be discovered.

In a study conducted in 2016, 25 women with orgasm problems between the ages of 21 and 65 years underwent monopolar RF treatment across the vagina and vulva three times at intervals of 1 month, and in later consultations, it was observed that the time to orgasm in patients was shortened by 50% [7].

Energy-based treatments have positive effects on sexual pleasure, arousal, lubrication, and reducing sexual pain.

In a prospective, multicenter, randomized, and controlled study (VIVEVE I), it was shown that the vaginal laxity levels and sexual functions of the patients in the study group improved significantly compared to the control group [10].

Vaseline is preferred as a lubricant in the applications of CO_2 and Erbium:YAG laser in the vaginal and vulvar area, and water-based gels are preferred for radiofrequency. In the table below, different energy-based technologies are compared (Table 18.3).

Table 18.3 Comparison of different energy-based technologies

Comparison	Monopolar RF	Bipolar RF	CO_2 laser	Er:YAG laser
Size	Portable	Usually not portable	Large, not portable	Large, not portable
Probe size	Disposable, small, ergonomic	Long and thick for vagina, small for introitus	Larger, with special cover	Larger, with special cover
Penetration depth	4 mm	0.5 mm	0.6 mm	0.2 mm
Protective equipment	No need	No need	Goggles, mask, and garment	Goggles, mask, and garment
Sessions	3–4 sessions a month	4–6 sessions, 2–3 weeks apart	3 sessions, 1–1.5 months apart	Protocol varies by device
Pain degree and anesthesia	(−) No pain and no anesthesia	(+) May be slightly painful in introitus, anesthetic cream can be applied	(++) There may be pain in introitus, anesthetic cream can be applied	(−) There is little to no pain
Sexual abstinence	No	No	7 days	3 days

18.10 Histological Studies

According to the results of a recent study, an increase in small nerve fibers was observed after RF treatments [11]. In a biopsy study, Leibaschoff et al. showed that neocollagenesis and neoelastogenesis increased in the submucosa after RF treatments [12].

18.11 Combined Procedures

RF rejuvenation can be performed simultaneously with all genital surgical procedures. It can also be combined with genital PRP for sexual enhancement. In such a combined treatment, first RF and then PRP injections should be performed.

Laser-PRP or RF-PRP combined regimes give very successful results for the treatment of lichen sclerosus et atrophicus disease.

Energy-based treatments such as laser and RF can be applied in some patients to relieve the complaints of vaginal dryness and dyspareunia that may develop after vaginoplasty operations. These treatments also increase the elasticity of the skin. Unlike vaginoplasty, the ability to treat all vaginal walls is also advantageous.

18.12 Complications

No major complications were observed after RF. In cases where the application is long, mild redness, blistering, and edema may be seen in the vestibular area. If the grounding plate is not fully contacted with the skin and the patient is under anesthesia due to a different surgical procedure, up to third degree burns may occur.

18.13 Post-procedure Term

The procedure is completely non-invasive and is referred to as a "*lunch time management*." Patients can return to their social life immediately after the treatment without downtime. Since it is non-ablative, there is no restriction for the intercourse on the same day. It is normal to have clear vaginal discharge in the first few days after the application. In addition, it is beneficial to recommend pelvic floor muscle exercises to patients. The desired tightening, lubrication, and pleasure effects begin three weeks after the treatment.

In order to relieve the concerns, it is beneficial to give the patients a written paper stating the expected situations and what to do after the procedure.

Appendix

With the purchase of this book, you can use our "SN Flashcards" app to access questions free of charge in order to test your learning and check your understanding of the contents of the book.

To use the app, please follow the instructions below:

1. Go to https://flashcards.springernature.com/login
2. Create a user account by entering your e-mail address and assigning a password.
3. Use the following link to access your SN Flashcards set: ▶ https://sn.pub/tvlq7Q

If the link is missing or does not work, please send an e-mail with the subject "SN Flashcards" and the book title to customerservice@springernature.com.

References

1. Desai SA, Kroumpouzos G, Sadick N. Vaginal rejuvenation: From scalpel to wands. Int J Womens Dermatol. 2019;5(2):79–84.
2. Pauls RN, Fellner AN, Davila GW. Vaginal laxity: a poorly understood quality of life problem; a survey of physician members of the International Urogynecological Association (IUGA). Int Urogynecol J. 2012;23(10):1435–48.
3. ACOG. ACOG practice bulletin No. 119: female sexual dysfunction. Obstet Gynecol. 2011;117(4):996–1007.
4. Görgü M, Gökkaya A, Kızılkan J, Karanfil E, Doğan A. Radiofrequency: review of literature. Turk Plast. 2019;27(2):62–72.

5. Dillon B, Dmochowski R. Radiofrequency for the treatment of stress urinary incontinence in women. Curr Urol Rep. 2009;10(5):369–74.
6. Sadick NS, Malerich SA, Nassar AH, Dorizas AS. Radiofrequency: an update on latest innovations. J Drugs Dermatol. 2014;13(11):1331–5.
7. Alinsod RM. Transcutaneous temperature controlled radiofrequency for orgasmic dysfunction. Lasers Surg Med. 2016;48(7):641–5.
8. Tadir Y, Gaspar A, Lev-Sagie A, Alexiades M, Alinsod R, Bader A, Calligaro A, Elias JA, Gambaciani M, Gaviria JE, Iglesia CB, Selih-Martinec K, Mwesigwa PL, Ogrinc UB, Salvatore S, Scollo P, Zerbinati N, Nelson JS. Light and energy based therapeutics for genitourinary syndrome of menopause: consensus and controversies. Lasers Surg Med. 2017;49(2):137–59.
9. Rosen R, Brown C, Heiman J, Leiblum S, Meston C, Shabsigh R, Ferguson D, D'Agostino R Jr. The female sexual function index (FSFI): a multidimensional self-report instrument for the assessment of female sexual function. J Sex Marital Ther. 2000;26(2):191–208.
10. Krychman M, Rowan CG, Allan BB, DeRogatis L, Durbin S, Yacoubian A, Wilkerson D. Effect of single-treatment, surface-cooled radiofrequency therapy on vaginal laxity and female sexual function: the VIVEVE I randomized controlled trial. J Sex Med. 2017;14(2):215–25.
11. Gold M, Andriessen A, Bader A, Alinsod R, French ES, Guerette N, Kolodchenko Y, Krychman M, Murrmann S, Samuels J. Review and clinical experience exploring evidence, clinical efficacy, and safety regarding nonsurgical treatment of feminine rejuvenation. J Cosmet Dermatol. 2018;17(3):289–97.
12. Leibaschoff G, Izasa PG, Cardona JL, Miklos JR, Moore RD. Transcutaneous temperature controlled radiofrequency (TTCRF) for the treatment of menopausal vaginal/genitourinary symptoms. Surg Technol Int. 2016;29:149–59.

19 G-Spot Augmentation by Hyaluronic Acid

No, science is not a dream; but it's a dream to think we'll find what he didn't give us somewhere else.

Sigmund Freud

For centuries, there has been mention of the existence of an important region of high erotic sensitivity and engagement in the anterior vaginal wall. Although a large survey has shown that 84% of women believe there is such a sensitive area in their vagina [1], G-spot still remains as an "*anatomical UFO*."

19.1 Historical Background

This area on the anterior vaginal wall, close to the bladder and urethra, between the pelvic bone and cervix, is sensitive to mechanical stimulation. This erogenous zone of 1–2 cm was first described in 1950 by the German gynecologist Dr. Ernst Gräfenberg. He notified these sentences in his article "*Innumerable erotogenic spots are distributed all over the body, from where sexual satisfaction can be elicited; these are so many that we can almost say that there is no part of the female body which does not give sexual response, the partner has only to find the erotogenic zones… An erotic zone always could be demonstrated on the anterior wall of the vagina along the course of the urethra. Even when there was a good response in the entire vagina, this particular area was more easily stimulated by the finger than the other areas of the vagina… During orgasm this area is pressed downwards against the finger like a small cystocele protruding into the vaginal canal… Analogous to the male urethra, the female urethra also seems to be surrounded by erectile tissues like the corpora cavernosa. In the course of sexual stimulation, the female urethra begins to enlarge and can be felt easily. It swells out greatly at the end of orgasm. The most stimulating part is located at the posterior urethra, where it arises from the neck of the bladder…*"

"G-spot" (Gräfenberg spot) is a term meaning "erotic sensitive zone" first used in 1981 by Dr. Addiego and Nurse Whipple, 24 years after the death of Dr. Gräfenberg. While the correct terminology should be a G-zone (or G-area), generally the term of G-spot is used, and so we chose to use the same terminology in this book. Another interesting issue is that this region was first identified by Reignier deGraff in the seventeenth century. DeGraff defined this area as the "female prostate" or "corpus glandulosum."

In his article, Addiego found that the digital palpation of the anterior vaginal wall of a multiparous patient who presented with the complaint of urinary incontinence and had mild

S. Eserdağ, *Aesthetic and Functional Female Genital Surgery*,
https://doi.org/10.1007/978-3-031-16019-6_19

cystocele had a feeling of urine first, and then a feeling of pleasure, and simultaneously this area grew by 50% on examination [2]. Addiego et al. defined the term "female orgasm" as a sudden discharge from the urethra, and they thought that the glands and ducts around the urethra were homologous to the male prostate.

In 1981, Perry and Whipple defended the hypothesis that women who ejaculate during orgasm under voluntary control have stronger pelvic muscle contraction than those who do not. According to them, female ejaculation was a component of the uterine orgasm [3].

19.2 Scientific Data

Opinions about female ejaculation are quite contradictory physiologically. In 2009, Shafik et al., in the results of their study involving 38 patients, argued that ejaculation did not accompany female orgasm.

Skene's glands secrete some fluid by activating sexual stimulation and especially orgasm. The rapid discharge of this fluid is called ejaculation. However, the relationship between female ejaculation and the G-spot is not clear. Their only relationship is that G-spot and Skene's glands are anatomically close to each other. Also, there is no receptor on the Skene's glands to transmit sensory nerves. According to many studies, Skene's glands in the periurethral region in women are analogous to the prostate gland in men, and they drain their secretions into the urethra through their long duct. Conversely, the fluid that spreads during orgasm has all the biochemical properties of prostate fluid. In 2001, the Anatomical Terminology Federative Committee acknowledged that the term female prostate can also be used instead of the Skene's gland.

Skene's glands are located in the urethral sponge surrounding the urethra. This spongy region surrounding the urethra is a tissue rich in sensitive nerve endings, located between the pubic bone and the vagina. The urethral sponge also surrounds the clitoral nerves. Therefore, during sexual intercourse, especially in positions where the man is behind the woman, the urethral sponge and clitoral nerve endings on the anterior wall can be stimulated more intensely. The G-spot is also located in the urethral sponge area.

Shafic et al. demonstrated the presence of a pacemaker in the anterior distal vaginal wall in their electrovaginogram in vivo study. This region in the anterior distal vaginal wall produced low voltage electrical waves. In addition, increased pressure on the anterior vaginal wall increased pacemaker activity and caused vaginal muscle contraction. According to the study results, it was a small, erotic sensitive area in the vagina with a pacemaker feature (i.e., G-spot) [4].

In another study, blood flow in the vaginal wall increased during sexual arousal [5]. Some women report that the sensations of clitoral orgasm and intravaginal (G-spot) orgasm are different. While it is claimed that the G-spot orgasm is felt deeper into the body, a feeling similar to the Valsalva maneuver occurs and the cervix exerts pressure on the vagina; in clitoral orgasm, mostly the distal of the vagina becomes balloon-like (swells). Many women experience mixed orgasm with both vaginal and clitoral stimulation. Also, not every woman likes stimulation of the anterior vaginal wall.

Ostrzenski claimed to have discovered the existence of the anatomical structure of the G-spot in 2011 and published histological findings in 2012 [6]. However, Ostrzenski, who defines the G-spot as a new anatomical discovery, has been the target of many different criticisms. In his article, the G-spot on an 83-year-old cadaver was defined as a sac with a wall resembling fibroconnective tissues, easily observed and with clear borders. However, this article lacks a study of histological sampling.

The G-Spot International Working Group confirmed the anatomical existence of the G-spot and published its data in 2014 by discovering its microscopic features separating it from the vaginal wall [6].

In another fresh female cadaver study, Ostrzenski also stated that making natural or artificial fillers here may be harmful due to the anatomical role of the G-spot in anterior vaginal engagement [7]. In a series of three patients published in 2018, Ostrzenski stated that repairing the anterior vaginal wall with a simple surgical method called "G-spotplasty" increases sexual activity, sexual behavior, and sexual interest [8].

Ting Li et al. took biopsies from different parts of the vagina and examined them histomorphologically. They observed that the distal 1/3 of the vagina was significantly richer in nerve and microvessel density, and they associated this with the histomorphological basis of the G-spot [9].

19.3 Conflicting Thoughts

Buisson et al. showed that the clitoral body descends and closes the distal anterior vaginal wall by contractions of the levator muscles during sexual stimulation.

Alzate et al. showed that orgasm can occur with manual stimulation of the posterior vaginal wall [10].

In many ultrasound and MRI scans, an anatomical region that could be the G-spot was not detected. In a single study, Jannini et al. found that women with vaginal orgasm had a thicker urethravaginal gap than those without [11].

Komisaruk et al. showed that the self-stimulated sensory cortex areas of the clitoral, vaginal, or cervical areas can be separate from each other, although they overlap somewhat. The fact that there is a significant separate region belonging to each genital area in the sensory cortex suggests the possibility of a separate area belonging to the G-spot.

Studies on G-spot injection are based on the observation that sexual function in women increases after the adaptation of collagen injections to the anterior vaginal wall for urethral sphincter insufficiency.

19.4 G-Spot Dermal Filler Injections

G-spot injections are among the applications in cosmetic gynecology. Dermal fillers and injections of collagen-like materials are among the most common applications in this area. The enlargement of G-spot area is known by name "G-spot Augmentation." The terms "G-spot Amplification©" (GSA) and "G-Shot©" describe augmentation of G-spot area by the injections of hyaluronan, but these terms are registered by its inventor Dr. David Matlock. He describes G-shot© as a short office based, simple, nonsurgical procedure for sexual arousal and gratification.

G-spot augmentation is a minimally invasive method and is applied in order to provide sensitivity and increase satisfaction with friction from the penis during sexual intercourse. The injection is usually done intradermally to the area between the bladder neck and vagina. There is still not enough scientific evidence regarding its necessity, safety, or efficacy. The FDA has not approved G-spot amplification© and defines injection as an off-label application. In its committee decisions published in 2007, ACOG reported that vaginal rejuvenation, designer vaginoplasty, hymenoplasty, and G-spot Amplification© are procedures that do not have medical indications and there is no documentation about their safety and efficacy. It was also underlined that there are not enough studies in terms of long-term satisfaction, safety, and complication rates. G-spot dermal injection is seen as a money trap by many physicians [12, 13]. Even today, it is completely commercial and misleading for physicians to use terms such as A-spot, C-spot, U-spot, K-spot by taking advantage of media support.

19.5 G-Spot Augmentation Indications

All information should be given to the patient who will undergo G-spot dermal application, the consent paper should be signed, and then the process should be started. The only purpose of the procedure is to increase sexuality. G-spot augmentation is recommended by some physicians only for those who have problems with orgasm during sexual intercourse (coital anorgasmia). No test is required before the procedure. It can be reserved for the group of patient who has the complains or queries such as "I have lost the sensitivity over time during the sexual penetration", "I have difficulty in orgasm during sexual intercourses", "I force myself too much to have orgasm during sex", or "I want to enhance my sexuality and feel better".

19.6 Contraindications

G-spot augmentation should not be done in the following situations:

- Those with excessive vaginal width or POP
- During pregnancy
- Those with hyaluronic acid allergy
- Those who have never had an orgasm in their lifetime
- Those who lack knowledge about sexuality
- Patients with overly high expectations

19.7 How is G-spot Augmentation Performed?

First, gynecological examination is performed in the lithotomy position. The vagina and cervix are evaluated with external genital area and speculum examination. The anterior vaginal wall is checked by palpation. After making sure that there is no pelvic pathology or infection, the patient, who is left alone in a private room, is asked to stimulate the anterior wall of the vagina for 5–10 min using one or two fingers by herself on the gynecological examination table.

After self-stimulation, the enlarged and swollen area on the anterior vaginal wall is detected by palpation and speculum examination. While the speculum is inserted, the vaginal walls are wiped with iodized solution, dried, then the speculum is rotated 90° counterclockwise in the vagina, and the circumference of the detected area is marked with a marker pen. Marking will provide convenience for injection. Later, some anesthetic cream is applied here and a few minutes wait. After mild numbness is achieved, 2 cc of local anesthetic is injected subcutaneously at the marked area with a 30 G needle. Afterward, hyaluronic acid (HA) injection is applied intradermally to the numbed area (Fig. 19.1).

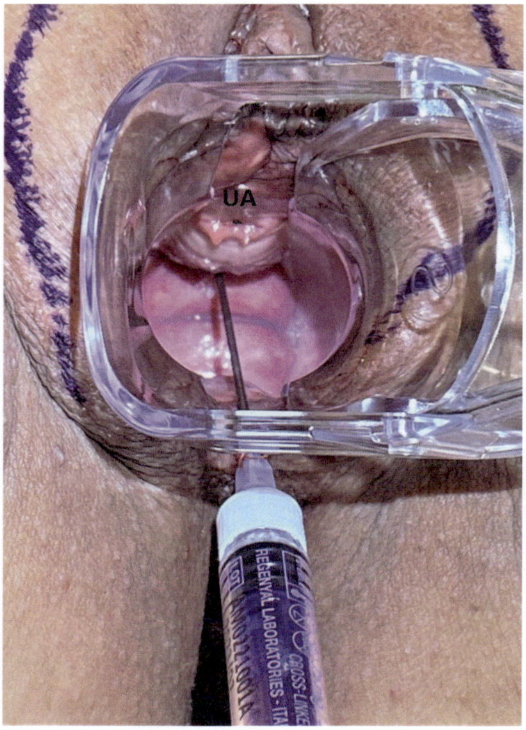

Fig. 19.1 G-spot augmentation by filler. After the anterior vaginal wall exposition by the vaginal speculum undergoing 90° of rotation, the blades are opened. UA: Urethral Orifice

In order to avoid urethral damage and obstruction, I suggest a total of 2 cc of HA injection slightly lateral of the marked area, 1 cc each at 11 and 1 o'clock positions. There is a needle for injection in the commercially purchased HA box, and HA is usually injected with the needle in the box. Deep injection should be avoided, and the injection area should be felt when palpated after the procedure.

19.8 Complications

HA injections into the anterior vaginal wall may not be as innocent as they seen. Although rare, complications such as hypersensitivity, inflammatory reaction, urinary tract infection, urinary retention, fistula formation, erosion, infection, and wound formation may occur.

Park et al. reported a non-thrombotic pulmonary embolism that developed as a result of the injection of HA at a high volume of 5 cc for G-spot augmentation in a patient [14].

19.9 Post-Procedure Term

After G-spot augmentation, bleeding in the form of leakage, mild pain that does not require painkillers, and discharge are normal. There is no need for any dressing or special care after the procedure. No sexual avoidance is needed. Depending on the hyaluronic acid cross-link and viscosity, the effect generally lasts between 4 and 9 months. The procedure can be repeated in satisfied patients. Nowadays, G-spot HA applications have been mostly replaced by genital PRP treatments.

Appendix

With the purchase of this book, you can use our "SN Flashcards" app to access questions free of charge in order to test your learning and check your understanding of the contents of the book.

To use the app, please follow the instructions below:

1. Go to https://flashcards.springernature.com/login
2. Create a user account by entering your e-mail address and assigning a password.
3. Use the following link to access your SN Flashcards set: ▶ https://sn.pub/tvlq7Q

If the link is missing or does not work, please send an e-mail with the subject "SN Flashcards" and the book title to customerservice@springernature.com.

References

1. Darling CA, Davidson JK Sr, Conway-Welch C. Female ejaculation: perceived origins, the Grafenberg spot/area, and sexual responsiveness. Arch Sex Behav. 1990;19(1):29–47.
2. Addiego FBE, Comolli J, Moger W, Perry JD, Whipple B. Female ejaculation: a case study. J Sex Res. 1981;17:13–21.
3. Perry JDWB. Pelvic muscle strength of female ejaculators: evidence in support of a new theory of orgasm. J Sex Res. 1981;17:22–39.
4. Shafik A, El Sibai O, Shafik AA, Ahmed I, Mostafa RM. The electrovaginogram: study of the vaginal electric activity and its role in the sexual act and disorders. Arch Gynecol Obstet. 2004;269(4):282–6.
5. Woodard TL, Diamond MP. Physiologic measures of sexual function in women: a review. Fertil Steril. 2009;92(1):19–34.
6. Ostrzenski A, Krajewski P, Ganjei-Azar P, Wasiutynski AJ, Scheinberg MN, Tarka S, Fudalej M. Verification of the anatomy and newly discovered histology of the G-spot complex. BJOG. 2014;121(11):1333–9.
7. Ostrzenski A. Anatomic documentation of the G-spot complex role in the genesis of anterior vaginal wall ballooning. Eur J Obstet Gynecol Reprod Biol. 2014;180:186–91.
8. Ostrzenski A. G-Spotplasty: a new surgical plastic intervention-the preliminary study. Aesthet Plast Surg. 2018;42(4):1126–32.
9. Li T, Liao Q, Zhang H, Gao X, Li X, Zhang M. Anatomic distribution of nerves and microvascular density in the human anterior vaginal wall: prospective study. PLoS One. 2014;9(11):e110239.
10. Alzate H. Vaginal eroticism: a replication study. Arch Sex Behav. 1985;14(6):529–37.
11. Gravina GL, Brandetti F, Martini P, Carosa E, Di Stasi SM, Morano S, Lenzi A, Jannini EA. Measurement of the thickness of the urethrovaginal space in women with or without vaginal orgasm. J Sex Med. 2008;5(3):610–8.
12. Kilchevsky A, Vardi Y, Lowenstein L, Gruenwald I. Is the female G-spot truly a distinct anatomic entity? J Sex Med. 2012;9(3):719–26.
13. Puppo V, Gruenwald I. Does the G-spot exist? A review of the current literature. Int Urogynecol J. 2012;23(12):1665–9.
14. Park HJ, Jung KH, Kim SY, Lee JH, Jeong JY, Kim JH. Hyaluronic acid pulmonary embolism: a critical consequence of an illegal cosmetic vaginal procedure. Thorax. 2010;65(4):360–1.

Part IV

Regenerative Treatments

Hyaluronic Acid Applications to Genital Area

20

It is science and knowledge that guides everything in the world, for materiality, for spirituality, for life, for success. Seeking a guide other than science and knowledge is heedlessness, ignorance, deviation from the right path.

Mustafa Kemal Atatürk

Dermal fillers, also known as "injectable implants," "soft tissue fillers," or "wrinkle fillers" are medical device implants approved by the FDA for use in helping to create a smoother and/or fuller appearance in the face, including nasolabial folds, cheeks, chin, lips, and the backs of the hands. Hyaluronic acid fillers are the most preferred in cosmetic and regenerative medicine.

Hyaluronic acid (HA), or hyaluronan, is a linear, high molecular weight (between 0.1 and 10 million Daltons) type of sugar with a polysaccharide structure formed by D-glucuronic acid and N-acetyl-D-glucosamine (Fig. 20.1). This kind of sugar is found in the dermis, epidermis, and cartilage in mammals. The name is derived from the Greek term "*Hyalos*" (glassy, transparent) and uronic acid. It is also the basic building block of the connective tissue extracellular matrix.

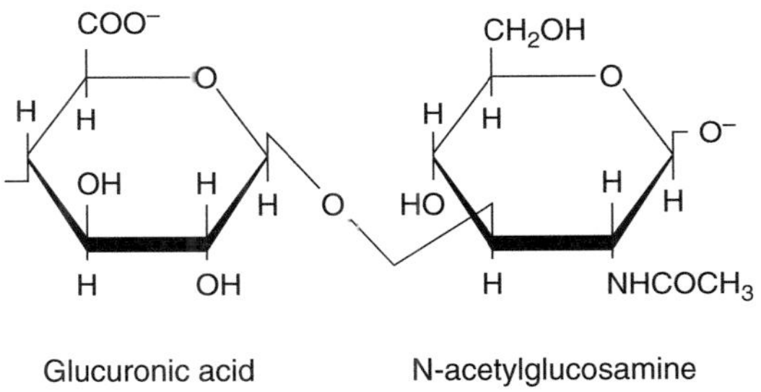

Fig. 20.1 Hyaluronic acid—glycosaminoglycan (GAG) structure

S. Eserdağ, *Aesthetic and Functional Female Genital Surgery*,
https://doi.org/10.1007/978-3-031-16019-6_20

20.1 Where Is Hyaluronic Acid (HA) Found?

Most HA is found in the dermis in mammals. In humans, there are 15–20 g of HA in the dermis, which is one-third of all HA in the body.

HA is primarily found in the vitreous fluid of the eye, hyaline cartilage, synovial fluid, dermis, and epidermis [1]. It is one of the most important components of synovial fluid. It is also found in significant amounts in lung, kidney, brain, and muscle tissue. The lowest levels are in blood serum.

HA increases the volume in the vitreous fluid, provides a lubricating effect on tendons and muscles, and provides lubrication around chondrocytes in joints. For example, in osteoarthritis, loss of function is observed as the amount of HA in the joints decreases. It is used in the treatment of osteoarthritis because of the improvement in symptoms of high-density purified HA injections into the joint. Intra-articular HA application to the knee joint has been FDA approved since 1997 [2]. HA is frequently used in cataract surgery in ophthalmology, rheumatoid arthritis treatment in rheumatology, and temporomandibular joint problems in dentistry.

While HA is found in large amounts as a component of the skin of the fetus, this amount decreases with age. HA also plays a role in the maternal–fetal relationship in the umbilical cord.

The regulatory roles of HA on cell motility, cellular proliferation, morphogenesis, embryological development, cancer metastasis, and inflammation have also been demonstrated.

HA is synthesized in the skin of mammals. It has been determined that this synthesis rate in the skin is affected by various factors. Environmental and biological factors can change the amount of HA in the body. Sunlight, cytokines, low pH, fruit acids, and lipopolysaccharides increase the synthesis rate of HA, while glucocorticoids, estrogen, and low temperature decrease the synthesis rate of HA. When our skin is exposed to excessive ultraviolet B rays and inflammation develops due to sunburn, HA production stops in the dermis and destruction increases. It has been observed that aging does not the rate of synthesis [3].

HA is also very effective in tissue repair and regeneration. For this reason, it also allows wounds to heal without leaving any scars. It is very effective in the treatment of many skin diseases such as skin ulcers, atopic dermatitis, dryness, and redness [4]. Additionally, it has a protective effect and anti-inflammatory properties against oxidative damage caused by free radicals.

20.2 Historical Background

The first HA was obtained from the vitreous fluid of the bovine eye in 1934 by biochemists Karl Meyer and John Palmer at Columbia University. Meyer et al. discovered its chemical structure in the 1950s. The first medical application of HA for humans was as a vitreous substitution/replacement during eye surgery in the late 1950s. Its use for treatment purposes began to increase in the 1970s. Later, it found a place in many areas including osteoarthritis treatment, percutaneous embolization treatment, arteriovenous malformation treatment, vascular tumor treatment, and hemorrhage treatment.

20.3 Obtaining of HA

HA is generally obtained by direct isolation from animal sources or by fermentation from bacteria. Animal sources include rooster comb, spinal cord, skin, and joint fluid. Sea animals have also been used in production in recent years [5]. The HA obtained from microorganisms by the fermentation method is of high purity. It can be obtained from streptococci by bacterial expression. Its molecular size also changes according to the source from which it is isolated [6].

Hyaluronan is a commonly found natural substance, from the simplest bacteria to the most developed organisms. It is critical in the formation of the organism. Even the fertilization of the egg, 98% of which is surrounded with a layer of

HA, by the sperm takes place, thanks to the hyaluronidase enzyme.

The hyaluronidase enzyme reduces HA's viscosity by catalyzing the hydrolysis of HA, which is an important component of the interstitial barrier. Thus, it increases tissue permeability. Therefore, hyaluronidase can be used in addition to treatment in order to increase the distribution of some drugs and accelerate their reaching to the tissues. For example, hyaluronidase is commonly used in combination with local anesthetics in ophthalmic surgery. Conversely, some bacteria even produce hyaluronidase to increase their mobility in body tissues.

20.4 Indications of HA in Cosmetic Dermatology

HA is widely used in dermatology and cosmetology for its plumping, moisturizing, collagen production stimulating, antiaging, anti-inflammatory, and anti-edema properties. Its water retention feature plays an important role in providing turgor to the skin. It is one of the most hydrophilic molecules in nature; 1 g of HA can absorb 6 liter of water. Fillers containing HA are used extensively in the cosmetic field. Cosmetic indications of HA fillers are:

- Elimination of signs of aging (antiaging),
- Treatment of wrinkles around lips and eyes,
- Lip enlargement,
- Revealing facial lines.

20.5 FDA Declaration on Dermal Fillers (2020)

The FDA stated in its declaration dated 11 September 2020 that dermal fillers can be used in adults 22 years of age or older [7]:

- Absorbable (temporary) fillers can be used for moderate to severe facial wrinkles and skin tags, such as nasolabial folds and perioral lines.
- They can be applied to lips, cheeks, chin, and back of the hand to increase the volume (augmentation).
- Non-absorbable (permanent) fillers are approved for only nasolabial folds and cheek acne scars.
- The restoration and correction of signs of facial fat loss (lipoatrophy) in people with human immunodeficiency virus (HIV).
- Correction of contour deficiencies, such as wrinkles and acne scars.

The FDA is against all dermal fillers or all injectable fillers for:

- Breast augmentation
- Buttocks augmentation
- Increasing fullness of the feet
- Implant into bone, tendon, ligament, or muscle
- Injecting the glabella, nose, periorbital area, forehead, or neck

Injectable silicone is not approved for any aesthetic procedure including facial and body contouring or enhancement. Silicone injections can lead to long-term pain, infections, and serious injuries, such as scarring and permanent deformity, embolism, stroke, and death.

20.6 Applications in Genital Area

HA application set consists of HA in a screwed injector, puncture needle, cannula, and local anesthetic solution (Fig. 20.2).

Dermal fillers can be applied anterior, posterior, and lateral walls of the vagina as well as submucosal tissue. They are applied to the 1/3 proximal anterior vaginal wall for G-spot enlargement. They can also be applied to the perineum, vestibular area, and labia majora. However, it is not recommended to apply volumizing HA to the

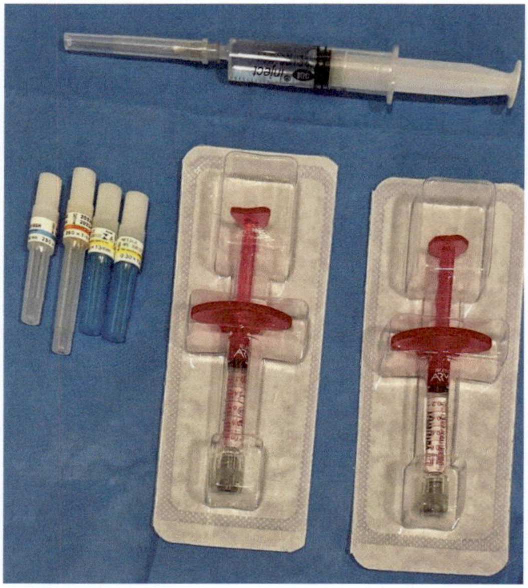

Fig. 20.2 HA application set

clitoris, labia minora, or clitoral hood area. Since it is an expensive substance, it is important to use it effectively.

20.7 Use of HA in Gynecology

HA has been used in the genital area for aesthetic and functional purposes, especially in recent years.

20.7.1 Functional Purposes

20.7.1.1 Vaginal Dryness Treatment

Vaginal dryness, caused by the effect of estrogen hormone decreasing after menopause, is an important cause of sexual problems. Menopausal complaints are more intense after surgical menopause. The first-line treatment for vaginal dryness is local estrogen preparations. However, estrogen therapies, even if locally effective, are not recommended for those undergoing breast cancer treatment or who are at risk of cancer. Vaginal laser, radiofrequency, PRP, and HA treatments can be recommended as alternative approaches for these patients. For vaginal dryness, HA injection can be applied alone or in combination with energy-based treatments. According to our observations, the success rate is higher in combined treatments.

HA can provide hydration of the vaginal mucosa due to its water-retaining feature. It also provides symptomatic treatment by stimulating collagen production, especially in cases of atrophic vaginitis.

In intravaginal injections, it is appropriate to administer HA to a submucosal depth between 2 and 4 mm.

20.7.1.2 Vulvar Vestibulitis Treatment

HA applied to the vestibular submucosa both stimulates collagen synthesis and provides an anti-inflammatory effect for the treatment of vulvar vestibulitis, which is characterized by the problem of not having intercourse or having painful intercourse due to hyperesthesia at the vaginal entrance (vestibular region) (Fig. 20.3). In a preliminary study, it's been demonstrated that FSFI scores and VAS scores were improved in provoked vestibulodynia patients by submucosal vestibular HA injections [8].

20.7.1.3 G-spot Injection

G-Spot hyaluronic acid injections are intended for sexual enhancement. The purpose of fillings made to enlarge the G-spot area is to increase sexual pleasure. This subject is discussed in detail in the "G-Spot Augmentation by Hyaluronic Acid " section (Chap. 19).

20.7.1.4 Perineal Lifting

Slightly elevating the perineum area with HA injection can positively affect sexuality by increasing the stimulation of the anterior wall during coitus and slightly tightening the vaginal entrance.

20.7.1.5 Perineal Scar Treatments

These are treatments aimed at relieving sexual pain by filling atrophic scars. These treatments provide aesthetic and functional benefits. Nowadays, atrophic and hypertrophic scar treatments can be successfully applied with high-density HA preparations containing collagenase enzyme.

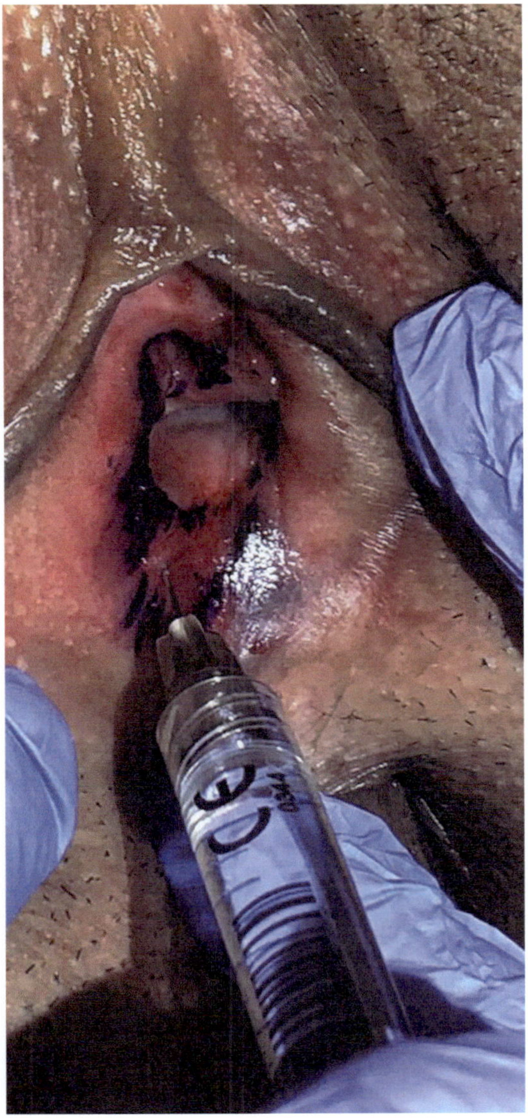

Fig. 20.3 Vulvar vestibulitis. Injection of HA into subcutaneous tissue after the painful area is marked

20.7.2 Aesthetic Purposes

20.7.2.1 Correcting Labium Majus Hypotonicity and Hypotrophy

The aesthetic problems of the labia majora can be solved quickly with HA injection on an outpatient basis. The most common areas of application:

- Labial augmentation: performed to enlarge the labia majora in those that are smaller than normal or to hide the deformations in labia minora behind enlarged labia majora.
- Labial collapse: applied to remove depressions and wrinkles on the labia majora.
- Labial asymmetry: preferred to provide balancing if one labium is bigger or smaller than the other.

Loss of tonus and trophism may develop due to collagen loss due to reasons such as rapid weight gain, smoking, stressful life, and genetic predisposition. In addition, the effects of aging and menopause increase these losses. In this case, functional and aesthetic HA application can be applied to the labia majora. With rejuvenation of the labia majora, the genital area will have a fuller, brighter, and younger appearance.

Labia majora hypotrophy is classified into three separate groups (Table 20.1).

In a retrospective study, a significant improvement was detected in the Global Aesthetic Improvement Scale (GAIS) after one-session HA application of 19 mg/mL to 31 patients with mild-moderate hypotrophy and 21 mg/mL to 23 patients with severe hypotrophy. Improvement was more pronounced and no complications were

Table 20.1 Classification of labia majora hypotrophy [9]

	Subcutaneous layers	Cutaneous layer	Symptoms
Stage 1 mild (early)	Mild hypotrophy. Distribution of adipose tissue is usually symmetrical	None to mild cutaneous hypotrophy. Thin wrinkles may be visible	Usually asymptomatic. Possible consequence of weight loss
Stage 2 moderate	Moderate hypotrophy. Possible asymmetric distribution of adipose tissue	Moderate cutaneous laxity, dermatochalasis. Wrinkles are visible	Dryness, dispareunia, soreness could be observed
Stage 3 severe	Severe hypotrophy. Frequent asymmetric distribution of adipose tissue	Severe dermatochalasis and deep wrinkles	Usually associated to symptoms like dryness, dispareunia, soreness

encountered, especially in patients with severe hypotrophy [9].

Linear retrograde application is mostly preferred in labia majora augmentation.

20.8 HA Application Techniques

HA applications can be made in different ways according to the region and purpose (Fig. 20.4). These include:

- *Linear threading technique*
- *Point-by-point application (serial puncture) technique*
- *Fanning technique*
- *Cross-hatching (cross radial) technique*

20.8.1 Linear Threading Technique

The filler is given along the linear line during pushing when the cannula is inserted or during withdrawal after the cannula is inserted. This technique is especially preferred to fill wrinkles.

20.8.2 Point-by-Point Application (Serial Puncture) Technique

Particularly preferred in low viscosity fillings are intermittent, serial, heaps of point applications.

20.8.3 Fanning Technique

This is the scanning of the area in the form of a fan, clockwise or counterclockwise, by entering from different areas.

20.8.4 Cross-Hatching (Cross Radial) Technique

This is a series of linear applications in the form of a cage made to fill large areas.

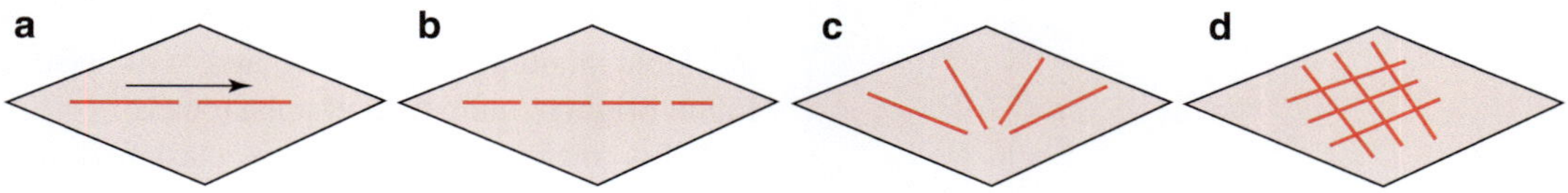

Fig. 20.4 HA filler application techniques. (**a**) Linear threading, (**b**) point-by-point application, (**c**) fanning, (**d**) cross-hatching

20.9 Some Fillers in the Market

- Juvéderm™ (Allergan—Ireland)
- Surgiderm™ (Corneal—France)
- Belotero™ (Merz—Germany)
- Radiesse™ (Merz—Germany)
- Teosyal™ (Teoxane—France)
- Stylage™ (Vivacy—France)
- Filorga/FillMed™ (Filorga—France)
- Neauvia™ (Matex Lab—Switzerland)
- Sculptra™ (Galderma—Switzerland)
- Restylane™ (Galderma—Switzerland)
- Aquashine™ (Caregen—Korea)
- Dermaheal™ (Caregen—Korea)
- DR.CYJ Hair Filler™ (Caregen—Korea)
- Profhilo™ (IBSA—Italy)
- Goldfill™ (Dermaqual—France)
- Desirial™ (Vivacy—France)
- Armonia™ (Regenyal—Italy)

Some filler materials also contain lidocaine to prevent pain during injection.

CE (abbreviation of "*Conformité Européenne*," as the logo CE) marking is an administrative marking that indicates conformity with health, safety, and environmental protection standards for products sold within the European Economic Area (EEA). It is not a quality indicator or a certification mark. The CE marking is also found on products sold outside the EEA that have been manufactured to EEA standards. This makes the CE marking recognizable worldwide even to people who are not familiar with the EEA. It is, in that sense, similar to the FCC Declaration of Conformity used for selling certain electronic devices in the USA. The CE marking is the manufacturer's declaration that the product meets EU standards for health, safety, and environmental protection and indicates that the product may be sold freely in any part of the European Economic Area, irrespective of its country of origin.

There are only a few HA fillers having CE marking for indications in genital area so far: Armonia™ and Armonioso™ (from Regenyal company) and Desirial™ and Desirial Plus™ (from Vivacy company). Most of the fillers used are off-label applications. Off-label fillers should not be preferred in order to avoid legal problems in case of any complications.

CE marked filler, Armonia™ is an injectable biorivolumetric gel, containing 25 mg/mL cross-linked hyaluronic acid with a 12% intercalated multifractional component. It is a class III CE medical device, biocompatible, bio-resorbable (sterile, apyrogenic, isosmotic, and isotonic gel) to be used on the external male and female genitals. Armonia is applied for different indications in the female genital area such as compactness, volume, and hydration of labia majora and vulva, reducing vaginal dryness, and correction of episiotomy scars. Armonioso™ is also containing 25 mg/mL cross-linked hyaluronic acid, but has more molecular weight compared to Armonia™ and 7% intercalated multifractional component, so it is recommended especially for labia majora augmentation indications.

The other CE marked filler, Desirial™ contains 19 mg/mL HA and is used for vaginal complaints such as genital dryness and relief of chronic irritation. It provides hydration of the vulvovaginal area, softens irritated areas, and increases the quality of the genital mucosa. In the treatment of vaginal dryness, atrophy, and chronic irritation, Desirial™ can be applied with 30 G needles for hydration, reducing irritation, and increasing mucosal tissue quality. The other form, Desirial Plus™ contains 21 mg/mL HA and is used for labia majora augmentation. In labia majora hypotrophy, it can be applied with 25 G or 27 G cannulas to provide volume replacement and rejuvenation.

20.10 HA Filler Applications for Labia Majora Augmentation

The steps of labia majora augmentation by HA are described in Table 20.2.

Table 20.2 Step-by-step labia majora augmentation by HA

- Inform the patient and obtain the consent form
- Clean the vulva with an antiseptic solution in lithotomy position and then dry
- Examine the external genital area, and determine the wrinkled or collapsed areas
- Mark the area to be augmented with a skin marker (optional)
- Insert the cannula subcutaneously. Cannula insertion can be from the top (superior) to the bottom (inferior) or from bottom to top. The puncture point can be at the clitoral level for top to bottom applications. For bottom to top applications, it can be fourchette level. However, it can be determined along with the wrinkled locations
- Inject the local anesthetic solution into the determined insertion point as a single papule (intradermally)
- Make a small hole with a spinal needle or perforator needle (in the package)
- Place the blunt-tipped filler cannula subcutaneously, and be sure that you passed the dartos layer. It should be removing both sides easily
- Fix the hyaluronic acid syringe to the cannula by rotating
- Inject the hyaluronic acid by linear retrograde infiltration, that is, with the retraction of the cannula while the HA is injected, or as a retrograde zigzag scan
- Massage gently to distribute the HA homogeneously into the tissue
- Inspect the tissue for a few minutes for any allergic reaction (hyperemia and local temperature increase)

HA injection is performed just beneath the dartos layer. The cannula is movable toward the sides in this layer, as shown in Fig. 20.5. Deeper applications may cause loss of volume, and more superficial applications may cause surface irregularities or Tyndall effect.

HA application in the labia majora should be performed superficially between the dartos fascia and the fibrous tunic (elastic sac) (Fig. 20.6). If the filler is placed into the adipose tissue, it will disappear, the effect will not be noticed, and the volume will be wasted. In deep applications, the filler can also go down through the passage in the adipose tissue to the ischiorectal fossa. Conversely, if it is too superficial, it may cause palpable lumps on the skin.

Below is the passage descending through the adipose tissue on a cadaver (Fig. 20.7).

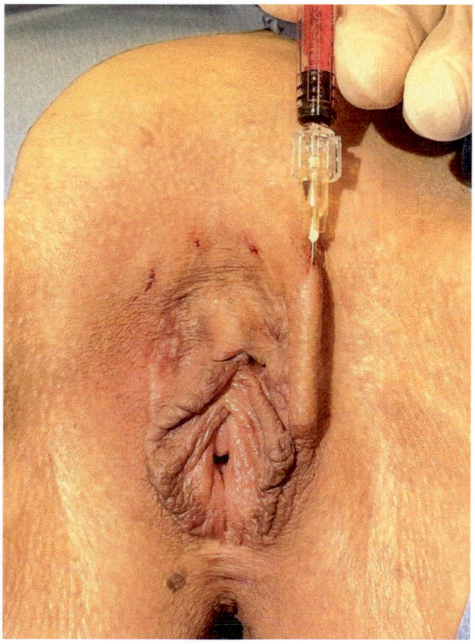

Fig. 20.5 Subcutaneous application of cannula just beneath the dartos layer

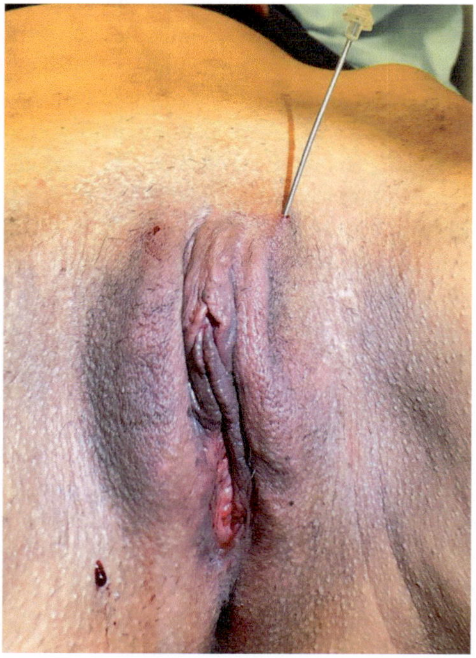

Fig. 20.6 Labia majora HA injection. It has been applied to the right side; it is currently being applied to the left

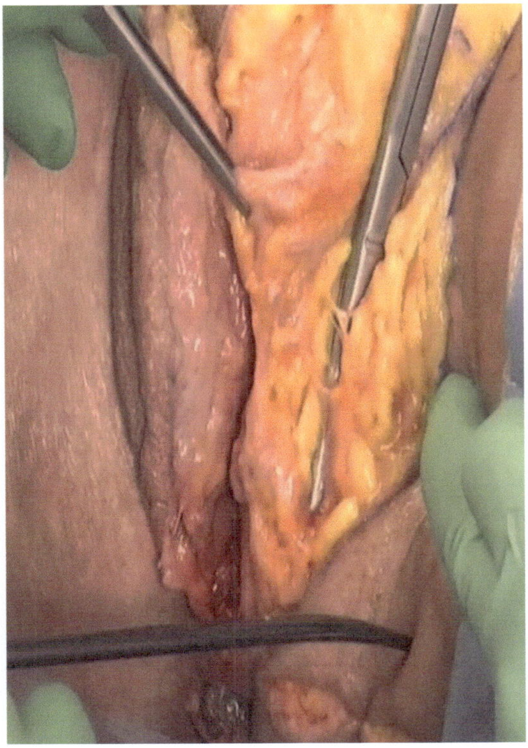

Fig. 20.7 Longitudinal passage in the labia majora adipose tissue (cadaver study)

20.11 Vaginal and Vestibular HA

20.11.1 Fillers

Low viscosity fillers are generally preferred. Point-by-point or linear threading technique can be chosen. Injections can be made into the vagina or vestibule with a needle point-by-point technique at 1 cm intervals. In the linear threading technique, after the cannula is inserted into the vagina and checked with negative aspiration, the entire vagina can be scanned along linear lines. Generally, a total of 2 cc of application is sufficient. Deep applications should be avoided to prevent complications due to vascular damage.

20.11.2 Features in HA Selection: HA Rheology

First, it should be known for which indication (augmentation, lifting, regeneration) the HA will be used. The "HA rheology," i.e., elasticity and viscosity, to be injected is important. It is also important to know how long the filler material will remain because the more permanent the filler material, the lower the cost.

The permanence of the filler is generally related to the cross-link structure. The retention period can be short-, medium-, or long-term. Long-lasting ones are those with more cross-links. These are more economical for patients. As the number of cross-links decreases, the permanence decreases. Generally, butanediol diglycidyl ether (BDDE) active ingredient is used as a cross-linker. However, due to its toxic effects, the BDDE content should be as minimal as possible. Another cross-link alternative is polyethylene glycol diglycidyl ether (PEGDGE). The purpose of both cross-link formulations is to prolong the persistence of hyaluronic acid by creating resistance to the rapid degradation effect of the hyaluronidase enzyme.

20.11.3 Contraindications

- Vaginal inflammation or infections
- Active HSV infection
- Unidentified vulvar pathologies
- Genital cancer or cancer suspicion
- Pregnancy or pregnancy suspicion
- Lactation period
- Autoimmune diseases
- Under immunosuppressive therapy
- Local or systemic infections
- Allergic reactions to HA or additives
- Bad bleeding profile or using anticoagulants

20.11.4 Comparison with Autologous Fat Transfer

Labia majora augmentation can also be provided via autologous fat grafts. Both processes have advantages and disadvantages compared to each other as shown in Table 20.3.

20.11.5 Combined Therapies

HA injection can be combined with different treatments depending on the application area and purpose. It can be combined with laser, RF, and carboxytherapy treatments to reduce vaginal dryness and eliminate atrophy problems, especially during menopause. In these cases, applying energy-based treatments first and then HA injection at least 3–4 weeks later is recommended. Conversely, some physicians recommend the application of HA by mixing it with PRP. However, the PRP content may disrupt the HA formulation, reducing the effect of the procedure. Vulvar laser bleaching and HA injection in majora should not be applied in the same session because it can cause severe inflammation and spoiling of the HA.

Table 20.3 Comparison of HA injections and autologous fat transfer

Comparison	HA injections	Autologous fat transfer
Difficulty	Easy	Difficult, requires experience
Application	Non-surgical	Surgical
Facility	Office	Office/hospital
Anesthesia	Local	General, sedation, regional
Duration	5–10 min	45 min
Step(s)	Single	Three steps (lipoaspiration, processing, and lipofilling)
Application area for majora	Superficial. It is injected between dartos and fibrous tunic (elastic sac)	Superficial and deep. It is given to superficial and deep (adipose tissue) areas within different passages
Complication risk	Minimal	(+)
Source	Heterologous (xenologous)	Autologous
Downtime	No	7 days
Stem cell content	No	Yes
Water absorbtion (hydration)	Yes	No
Repeat	6–9 months	3–5 years
Fee	Cheaper	Expensive. However, it might be cheaper if we consider it in terms of repetition, time, volume, and efficiency

20.11.6 Complications and Undesirable Effects

HA is a natural component found in all living things and has biocompatible, degradable, viscoelastic, and suitable hygroscopic properties. Complications are rare. Among the undesirable effects, the most common in the early period in the application area are allergic reactions, tissue necrosis, edema, rash, itching, and localized pain. Although topical anesthetics can be used to prevent pain, the contact reaction property of these substances should also be known. Side effects can be eliminated by using the hyaluronidase enzyme in complications related to HA injection. In very rare cases, there are risks such as anaphylaxis, shock, filler migration, leakage of the filler from the injection site, and nodule formation.

Rare but quite severe complications of HA injections include pulmonary embolism, vascular occlusions, and death. In the literature, pulmonary embolism has been reported in two patients so far. In order to minimize these risks, the practicing physician should have information about the localization of the anterior labial artery, the branches of the external pudendal artery, the posterior labial artery, and the branches of the internal pudendal artery that provide circulation to the vulva. In order to minimize the risk of embolism, the injection cannula should be thin (27–28 G), it should be checked whether it is in the vessel with negative pressure before injection, and a linear retrograde injection should be made as much as possible.

Aseptic conditions should be followed and organ injuries should be avoided to minimize the risk of infection.

One of the undesirable effect of HA fillers is "Tyndall effect." Tyndall effect, also known as the "Tyndall phenomenon," that is named after an Irish Physicist John Tyndall, is the scattering of a light beam by a medium containing tiny suspended particles which makes a light beam entering a window visible. Short-wavelength blue light is scattered about 10 times more than long-wavelength red light when passing through very small particles. This is why the sky appears blue. In cosmetic medicine, the Tyndall effect is used to describe the bluish hue that is visible within the skin caused by too superficial placement of hyaluronic acid (HA) filler. That is why very superficial placement of HA should be avoided.

The Tyndall effect is more commonly referred to as "Rayleigh scattering" by physicists after Lord Rayleigh who elaborated the process. The principle of the Tyndall effect is that different wavelengths of light do or do not scatter depending on the size of the substance they encounter. A greater amount of small particles within a substance, the greater the scattering and the more obvious discoloration. This is the reason the Tyndall effect is more common with more particulate dermal fillers.

The Tyndall effect can be distressing for patients and gives a poor aesthetic outcome leading to anxiety and dissatisfaction. It may be visible immediately after treatment although it may appear after a few days and, without corrective measures, may last for months or years [10].

Among the long-term complications of HA, there are delayed hypersensitivity reactions that can be seen within a few weeks to a few months, and inflammatory granulomas that can develop in a few months to a few years due to the introduction of foreign substances under the skin (Fig. 20.8). Intralesional steroids are the most commonly used agents in the treatment of such complications. Rarely, surgical excision of the nodule may be required.

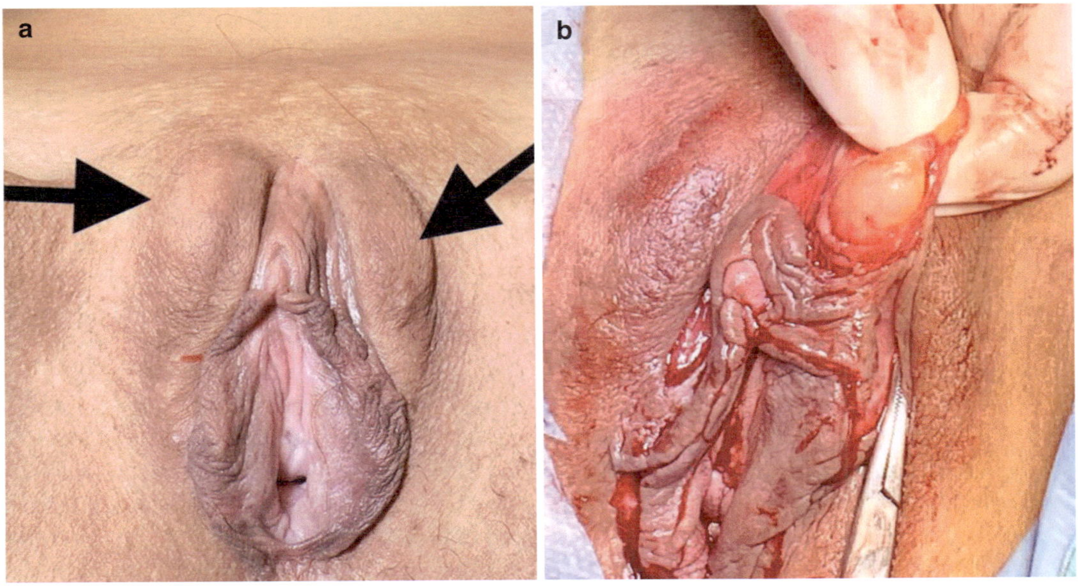

Fig. 20.8 Bilateral granuloma formations in majora due to HA injections 3 months ago (**a**) and surgical extirpation (**b**). Pathology confirmed "granulomatous inflammation"

20.11.7 Hyaluronidase Enzyme

Hyaluronidase is a family of enzymes that degrade hyaluronic acid. It increases vascular permeability and temporarily disrupts the extracellular matrix, promoting the diffusion of substances through tissues. Human hyaluronidase is present both in organs (testis, spleen, skin, eyes, liver, kidneys, uterus, and placenta) and in body fluids (tears, blood, and semen) [11]. There are six known types (hyaluronidase 1–4, PH-20, and HYALP1). PH-20 exerts the most vital biologic activity, is found in high concentrations in the testicles, and can be localized on the head and the acrosome of human spermatozoa. Initially discovered in bacteria, hyaluronidases are widely distributed in nature and found in many classes, including insects, snakes, fish, and mammals.

Medical hyaluronidase, which also breaks down hyaluronic acid, has been used for unsatisfactory conditions after filler injection. For hyaluronidase to dissolve a hyaluronic acid filler, it must interact with its binding sites within the hyaluronic acid. The reaction of a filler to hyaluronidase depends on the hyaluronic acid concentration, the number of cross-links, and the form of the filler. The more cross-linking, the more difficult it is for hyaluronidase to access its binding sites inside the hyaluronic acid filler. Thus, highly cross-linked fillers require a long time to dissolve with hyaluronidase. In addition, the higher the concentration of hyaluronic acid, the slower it will be dissolved by hyaluronidase [12].

Hyaluronidase is rapidly degraded and deactivated in the body. Therefore, to dissolve a hyaluronic acid filler, a sufficient amount of hyaluronidase must be injected close to the filler. Hyaluronidase injection into the filler itself may help if the filler is placed subcutaneously. However, if the filler is placed within a blood vessel, it is sufficient to inject hyaluronidase in the vicinity of the vessel instead of into the filler itself.

Subcutaneous injections of hyaluronidase are more effective than intravascular injections for preventing skin necrosis caused by hyaluronic acid filler embolism. The amount of hyaluronidase is important when injecting hyaluronidase in the vicinity of a blood vessel to dissolve filler inside the vessel.

Several categories of hyaluronidases have been approved for clinical use from animal or recombinant production. The FDA has approved these enzymes for three purposes:

1. as an adjuvant to increase the absorption and dispersion of other injected drugs,
2. to produce hypodermoclysis (subcutaneous fluid infusion),
3. as an adjunct in subcutaneous urography for improving reabsorption of radiopaque agents.

Off-label uses include dissolving hyaluronic acid fillers for filler-related complications such as

- eliminating HA nodules,
- correcting unsightly HA overfilling,
- treating skin necrosis associated with filler injections,
- treating granulomatous foreign body reactions.

Moreover, hyaluronidase is used as an adjunct to local anesthetics in skin infiltration, skin graft harvesting, tumescent analgesia, treatment of extravasation injury, prevention and management of edema and hematoma absorption, treatment of ganglion, and management of scars.

Medical hyaluronidase has become an essential drug for correcting complications and unsatisfactory results due to hyaluronic acid fillers. Treatment of the affected area should be started with ultrasonographic evaluation to assess the lesion's depth, quantity, and extension. The areas to be treated should be marked, and infiltration by hyaluronidases should be extremely limited to the affected area. The doctor should adjust the quantity of hyaluronidase injected according to the type of hyaluronic acid and the extent of affected areas. Generally, a few units of the enzyme (10–20 units) are adequate to treat each affected area. In any case, the injection of more than 200 units of hyaluronidase per treatment should be avoided. A 30-gauge needle can be used perpendicularly to the skin, ranging from 3 to 13 mm in length. If multiple management is necessary, the treatments can be repeated every 3 weeks. These intervals can be shorter for high-density filler applications.

If inflammatory and painful nodules are formed after the HA, independent of using hyaluronidases, antibiotic therapy for two weeks should be advised (e.g., clarithromycin 500 mg/day). In some cases, mainly when large amounts of HA filler should be eliminated, an incision for drainage of the HA is suggested, along with enzyme injection. After careful evaluation, steroids could be employed when hyaluronidases are ineffective in dissolving the nodules (e.g., inflammatory nodules or long-lasting fillers). In these cases, steroids should be administered only after antibiotic therapy has been initiated. This treatment is not appropriate for early-onset inflammatory nodules before antibiotic treatment and before attempting treatment with hyaluronidase. However, surgical excision may be considered when a long-lasting filler has been employed and shows resistance to hyaluronidases.

HA may cause cutaneous ischemia due to arterial compression. The skin pales within a few hours in these patients, while necrosis and ulcers may occur within 24 h. Hyaluronidases may be effective when applied in the first 4 h. Injection of the enzymes in the following hours does not seem effective in eliminating tissue necrosis.

Local injections of hyaluronidase can cause side effects such as local pruritus and allergic reactions. The incidence of allergic reactions is less than 1%, and urticaria and angioedema have also been reported to occur at a low frequency (less than 0.1%) [13]. Allergic reactions are more likely to occur when the hyaluronidase dose is more than 100,000 IU through an intravenous injection. Allergic complications rise to 31.3% if the dose increases to 200,000 IU [13]. Overall, hyaluronidase appears to be a very safe, cheap, and effective medication for various uses.

20.11.8 Post-procedure Term

There are no restrictions for the patient after HA injections into the vagina and vestibulum. This includes sexual intercourse. It may take up to a month to see the desired effect in applications due to collagen stimulation or coital pain.

In labium majus HA augmentation, the patient should avoid hot water, thermal pools, saunas, and hot springs for seven days. Horse and bicycle riding are also prohibited for a week. Coitus should be avoided for 5 days, because of the stabilization of the HA. Since the visible effect occurs immediately after the labium majus augmentation, patient satisfaction is quite high. Drinking three liters of water per day for the first 2–3 days after the procedure will increase the water absorption of the filler.

20.12 Different Tissue Fillers

20.12.1 Absorbable (Temporary) Materials

20.12.1.1 Collagen

One of the most commonly used tissue materials other than HA is collagen. Composed of a kind of protein structure, collagen is the shortest-lived injectable filler material and disappears in an average of 3–4 months.

20.12.1.2 Calcium Hydroxyapatite

These fillers that are found in human bone and tooth structures are especially used in the treatment of wrinkles in the face and hand areas, and the effect can last up to 18 months. It can hide underlying pathologies because it is visible on direct radiography.

20.12.1.3 Poly-L-Lactic Acid (PLLA)

This is a biodegradable, biocompatible polymer produced especially for use in absorbable sutures and bone screws. Its effect can continue for up to 2 years.

20.12.2 Non-absorbable (Permanent) Materials

20.12.2.1 Polymethylmethacrylate (PMMA Microspheres)

They are non-biodegradable, biocompatible, non-absorbable synthetic volumizing materials used especially in bone cement and intraocular lenses.

Liquid silicone or silicone gels should never be injected into any part of the body for augmentation or wrinkle treatment, and they do not have FDA approval. Otherwise, complications such as long-term pain, infection, scar formation, granuloma formation (Fig. 20.9), embolism, stroke, and even death may be encountered.

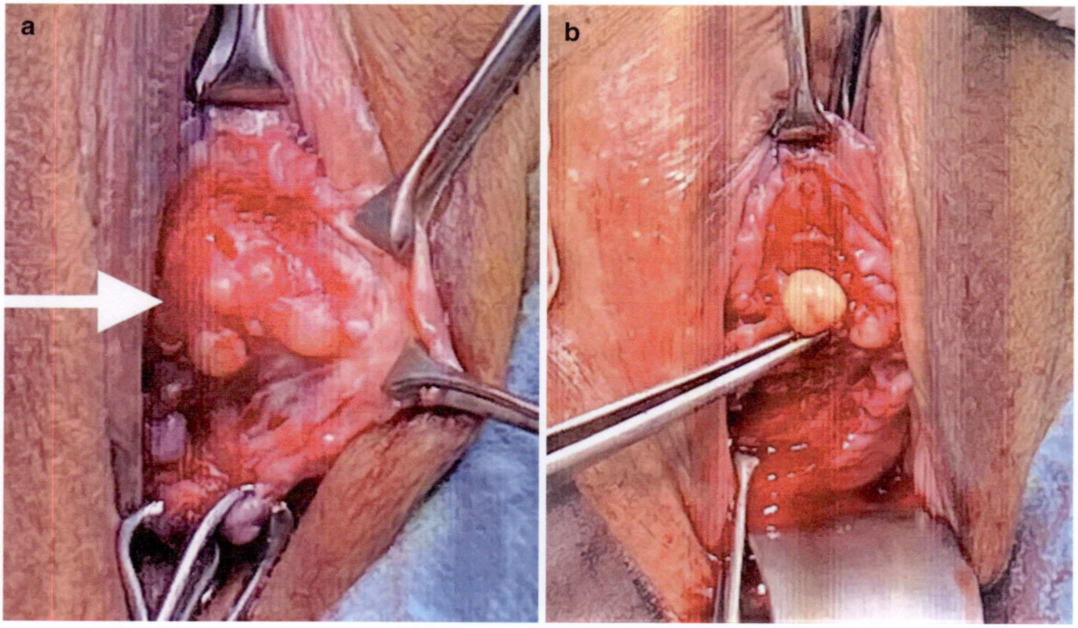

Fig. 20.9 Granuloma formation of a patient who had a permanent filler (?) injection into the vaginal anterior wall 6 years ago (**a**), and surgical excision (**b**)

Appendix

With the purchase of this book, you can use our "SN Flashcards" app to access questions free of charge in order to test your learning and check your understanding of the contents of the book.

To use the app, please follow the instructions below:

1. Go to https://flashcards.springernature.com/login
2. Create a user account by entering your e-mail address and assigning a password.
3. Use the following link to access your SN Flashcards set: ▶ https://sn.pub/tvlq7Q

If the link is missing or does not work, please send an e-mail with the subject "SN Flashcards" and the book title to customerservice@springernature.com.

References

1. Beasley KL, Weiss MA, Weiss RA. Hyaluronic acid fillers: a comprehensive review. Facial Plast Surg. 2009;25(2):86–94.
2. DIraçoğlu D. Osteoartritte intraartiküler Hyalüronik Asit Tedavisi. Türk Fiz Tıp Rehab Derg. 2007;53:154–9.
3. Bernstein EF, Underhill CB, Hahn PJ, Brown DB, Uitto J. Chronic sun exposure alters both the content and distribution of dermal glycosaminoglycans. Br J Dermatol. 1996;135(2):255–62.
4. Kavasi RM, Berdiaki A, Spyridaki I, Corsini E, Tsatsakis A, Tzanakakis G, Nikitovic D. HA metabolism in skin homeostasis and inflammatory disease. Food Chem Toxicol. 2017;101:128–38.
5. Giji S, Arumugam M. Isolation and characterization of hyaluronic acid from marine organisms. Adv Food Nutr Res. 2014;72:61–77.
6. Brown MB, Jones SA. Hyaluronic acid: a unique topical vehicle for the localized delivery of drugs to the skin. J Eur Acad Dermatol Venereol. 2005;19(3):308–18.
7. https://www.fda.gov/medical-devices/aesthetic-cosmetic-devices/dermal-fillers-soft-tissue-fillers.
8. Eserdag S, Akdag Özkok B, Süphan Ersahin S, Zeynep Yilmaz E. Vestibular hyaluronic acid injection in provoked vestibulodynia patients and its effect on pain and sexual function: A preliminary report. Eur J Obstet Gynecol Reprod Biol. 2023;280:64–7.
9. Fasola E, Gazzola R. Labia majora augmentation with hyaluronic acid filler: technique and results. Aesthet Surg J. 2016;36(10):1155–63.
10. King M. Management of Tyndall effect. J Clin Aesthet Dermatol. 2016;9(11):E6–8. Epub 2016 Nov 1.
11. Menzel EJ, Farr C. Hyaluronidase and its substrate hyaluronan: biochemistry, biological activities and therapeutic uses. Cancer Lett. 1998;131:3–11.
12. Jung H. Hyaluronidase: an overview of its properties, applications, and side effects. Arch Plast Surg. 2020;47(4):297–300.
13. Cavallini M, Gazzola R, Metalla M, et al. The role of hyaluronidase in the treatment of complications from hyaluronic acid dermal fillers. Aesthet Surg J. 2013;33:1167–74.

21 Genital PRP, PRF, and ACRS

The greatest mistake in the treatment of diseases is that there are physicians for the body and physicians for the soul, although the two cannot be separated.

Plato

Another of the aesthetic and functional applications of the genital area is genital platelet-rich plasma (PRP) injection.

Throughout our entire education, we were all informed that thrombocytes are blood platelets, involved in the coagulation mechanism. However, in subsequent years, we saw that platelets also have incredible functions in wound healing and tissue regeneration. These very special functions have enabled them to be used in medical and cosmetic treatments. The advantages of genital PRP are that it is autologous, non-allergenic, effective, and can be performed without anesthesia under office conditions.

21.1 What is the Platelet-Rich Plasma (PRP) Procedure?

The PRP procedure is the injection of PRP extracted from the components formed after centrifugation, after the venous blood drawn from the person is passed through a special centrifugation process.

Platelets are effective in wound healing due to their growth factors (GF). With the release of GF into the environment, the healing and regeneration process begins with the stimulation of collagen production and angiogenesis. Platelets are the main source of the GF complex that plays a fundamental role in the wound healing process. The idea of using PRP for therapeutic purposes is also due to the high GF content in platelets.

PRP in the literature is also referred to as platelet-enriched plasma, platelet-rich concentrate, autologous platelet gel, platelet releasate, and plasma-rich growth factors (PRGFs) [1].

The regenerative effect of platelets *in vitro* was first shown in 1970 by Ross et al. [2]. The first PRP application was used in 1987 by cardiovascular surgeon Dr. Ferrari and colleagues to prevent excessive bleeding during an open-heart surgery.

21.2 Platelet-Rich Fibrin (PRF)

21.2.1 What is Platelet-Rich Fibrin (PRF)?

Another regenerative application different from PRP as a preparation method is PRF, which is platelet-rich fibrin. PRF is a second-generation platelet-

S. Eserdağ, *Aesthetic and Functional Female Genital Surgery*,
https://doi.org/10.1007/978-3-031-16019-6_21

rich concentrate in which autologous platelets and leukocytes are contained in a complex fibrin matrix. The aim is to ensure regeneration by releasing supraphysiological platelets into the environment.

PRF is prepared by centrifugation of peripheral blood transferred to a tube without anticoagulant. Platelets are activated during centrifugation and their massive degranulation causes significant cytokine release. Among the known cytokines and GF, there are the greatest amounts of TGF-β1, PDGF-AB, and VEGF in PRF. In addition, interleukin 1 β (IL-β), IL-4, tumor necrosis factor α, PDGF α and β, and insulin-like growth factor 1 exist [3]. All these growth factors stimulate the production of collagen in soft and hard tissues, increase the strength of the wound area, and provide callus formation. PRF also includes platelets, leukocytes, and circulating stem cells.

The fibrin obtained in PRF is the activated form of fibrinogen and is the last substance in the coagulation reaction. Soluble fibrinogen becomes insoluble by thrombin effect. Also, leukocytes in PRF are responsible for the immune response for defense mechanisms.

PRF differs from PRP in terms of preparation, GF release rate, and clot formation pattern.

Table 21.1 Differences between PRP and PRF

Comparison	PRP	PRF
Used tube	Anticoagulant (+)	Anticoagulant (−)
Centrifuge speed	Fast	Slow
Method of application	27–30 G needle	Cannula
Activation	Induced by thrombin or CaCl	Coagulation and fibrin formation occur naturally
Autologous feature	Can sometimes cause the opposite immune response due to anticoagulant substances	It is completely autologous
GF release rate	Rapid GF release within the first 24 h	GF release prolonged up to 7–10 days
Leukocyte content	Is between 0 and 50%	Is around 65%
Effect on mesenchymal stem cell migration	Yes	Yes
Desired effect	Regeneration	Regeneration and volume
Lifespan	Short term	Longer term
Preparation and application	More troublesome and more expensive	Easier and cheaper

21.2.2 Comparison with PRP

Wound healing and spreading of regenerative signals over a longer period are among the advantages of PRF [4]. It has been shown in many studies that PRF is more effective than PRP (Table 21.1).

21.2.3 How to Prepare PRF?

In order to obtain PRF, the blood drawn into a 10 cc glass or glass-covered tube is centrifuged at 3000 rpm for 10 min without delay. After centrifugation, cellular plasma is formed in the top layer of the tube, PRF in the middle, and a red area with red blood cells at the bottom. PRF is a dense fibrin rich in leukocytes, cytokines, structural glycoproteins, and GFs. The reason for the formation of dense fibrin is the coagulation of blood that hits the glass surface rapidly, as there are no anticoagulants during centrifugation. For PRF formation, it is necessary to use a glass tube or a tube covered with glass inside. It is important to draw blood quickly, transfer it into a tube immediately after it is drawn, and centrifuge. The PRF formed in the tube is removed and made ready for use (Fig. 21.1). Since the product obtained after PRF is not fluid like PRP, cannulas are used in the administration process. Since it has a solid consistency, it also creates a volume effect.

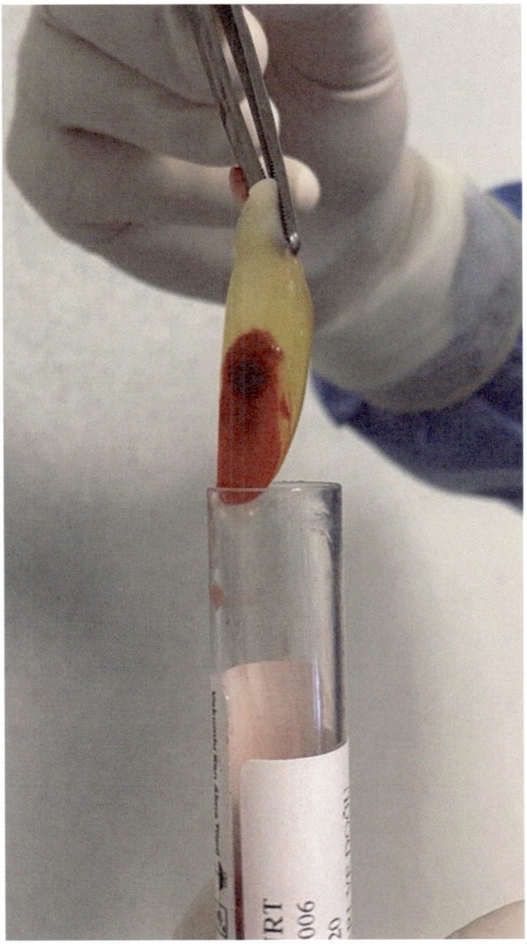

Fig. 21.1 PRF obtained after centrifugation

The PRF process is generally performed in areas where volume and regenerative effect are desired together. The G-spot injections can be a good option in this regard. It can also be applied to the labia majora for giving volume and rejuvenation. The application steps are as follows: after centrifugation, the fibrin formed in the tube is held with forceps and transferred into a 5 cc injector whose plunger has been removed. An 18 G blunt tip cannula is attached to the injector tip and the injector plunger is re-attached. Later, after the area where PRF is to be applied is anesthetized with local anesthesia, a hole is made with a thick needle, and then the cannula is inserted through this hole and the PRF is injected inside. Urethral damage should be avoided, especially in anterior vaginal wall applications.

Besides cosmetic gynecology, PRF is used in areas such as maxillofacial surgery, periodontal regeneration, and tissue engineering, especially in dentistry. It is also widely used in some orthopedic problems and medical aesthetics.

21.3 Autologous Cytokine-Rich Serum (ACRS)

Another alternative treatment for inflammation and wound healing is autologous cytokine-rich serum (ACRS) or autologous conditioned serum (ACS). The products of the companies have been marketed in orthopedics, sports medicine, physical rehabilitation, pain management, aesthetic medicine, dentistry, and oral and maxillofacial surgery. The focus here is on the increase of cytokines (interleukins and growth factors), which decisively intervene in the pain cascade, regulate it, and then trigger regeneration. With the serum obtained, the physician can treat pain and inflammation in the area of gynecology and, at the same time, activate regeneration processes.

21.3.1 How to Prepare Autologous Cytokine-Rich Serum?

Peripheral blood is withdrawn aseptically into the 10 mL of a syringe. The blood is transferred to the tubes, and then the tubes are stored at 37 °C in the incubator for up to 3 h. After incubation, the blood collection tube is centrifuged for 5 min at 4000 rpm. Then blood collection tube is removed from the centrifuge (Fig. 21.2). The serum is separated from the coagulated blood with the help of a 5 mL Luer-Lock syringe and pipetted off (approx. 3–5 mL) aseptically into a second cannula from the blood collection tube. Then, it is injected subcutaneously (Fig. 21.3).

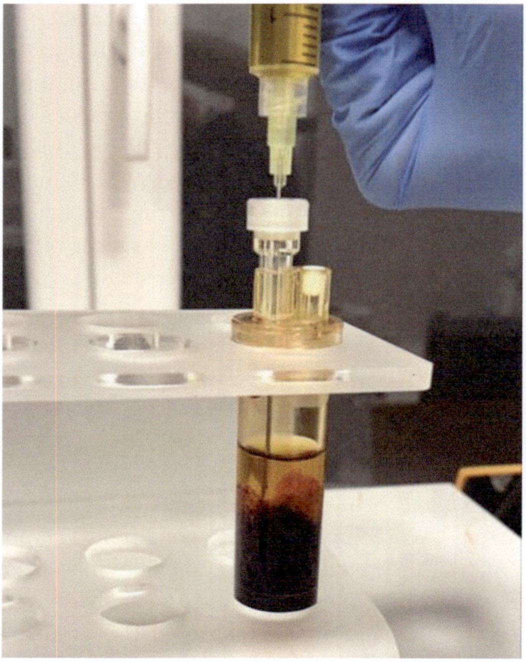

Fig. 21.2 Extraction of serum. The coagulated blood remains in the blood collection tube and is then disposed of (Prep. of Sanakin™)

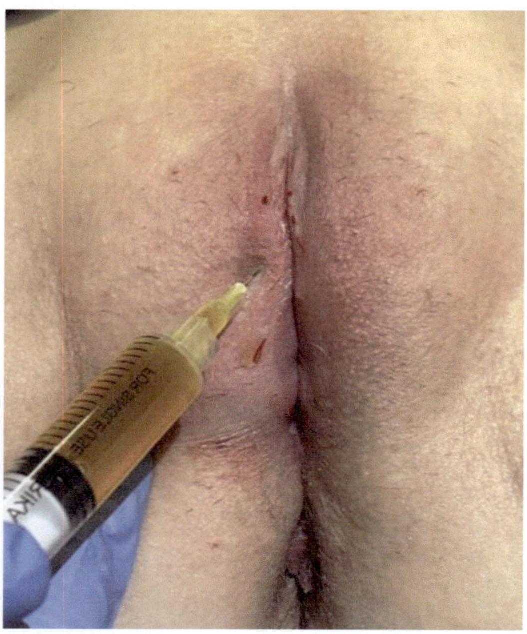

Fig. 21.3 Autolog serum injection. Then, autologous cytokine-rich serum in the syringe is injected

21.3.2 Action of Mechanism

The monocytes release growth factors in the form of peptides in the serum. In the ACRS tube, inflammation will be simulated, and anti-inflammatory cytokines will be released. Blood cells will be activated to produce cytokines and release them simultaneously. From the beginning, the serum contains exponentiated, activated, and released cytokines that have anti-inflammatory and antimicrobial effects.

21.3.3 Difference from the PRP

Both PRP and ACRS treatments can be used for many medical and aesthetic indications. ACRS has no additional substances or anticoagulants in the serum, and it is completely autologous. Conversely, although PRP is rich in thrombocyte cells that secrete growth factors, ACRS provides a platelet-poor solution but is rich in growth factors and anti-inflammatory cytokines.

21.3.4 Possible Indications

ACRS can be used for the regenerative effect with the similar indications of PRP in the skin that include:

- acne,
- psoriasis,
- Behçet's disease,
- menopausal vulvovaginitis,
- lichen sclerosus,
- neurodermatitis,
- scar damage,
- alopecia, and
- intertrigo.

Intra-articular administration of ACS demonstrated some clinical effectiveness in the treatment of osteoarthritis. A comparative analysis of the effectiveness of local therapy with PRP and ACS in patients with osteoarthritis of the knee demonstrated the local therapy with ACS is superior to PRP [5]. Although it seems to be effective, highly well-tolerated, autologous, and safe, patient's own biological variability, limited data, and lack of standardization of the protocols for preparation and application are the limitations of this procedure.

21.4 Platelet Structure

Platelets are the cytoplasmic fragmentation of megakaryocytes that form in the bone marrow. They exert their effects by interacting with leukocytes, endothelial cells, and circulating bone marrow-derived progenitor cells [6]. They trigger inflammatory response, chemotaxis, atherothrombosis, coagulation, and cellular differentiation regulation by autocrine and paracrine self-activation [7]. They also contribute to the formation of the newly formed extracellular matrix.

Platelets have a discoid structure, 2–4 μm in diameter, without nuclei. They contain three types of granules. These are α, lysosomal, and dense granules. In particular, in α and dense granules, GF, cytokines, chemokines, and coagulation factors play a role in hemostasis and wound healing, which are essential tasks [8]. The secretory molecules known as coagulation factors, GF, cytokines, chemokines, and integrins are released by activation of platelets within approximately ten minutes after coagulation. These secretory substances are packaged in granules in the megakaryocyte before being transferred to platelets and subjected to fragmentation. Platelets have an average life span of 7–10 days. In this process, the release of growth factors continues.

The most important growth factors are found in α granules of platelets. There are 50–80 α granules in each platelet, with more than 30 bioactive substances in each α granule [9]. Mitogenic growth factors such as PDGF, TGF-β1-2, IGF, EGF, VEGF, PDF, PDEGF, PDAF adhesive proteins such as osteocalcin, osteonectin, fibrinogen, fibronectin, VWF, vitronectin, thrombospondin, coagulation factors and fibrinolytic factors, antiproteases, cytokines (IL-1β, SCD40L, β-thromboglobulin), chemokines, membrane glycoproteins, angiogenesis regulating proteins, and bactericidal proteins are some of these bioactive substances [9].

Lysosomal granules contain proteolytic enzymes and acid hydrolase enzymes. Dense granules contain platelet agonists such as ADP/ATP, calcium, serotonin, histamine, dopamine, and catecholamine.

Platelets are found in high concentration in the vessels and spleen. Normally there are 130,000–400,000/mL platelets in the circulating blood. After completing their life in the circulation, they are degraded by macrophages in the reticuloendothelial system. In their deficiency (thrombocytopenia), bleeding disorders occur.

21.5 Platelets in the Wound Healing Process

In order to understand PRP treatment, it is necessary to know the wound healing process well. Wound healing is a complex, multicellular process that includes inflammation, proliferation, and remodeling stages and aims to restore tissue integrity. There are mechanisms that are still not fully understood within this process. Wound healing is a process in which keratinocytes, fibroblasts, endothelial cells, macrophages, and platelets take part and work in coordination. The migration, infiltration, proliferation, and differentiation of these cells initially create an inflammatory response, and subsequently, the wound closes with the formation of new tissue. Platelets and GFs secreted by platelets play an active role in all phases of wound healing (Fig. 21.4).

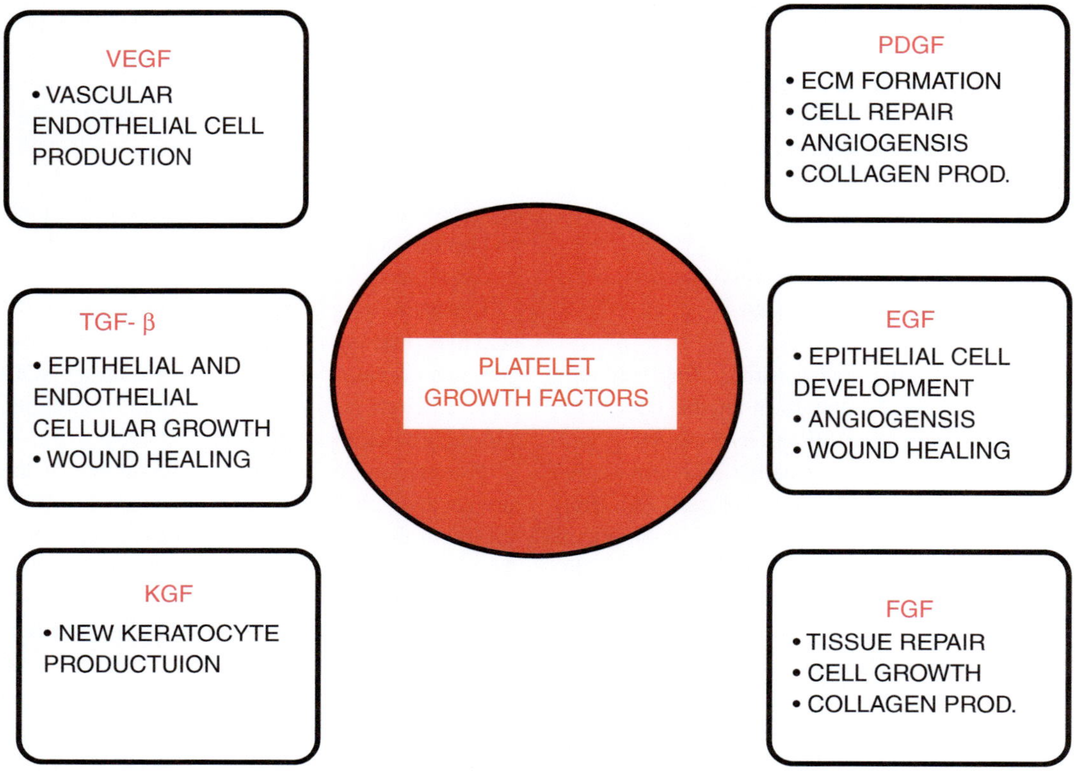

Fig. 21.4 Some growth factors released from platelets and their functions. *FGF* fibroblast growth factor, *PDGF* platelet-derived growth factor, *VEGF* vascular endothelial growth factor, *EGF* epidermal growth factor, *TGF-β* transforming growth factor beta, *KGF* keratinocyte growth factor

21.6 Growth Factors (GF)

PRP contains 7-fold increased TGF-β, 30-fold increased PDGF, and 10-fold increased EGF [10].

TGF-β is found in platelets and macrophages. It has mitogenic and morphogenic functions. Fibroblasts stimulate undifferentiated bone marrow cells and pre-osteoblasts. TGF-β takes part in the remodeling phase. It also has functions such as pro-osteoblast differentiation and osteoblast accumulation.

PDGF is found in both platelets and macrophages. It is a mitogen and chemoattractant for mesenchymal cells and provides extracellular matrix formation. It allows revascularization in the trauma site and plays a role in collagen synthesis, stem cell, and osteoblast mitogenesis. It stimulates fibroblasts and leukocytes such as neutrophils and macrophages. It is important for blood vessel maturation and collagen production.

VEGF and EGF play a role in angiogenesis, basement membrane formation, and endothelial differentiation. These growth factors bind to receptors on mesenchymal cells. Since they do not penetrate the cell and cell nuclei, they do not induce tumor formation.

TGF-α and β promote new collagen formation.

Leukocytes and antibodies present in PRP in small amounts also enable PRP to act as a physiological antibiotic. Hormones, biotransformed vitamins, and other nutrients are also included in the plasma.

The GF in PRP are important for tissue regeneration, new capillary formation, and epithelialization. PRP also contributes to the immune response, thanks to the small amount of leukocytes and globulins it contains. Some studies have shown antimicrobial and antifungal properties against *E. coli*, *S. aureus*, *C. albicans*, and *C. neoformans* [11].

There are studies in the literature showing that PRP treatment is particularly effective in chronic wounds. Unlike in acute wounds, proteinases, which occur as a result of intense bacterial and inflammatory activity in chronic wounds, delay the healing process by destroying GFs. Wound healing can be accelerated by eliminating this deficiency with thrombocytes, which are GF agonists.

Under optimum conditions, PRP should have at least 1,000,000/mL platelets [12]. Higher platelet counts may not affect wound healing positively, but may also negatively affect wound healing. Some studies have shown that high levels of TGF-β, EGF, and PDGF impair wound healing and increase scarring [13].

21.7 How to Prepare PRP?

For the procedure, approximately 15–20 cc of blood is drawn from the peripheral venous vessels in the arm. The volume drawn can be increased up to 50–60 cc, depending on the desired amount of PRP. The blood is then quickly transferred to tubes containing anticoagulants such as sodium citrate or acid phosphate dextrose, without hemolysis, and centrifuged. When performing centrifugation, it is important to comply with the number of cycles and minutes recommended by each PRP manufacturer. Centrifuge can be 12 min at 1200 rpm or 8 min at 3000 rpm. After centrifugation, three layers are formed in the tube:

- At the top is the clear platelet poor plasma (PPP),
- In the middle is the PRP part with platelets and white blood cells (slightly cloudy plasma part called "buffy coat"), and
- At the bottom is the red part with red blood cells.

21.8 Post-Centrifuge Values

The values obtained in PRP formed after centrifugation change in favor of platelets, unlike whole blood [14] (Table 21.2).

Table 21.2 PRP values obtained from peripheral blood

	Peripheral blood	PRP
Volume received	15 cc	1.5 cc
Red blood cell	93%	6%
Platelet	6%	93%
White blood cell	1%	1%

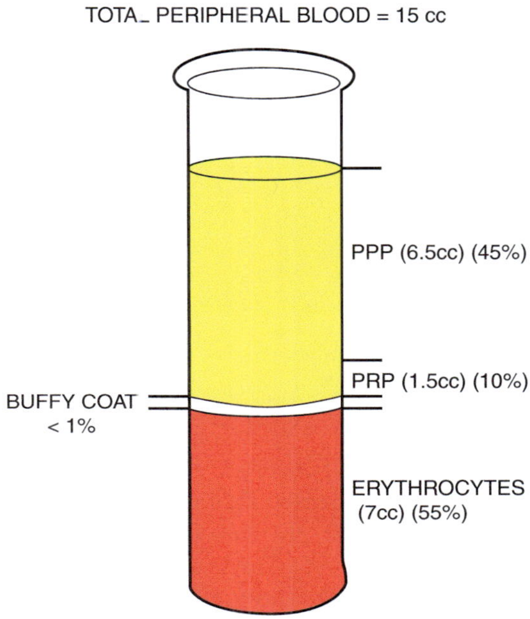

Fig. 21.5 Volumes and percentages of plasma obtained from 15 cc of centrifugated blood, after the first spin

PRP is extracted from approximately 10% of the blood drawn. Thus, approximately 1.5 cc of PRP is obtained from 15 cc of blood. PRP is extracted from the tube with a long-tipped needle (may be a spinal needle) just above the erythrocytes. Generally, a single centrifugation step (single spin) is sufficient for the process. However, if a higher platelet concentration is desired, a second centrifugation step (double spin) can be used. Thus, in the first spin, red blood cells are separated from plasma (Fig. 21.5). and in the second, PRP from platelet-poor plasma (PPP).

For a double spin, the plasma portion extracted from the first tube and transferred to a straight tube is centrifuged again. Sterility must be observed during transfer from tube to tube. After centrifugation, the cloudy plasma ("buffy coat") at the bottom of the tube, PRP and PPP

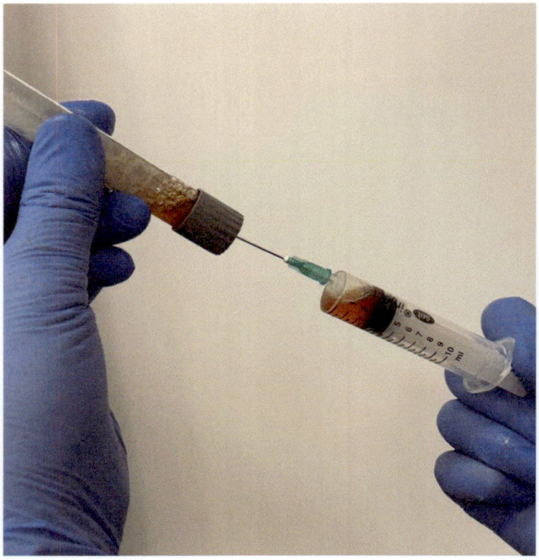

Fig. 21.6 Transferring the prepared PRP and PPP combination into the injector

are separately transferred to the injectors (Fig. 21.6). The reason for the cloudy appearance is that there are leukocytes along with platelets in this layer. There are some opinions that the anti-inflammatory effect of the leukocytes can be increased by photoactivation of plasma with UV light after centrifugation. Additionally, in some studies, it is recommended to mix blood with platelet agonists such as thrombin, batroxobin, or calcium chloride (CaCl) just before centrifugation to stimulate GF release and produce a rapid effect [15]. The PRP obtained afterward is injected into subcutaneous or/and submucosal tissue, just like in the mesotherapy application. Generally, 4 mm, 6 mm, or 13 mm long 30G needles are preferred for injections (Figs. 21.7 and 21.8).

Freshly prepared PRP should be injected within a maximum of 4 h. If the plasma is activated by thrombin or calcium, GF release starts in 10 min, and 95% of this release is completed within an hour [3].

Since PRP is prepared from the person's own blood (autologous), it does not contain any risk of allergies. Platelets and leukocytes dispersed in the tissue show a synergistic effect in the release of GFs.

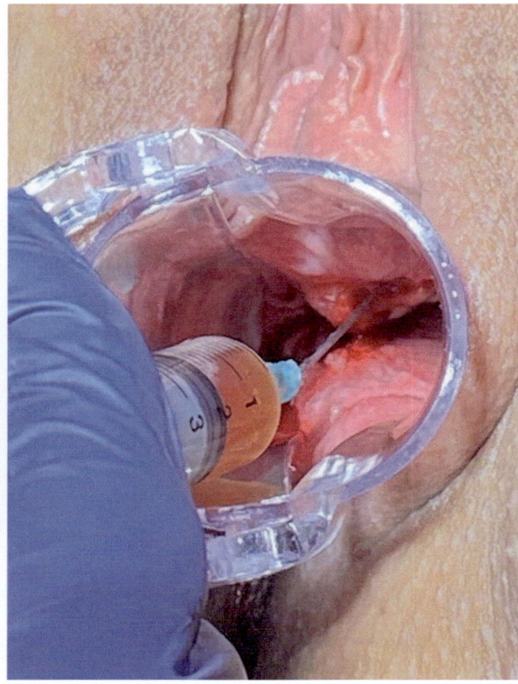

Fig. 21.7 PRP injection into the anterior wall. After rotating the speculum 90°, PRP is injected into previously marked areas. Bending the needle provides convenience

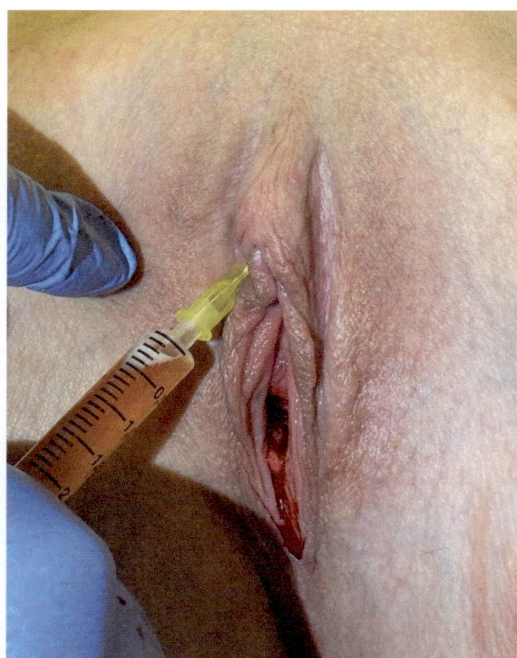

Fig. 21.8 Subcutaneous injections into the hood and vestibular areas with a 30 G needle

Studies have shown that a small amount of blood taken does not alter a person's hemoglobin, hematocrit, and platelet count [16].

21.9 Different Medical Applications of PRP

The procedure can be performed as a dermal or subdermal application. It provides an advantage in that it can be done under office conditions. PRP is a treatment method that has been used in different areas for years.

- *Orthopedic applications:* Spinal surgery, cartilage treatments, tissue defects
- *Dentistry:* Dental and oral surgical applications, maxillofacial surgery
- *Sports Medicine:* Traumas
- *Cardiovascular Surgery:* Surgeries requiring angiogenesis such as bypass
- *Eye:* Macular lesion, corneal epithelial defects
- *Orthopedics:* Surgery of bone, cartilage, and tissue defects
- *Plastic Surgery:* Flap rotating surgery and burn treatments
- *Urology:* Treatment of early Peyronie's disease (scientific data on its use for erectile dysfunction treatment are not yet sufficient)
- *Anesthesiology:* "Patch" treatment in dura mater perforations that manifest with complaints such as headache, dizziness, and nausea after epidural anesthesia
- *Dermatology:* Chronic ulcerated wounds, burn treatments, melasma, and lichen sclerosus treatment

There are quite contradictory results in the studies on PRP in the literature. Differences in results may be related to the tubes used, the protocols applied, patient-dependent factors, lesion-specific features, and the number of platelets injected. Insufficient standardization of the process seems to be a limiting factor for the use of PRP.

The FDA has approved the PRP extraction and collection systems of certain companies. Today, there are compact systems that completely cut off air contact and can perform the processes after blood collection completely automatically.

21.10 Use of PRP in Cosmetic Dermatology

PRP is frequently applied in different areas of cosmetic dermatology. Some of these are:

- skin rejuvenation (face, neck, décolleté, hand),
- treatment of fine lines and wrinkles,
- acne scars,
- after alopecia and hair transplantation,
- cellulite,
- stria, and
- wound healing.

Among the qualities generally sought in skin treatments are the high tolerability of the agent used, good tissue regeneration effect, long duration of the effect obtained with the agent, the treatment being easy and safe, and bio-stimulation of new and natural collagen production. PRP treatments meet these conditions.

Although the application protocols are not clear in cosmetic dermatological applications, 3 or 6 sessions every 2–4 weeks with the point-by-point technique in alopecia, 3 sessions every 2 weeks with the combination of nappage and point technique in skin renewal, and 2–3 sessions every 3 weeks with the linear tunnel technique in dermal filling [17].

Conditions such as the patient's age, gender, race, skin quality, systemic diseases such as concomitant diabetes, wound localization, wound depth, duration of formation, and the number of platelets in PRP content change the results of the application.

PRP injections can be performed simultaneously with laser, RF, vulvar HA injections, or botulinum toxin application [8].

21.11 Indications of PRP in Cosmetic Gynecology

PRP has been increasingly used in the gynecological field, especially in recent years. Since genital area applications are rather new, studies on this subject are also very limited.

21.11.1 Treatments for Functional Purpose

21.11.1.1 Sexual Pleasure Treatments

It was first claimed by Dr. Charles Runels in a pilot study involving 11 patients that intravaginal and intraclitoral PRP application could be used for the treatment of anorgasmia, sexual anorexia, and dyspareunia [17]. Later, this application was registered by him with the trade name "O-Shot©" (orgasm shot).

The genital PRP procedure may be a better alternative to hyaluronic acid procedures performed on the anterior vaginal wall. GFs in PRP provide a regenerative effect by stimulating angiogenesis and increasing collagen synthesis.

Before the PRP procedure for sexual pleasure, a general gynecological evaluation of the patient is made and anamnesis is taken. In suitable patients, 15–18 cc of venous blood is drawn from the arm, and PRP is prepared with a single spin. In this process, local anesthetic cream is also applied to the application area to provide a slight numbing. After the PRP is ready, the genital area is cleaned by wiping with a disinfectant. At this stage, if needed, half-diluted local anesthetic can be injected. Then, the prepared PRP and PPP fluid is injected into the 1/3 lower anterior wall of the vagina, around the clitoris, clitoral hood, and vestibular area with 27 G or 30 G needles. PRP procedure can be performed with a greater volume by taking 40–50 cc of blood from the patient.

The results of a study conducted in Turkey showed that PRP injections to the 1/3 lower anterior wall of the vagina and periclitoral areas positively affect sexual function [18].

21.11.1.2 Menopausal Genitourinary Syndrome (GSM)

The first step in the treatment of menopausal vulvovaginal atrophy complaints is locally used estrogen-containing drugs. However, as it is recommended that people who have been treated for breast cancer or those with cancer risk avoid estrogen-containing drugs, PRP treatment can be applied as an alternative method.

PRP injection can be done as point-by-point or infiltration injections to both the vulvar skin and the vaginal mucosa. Although there is no protocol in this regard, it may be recommended to repeat the application 3–5 times with 3–4 weeks intervals.

In postmenopausal women suffering from vulvovaginal atrophy, vaginal dryness, and dyspareunia, it was observed that with the combined treatment of PRP and HA, trophicity increased, vaginal dryness and dyspareunia decreased, and female sexual distress scores significantly decreased [19].

21.11.1.3 Lichen Sclerosus Treatment

Lichen sclerosus is an autoimmune skin disease with atrophy of the vulvar skin and vestibular mucosa. It is detailed in Chap. 5.

Lichen sclerosus causes complaints such as itching, burning, irritation when wearing trousers, and dyspareunia that disrupt the quality of life (Fig. 21.9). Complaints increase especially with the transition to the menopausal period. Symptom improvement can be achieved with PRP treatment applied to this area.

A study of a 67-year-old patient who received estrogen therapy due to menopausal atrophy and lichen sclerosus but did not respond to treatment found a decrease in the patient's complaints and

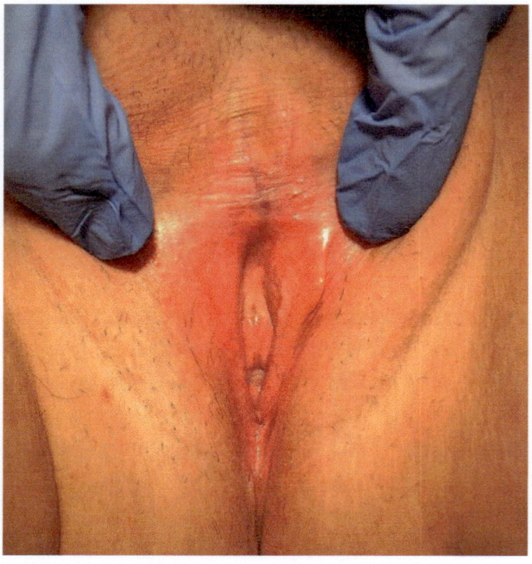

Fig. 21.9 Lichen sclerosus. Phimosis in the clitoral hood, obliteration of the glans, inflammation of the labia minora, and thin skin tissue are seen

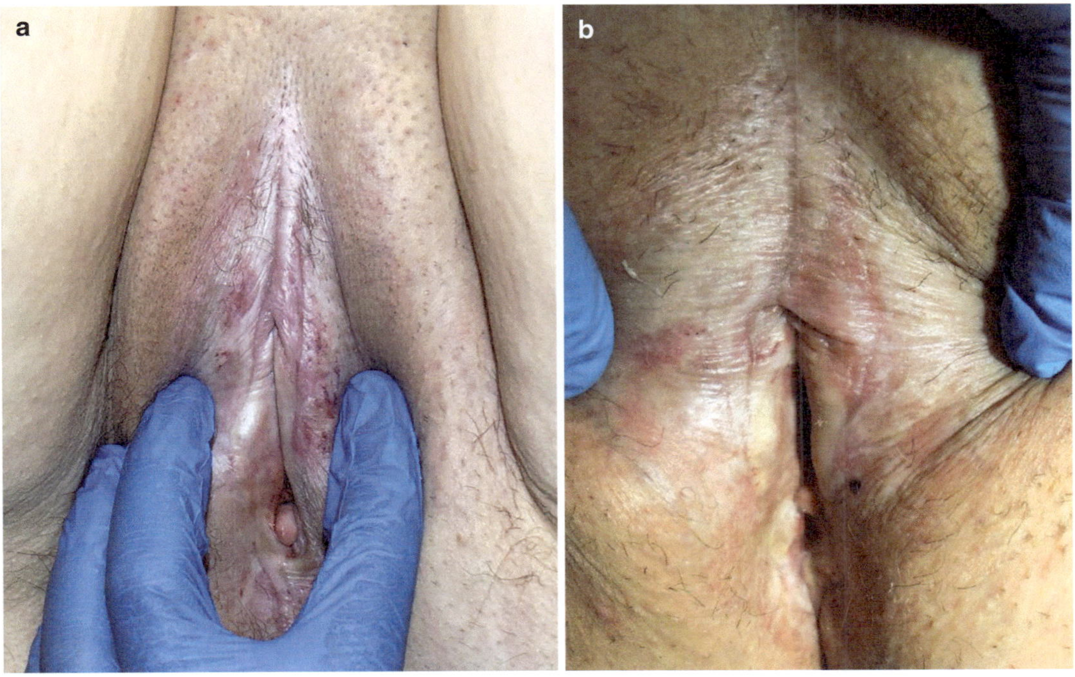

Fig. 21.10 Lichen sclerosus. The appearance before (**a**) and 4 months after (**b**) single session CO_2 laser and PRP treatment

improvement in vulvar atrophy after injecting a total of 40 cc of fat and PRP mixture into the labia majora [20].

In another study, it was stated that PRP could be a suitable alternative to topical steroids in the treatment of lichen sclerosus [21].

The combination of fractional carbon dioxide laser and PRP injection is quite effective in the symptomatic treatment of lichen sclerosus disease (Fig. 21.10). As a treatment protocol, 2–4 sessions can be applied every 3–4 months.

SVF (stromal vascular fraction) treatments may also be recommended in patients with resistant and highly active lichen sclerosis.

21.11.1.4 Other Indications

Although Charles Runels has stated on his website that genital PRP can be applied in stress incontinence, urge incontinence, interstitial cystitis, fecal incontinence, and chronic pain after mesh, scientific data on these issues are not yet sufficient.

In some studies in the literature, PRP injections are recommended to increase endometrial thickness and improve ovarian reserve in infertility treatments [22, 23].

21.11.2 Treatments for Aesthetic Purpose

21.11.2.1 Labium Majus Rejuvenation

PRP is not indicated for labia majora augmentation. However, vulvar PRP treatments performed in cases such as skin wrinkles, collapse, darkening, and hypotonicity in this area can provide aesthetic improvement by their regenerative effects. Vulvar rejuvenation treatments are often combined with energy-based technologies applied to this area. PRP procedures can be done by different methods such as point or retrograde injection into the subcutaneous tissue.

The process of inserting a thin needle into the skin alone (microneedling) increases collagen stimulation. Wound healing is stimulated with microneedling, growth factors are released, and neocollagenesis begins. Applying topical growth factors or PRP to the area after microneedling can accelerate the healing process.

21.11.2.2 Episiotomy Scar Treatment

PRP injections into and just below the scar in hypertrophic scars, and in the lower part of the scar in atrophic scars, can provide a certain improvement. Applications can be repeated 3–5 times with 3–4 weeks intervals, depending on the response.

Although some authors recommend injection of PRP to the wound site immediately after labiaplasty, vaginoplasty, and combined genital aesthetic operations in order to accelerate wound healing, there is no scientific data on this subject. However, it seems reasonable to use, especially in labiaplasty and vaginoplasty patients who have excessive intraoperative bleeding.

21.12 Different Indications of PRP in Gynecology

PRP and platelet-rich fibrin (PRF) are increasingly used for different indications in gynecology due to their regenerative effects. In an animal experiment on New Zealand rabbits, it was observed that PRP-coated mesh did not reduce adhesion parameters but decreased inflammation and oxidative stress and increased antioxidant values [24].

In another study, intralesional PRP was applied to a group of patients with symptomatic cervical ectopia twice, one week apart, and in the other group, Nd:YAG laser vaporization was applied to the lesion. The effects of both treatments were compared. Complete cure was observed in 93% of the PRP group and 92% in the laser group, and side effects such as vaginal discharge and bleeding were much less common in the PRP group. In addition, it was observed that the re-epithelialization time was shorter in the PRP group [25].

In a recent study, it was found that IVF results were positively affected by intrauterine PRP infusion 48 h before frozen embryo transfer in patients with recurrent implantation failure [26].

In another study, it was observed that PRP infusion positively affected endometrial thickness, pregnancy rates, and live birth rates, especially in recurrent pregnancy losses [27].

21.13 PRP Contraindications

- Platelet dysfunction syndrome
- Thrombocytopenia
- Hypofibrinogenemia
- Hemodynamic instability
- Sepsis
- Anticoagulant treatment
- Acute and chronic infections
- Presence of cancer or precancerous lesions in the application area
- Chronic liver pathology

21.14 Combined Therapies

PRP treatments can be combined with procedures such as botulinum toxin injection, HA, or autologous fat transfer. Mixing PRP with HA is not recommended, as PRP may disrupt the HA structure. However, they can be injected in succession. On the other hand, Cellular Matrix™ tubes (by Regenlab company) allow the preparation of autologous platelet-rich plasma combined with a non-crosslinked hyaluronic acid (HA) in a closed-circuit system. This technology is recommended especially in patients with osteoarthritis for giving better and longer-lasting results by combining the complementary clinical effects of PRP and HA. There are also some studies showing that when mixed with autologous fat, PRP increases adipocyte survival [28].

The use of PRP treatments together with thermal energy-generating technologies such as RF and laser is common among physicians. However, in a study conducted, VEGF, EGF, bFGF, IL-17, and IL-8 concentrations were examined after PRP was incubated at 37 °C, 23 °C, and 4 °C for 30 min, and it was observed that the highest concentrations were at 4 °C. Interestingly, PDGF values were not affected by temperature. As a result, low temperature accelerates platelet activation by increasing the release of α and dense granules. Conversely, there are opposing views that the regenerative effect will quickly disappear due to the rapid activity of platelets [29].

21.15 Complications

Generally, no major complications are expected after PRP. There is a risk of infection only if aseptic rules are not followed in the preparation process. However, it has been reported that PRP treatment may lead to life-threatening coagulopathy with the formation of antibodies against factor V, XI, and thrombin due to bovine thrombin used in treatment [30]. From this aspect, PRF seems more advantageous.

21.16 Post-procedure Term

The PRP application process is completely non-invasive, non-allergenic, safe, and has very minimal risk. If the indication is suitable for the person and it is done properly, the results are satisfactory.

After the genital PRP procedure, a mild pinkish vaginal discharge, burning, stinging, and skin edema are normal. PRP treatment does not require any maintenance or social restrictions. One day after the procedure, sexual intercourse is permitted. The expected effects are usually seen three weeks after the procedure.

After genital PRP application, NSAI or steroid-like drugs should not be used for 4 weeks, as an inflammatory reaction will begin. Only paracetamol group drugs should be recommended for any pain complaints. Combined procedures or different treatment options should be offered to patients whose complaints do not improve despite 2–3 applications.

Appendix

With the purchase of this book, you can use our "SN Flashcards" app to access questions free of charge in order to test your learning and check your understanding of the contents of the book.

To use the app, please follow the instructions below:

1. Go to https://flashcards.springernature.com/login
2. Create a user account by entering your e-mail address and assigning a password.
3. Use the following link to access your SN Flashcards set: ▶ https://sn.pub/tvlq7Q

If the link is missing or does not work, please send an e-mail with the subject "SN Flashcards" and the book title to customerservice@springernature.com.

References

1. Mehta S, Watson JT. Platelet rich concentrate: basic science and current clinical applications. J Orthop Trauma. 2008;22(6):432–8.
2. Ross R, Glomset J, Kariya B, Harker L. A platelet-dependent serum factor that stimulates the proliferation of arterial smooth muscle cells in vitro. Proc Natl Acad Sci U S A. 1974;71(4):1207–10.
3. Feigin K, Shope B. Use of platelet-rich plasma and platelet-rich fibrin in dentistry and oral surgery: introduction and review of the literature. J Vet Dent. 2019;36(2):109–23.
4. Pourang A, Rockwell H, Karimi K. New frontiers in skin rejuvenation, including stem cells and autologous therapies. Facial Plast Surg Clin North Am. 2020;28(1):101–17.
5. Khurana A, Goyal A, Kirubakaran P, Akhand G, Gupta R, Goel N. Efficacy of autologous conditioned serum (ACS), platelet-rich plasma (PRP), hyaluronic acid (HA) and steroid for early osteoarthritis knee: a comparative analysis. Indian J Orthop. 2020;55(Suppl 1):217–27.
6. Davì G, Patrono C. Platelet activation and atherothrombosis. N Engl J Med. 2007;357(24):2482–94.
7. Marx RE. Platelet-rich plasma (PRP): what is PRP and what is not PRP? Implant Dent. 2001;10(4):225–8.
8. Turan Y, Erbil H, Koç E. Plateletten Zengin Plazma ve Dermatoloji. Dermatoz. 2011;2:355–60.
9. Eppley BL, Pietrzak WS, Blanton M. Platelet-rich plasma: a review of biology and applications in plastic surgery. Plast Reconstr Surg. 2006;118(6):147–59.
10. Babbush CA, Kevy SV, Jacobson MS. An in vitro and in vivo evaluation of autologous platelet concentrate in oral reconstruction. Implant Dent. 2003;12(1):24–34.
11. Tang YQ, Yeaman MR, Selsted ME. Antimicrobial peptides from human platelets. Infect Immun. 2002;70(12):6524–33.

12. Mishra A, Woodall J Jr, Vieira A. Treatment of tendon and muscle using platelet-rich plasma. Clin Sports Med. 2009;28(1):113–25.
13. Barrientos S, Stojadinovic O, Golinko MS, Brem H, Tomic-Canic M. Growth factors and cytokines in wound healing. Wound Repair Regen. 2008;16(5):585–601.
14. Carlson NE, Roach RB Jr. Platelet-rich plasma: clinical applications in dentistry. J Am Dent Assoc. 2002;133(10):1383–6.
15. Crovetti G, Martinelli G, Issi M, Barone M, Guizzardi M, Campanati B, Moroni M, Carabelli A. Platelet gel for healing cutaneous chronic wounds. Transfus Apher Sci. 2004;30(2):145–51.
16. Floege J, Eitner F, Alpers CE. A new look at platelet-derived growth factor in renal disease. J Am Soc Nephrol. 2008;19(1):12–23.
17. Runels C, Melnick H, Debourbon E, Roy L. A pilot study of the effect of localized injections of autologous platelet rich plasma (PRP) for the treatment of female sexual dysfunction. J Womens Health Care. 2014;3:4.
18. Sukgen G, Ellibeş Kaya A, Karagün E, Çalışkan E. Platelet-rich plasma administration to the lower anterior vaginal wall to improve female sexuality satisfaction. Turk J Obstet Gynecol. 2019;16(4):228–34.
19. Hersant B, SidAhmed-Mezi M, Belkacemi Y, Darmon F, Bastuji-Garin S, Werkoff G, Bosc R, Niddam J, Hermeziu O, La Padula S, Meningaud JP. Efficacy of injecting platelet concentrate combined with hyaluronic acid for the treatment of vulvovaginal atrophy in postmenopausal women with history of breast cancer: a phase 2 pilot study. Menopause. 2018;25(10):1124–30.
20. Kim SH, Park ES, Kim TH. Rejuvenation using platelet-rich plasma and lipofilling for vaginal atrophy and lichen sclerosus. J Menopausal Med. 2017;23(1):63–8.
21. Behnia-Willison F, Pour NR, Mohamadi B, Willison N, Rock M, Holten IW, O'Shea R, Miller J. Use of platelet-rich plasma for vulvovaginal autoimmune conditions like lichen sclerosus. Plast Reconstr Surg Glob Open. 2016;4(11):e1124.
22. Sills ES, Wood SH. Autologous activated platelet-rich plasma injection into adult human ovary tissue: molecular mechanism, analysis, and discussion of reproductive response. Biosci Rep. 2019;39(6):BSR20190805.
23. Du J, Lu H, Yu X, Lü Z, Mi L, Zhang X. Efficacy and safety of platelet-rich plasma for the treatment of thin endometrium: a protocol for systematic review and meta-analysis. Medicine. 2020;99(3):e18848.
24. Belebecha V, Casagrande R, Urbano MR, Crespigio J, Martinez RM, Vale DL, de Almeida SHM. Effect of the platelet-rich plasma covering of polypropylene mesh on oxidative stress, inflammation, and adhesions. Int Urogynecol J. 2020;31(1):139–47.
25. Hua X, Zeng Y, Zhang R, Wang H, Diao J, Zhang P. Using platelet-rich plasma for the treatment of symptomatic cervical ectopy. Int J Gynaecol Obstet. 2012;119(1):26–9.
26. Zamaniyan M, Peyvandi S, Heidaryan Gorji H, Moradi S, Jamal J, Yahya Poor Aghmashhadi F, Hossein MM. Effect of platelet-rich plasma on pregnancy outcomes in infertile women with recurrent implantation failure: a randomized controlled trial. Gynecol Endocrinol. 2021;37(2):141–5.
27. Coksuer H, Akdemir Y, Ulas BM. Improved in vitro fertilization success and pregnancy outcome with autologous platelet-rich plasma treatment in unexplained infertility patients that had repeated implantation failure history. Gynecol Endocrinol. 2019;35(9):815–8.
28. Willemsen JC, Lindenblatt N, Stevens HP. Results and long-term patient satisfaction after gluteal augmentation with platelet-rich plasma-enriched autologous fat. Eur J Plast Surg. 2013;36(12):777–82.
29. Etulain J, Mena HA, Meiss RP, Frechtel G, Gutt S, Negrotto S, Schattner M. An optimised protocol for platelet-rich plasma preparation to improve its angiogenic and regenerative properties. Sci Rep. 2018;8(1):1513.
30. Kiran NK, Mukunda KS, Tilak Raj TN. Platelet concentrates: a promising innovation in dentistry. J Dent Sci Res. 2011;2:50–61.

22 Carboxytherapy

Medicine is not merely a science but an art. The character of the physician may act more powerfully upon the patient than the drugs employed.

Paracelsus

Carbon dioxide therapy, better known as "carboxytherapy", relates to percutaneous (intradermal and/or subcutaneous) infusion of medical carbon dioxide with therapeutic approaches. It has been suggested that by improving oxygenation, interacting with the tissue perfusion regulators, and disrupting the adipose cell membranes, the method can lead to notable improvements in different aesthetic and medical conditions. Conversely, carbon dioxide is currently the most frequently used gas for insufflation of the abdominal cavity (pneumoperitoneum).

CO_2 has antihypoxic, antioxidant, antiaging, vasodilatory, anti-inflammatory, analgesic, and spasmolytic activities; moreover, it improves blood viscosity and stimulates neoangiogenesis and regenerative processes. It is the most popular treatment that has been officially recognized worldwide and has become an alternative to pharmacotherapy for many diseases.

The technique originated in France in 1932, and initially, the treatment was carried out percutaneously by the so-called heated carbonated water baths or the application of water-saturated CO_2 directly to the skin of patients.

The multiple mechanisms of action of treatment (polymodal efficacy) make carboxytherapy a popular medical technology worldwide in cosmetology, aesthetic medicine, dermatology, angiology, orthopedics, cardiology neurology, pulmonology, gynecology, urology, proctology, plastic, and general surgery. Carboxytherapy provides a perfect example of off-label usage in medicine, making it one of the most extensively applied medical technologies for treating various diseases despite the lack of preclinical data and scarce relevant information.

22.1 Mechanism

Carbon dioxide is a sort of biochemical "peacemaker" in tissue oxygenation: when blood cells are exposed to high CO_2 concentrations, it will reduce the oxygen affinity of hemoglobin. So, the hemoglobin will release oxygen into the tissue. The administration of CO_2 in the tissues promotes hydration by forming erythrocytes of carbonic acid H_2CO_3, which dissociates into H + ion and bicarbonate HCO_3, known as the "Bohr effect." Since the human organism interprets carboxytherapy (local hypercapnia) as oxygen deficiency and responds to it by boosting the blood flow, the vascular endothelial growth factor (VEGF) stimulates neoangiogenesis, in the long run, enhances microcirculation, tissue oxygenation, and tissue tropism.

S. Eserdağ, *Aesthetic and Functional Female Genital Surgery*,
https://doi.org/10.1007/978-3-031-16019-6_22

Moreover, controlled administration of medical CO_2 into the subcutaneous tissue induces hypercapnia and decreases local pH, eliciting a strong vasodilator response by relaxing the pre-arteriolar smooth muscle on the site.

Studies showed that local application of CO_2 can improve peripheral circulation, increase tissue perfusion and oxygen partial pressure by reflex vasodilation, and stimulate neoangiogenesis [1].

Carbon dioxide is an odorless, colorless gas naturally produced by our bodies. Even in high doses, it is non-toxic and disposed of at the physiological level. After a single intradermal or subcutaneous treatment, the gas is absorbed in 5–10 min and diffuses at the skin microcirculatory level. Subsequently, the body will seek to restore an imbalance of oxygen/CO_2 levels, improving blood flow to supply oxygen and nutrients to the skin and vessels, eventually improving the skin appearance. One of the mechanisms of action of carboxytherapy might be due to the lysis of adipocytes resulting in the release of triglycerides into intercellular spaces, with subsequent improvement of skin elasticity. In addition, the vasodilatation produced by CO_2 gas permits the accumulation of inflammatory response and improves the healing process increasing collagen formation and reorganization and ultimately improving skin texture and tone.

The liquid carbon dioxide in the cylinder is turned into gas form by heating and transferred to a plastic cannula. After being filtered by a filter at the cannula's tip, it is injected transcutaneously with a fine needle. Some of the companies produced "carboxy-gun" as a handling probe, and some of them had a warming feature of the gas (up to +45°) to make the procedure less painful.

It is recommended to clean the area with 70% ethyl alcohol or any non-irritant antiseptics prior to the administration. 15 cc of carbon dioxide gas can spread intradermally and diffuse to cover an area of about 2–3 cm in diameter.

22.2 Cosmetic and Dermatologic Indications

In most studies, significant improvements in the mentioned conditions below have been obtained.

22.2.1 Stretch Marks

Stretch marks (striae distensae, striae atrophicans) are prevalent skin conditions that may cause a remarkable psychological influence on the patients. It was first described in 1889, and the frequency of it mentioned in publications differs significantly, ranging from 11 to 88% [2]. Simultaneously, anatomical affected areas vary, with sites mainly involved including the abdomen, breasts, thighs, and buttocks.

Two clinically different variants of stretch marks were reported; "striae rubrae" (the early erythematous or violaceous lesions) and "striae albae" (the wrinkled, hypopigmented, atrophic scar-like marks). The term "striae gravidarum" describes stretch marks occurring during pregnancy, frequently after the 24th week, and commonly affects the breast and abdomen [3].

Predisposing factors include:

- pregnancy,
- obesity,
- Cushing's disease,
- long-term use of oral and topical steroids,
- insufficient skin development (especially elastic and collagen fibers),
- mechanical stretching of the skin, and
- endocrinal imbalance.

The frequency and anatomical areas involved differ concerning gender and age. In adolescents, nearly 40% of males and 70% of females suffer from it. It is more prominent in the lower back and knees in adolescent males whereas thighs and calves in adolescent females [2].

Histologically, stretch marks are scars that show an atrophic flat epidermis with attenuated rete ridges, fraying, splitting with the horizontal organization of collagen bundles, dilatation of blood vessels, and clumping and fragmentation of elastic fibers.

For striae treatment, injections must be performed in two stages. In the first stage, with the formation of small papules: injection of CO_2 should be performed very superficially directly into the stretches (smaller), the angle of inclination of the needle is 15° while the bevel border is up, the dose is 5–10 mL, the length of the needle is 4–6 mm. Bulging caused by the gas injection could be seen and felt, which guarantees the injection of the whole area. Erythema, as well as tissue distension, was used as a clinical endpoint of CO_2 infusion. In the second stage, the linear method (more expressed stretches, wide and long ones), the zone is treated retrograde; the distance between injections depends on the length of the stretch. Both methods can be used simultaneously, but treating stretches systematically in two stages is recommended. There is a cosmetic effect, but stretches do not completely disappear (it is necessary to combine with other types of treatment).

The treatment protocol consisted of 8–15 sessions with an interval of 7 days. CO_2 infusion can be done with a 30 G or 32 G needle, 3 mm depth with 15° angulation. 15 cc of the gas can be applied and increased up to 45 cc in large areas. Then, a gentle massage was performed.

Different types of minimally invasive procedures such as skin needling, microdermabrasion, chemical peels, glycolic acid, ascorbic acid, topical treatments like tretinoin, platelet-rich plasma, stem cell therapy, soft tissue fillers, carbon dioxide, Er: YAG, diode, Q-switched Nd: YAG, pulsed dye and excimer laser, fractional photothermolysis, and radiofrequency are recommended or applied as a combined treatment to CO_2 therapy.

22.2.2 Cellulite and Local Adiposity Treatment

Cellulite (gynoid lipodystrophy) affects 80–90% of women, commonly in the buttocks and thighs, especially after puberty. Despite no morbidity, it causes excellent dissatisfaction and negatively influences the quality of life. Its etiology is multifactorial and involves complex issues. The accumulation of localized fat could contribute to increased local tissue compression, favoring the traction of fibrotic beams and herniation of adipocytes in the dermis, causing the appearance of the "orange peel skin" depressions, a characteristic feature of cellulite disorder [4].

Conversely, carboxytherapy effectively reduces localized fat in obese patients, which is mechanistically associated with altering the vasculature involved in VEGF [5]. The therapeutic effect of carboxytherapy lipolysis is obtained by temperature increase and VEGF-mediated vascularization.

In cellulitis and/or local fat deposition, the carboxytherapy course may include 8–15 procedures. It is held 3 times a week as an intensive course and up to 1 time a month as a supportive procedure. To treat cellulitis and reduce local fat deposits, the depth of CO_2 injections is from 4 mm to 8–10 mm, which allows for improving lymphatic drainage and outflow of cell decay products at the proper depth.

CO_2 infusion can be done with a 30 G needle (13 mm length) with 45° angulation and 10 mm depth. The dose is 10–20 mL. The procedure is carried out 1–2 times a week, with the hip approximately divided into 6–8 zones: 4 on the front side and 2–4 zones on the backside. In each zone, 4–8 injections are performed. When performing carboxytherapy in the hip area, it is necessary to know the location of large vessels.

Other recommended methods for cellulite and/or local adiposity treatments are a balanced diet, physical activity, massage, topical products, radiofrequency, mesotherapy, therapeutic ultrasound, and light-emitting diode therapy.

22.2.3 Face Rejuvenation

Carboxytherapy can be used for face rejuvenation like treating periorbital dark circles (periorbital hyperpigmentation) [6], lymphatic eye bags, acne scars, forehead, glabellar wrinkles, submental fat reduction, and jowl tightening for double chin appearance (Fig. 22.1).

Periorbital hyperpigmentation is a disturbing aesthetic concern for patients. Etiologies of the condition include pigmentary, structural, vascular, and mixed causes. For upper and lower eyelid processing, CO_2 injections must be done intracutaneously into the eyelid area, about 2 cm from the outer corner of the eye, with an inclination of 15°, dose 5–10 mL, needle length 4–6 mm. Despite visible swelling after the procedure, the patient does not feel pain. It is desirable to perform two injections at a distance of 2 cm from each other in the direction of the lower eyelid [7].

Effective treatments for periorbital hyperpigmentation include carboxytherapy, lasers, topical creams and serums, fillers, chemical peels, plasma-rich platelet injections, blepharoplasty, and normobaric oxygen. Soft tissue fillers and autologous fat grafting are most effective in treating dark circles due to volume loss. Blepharoplasty surgery is best when excessive skin laxity is the underlying cause. Various topical creams and chemical peels help treat pigment-based lesions, whereas lasers are mild to moderate beneficial for vascular and pigment types.

Injections in the forehead are recommended to begin along the line 1–2 cm above the upper eyelid. The distance between injections and lines is 3 cm. In the glabella area, injection is carried out over the wrinkle toward the root of the nose, sometimes in the upper eyelid region in the inner corner of the eye.

For the treatment of the cheek area, CO_2 injections must be only intradermal and be parallel along with the line, copying the shape of the face and lower jaw. The distance between injections is 3–4 cm; then, one injection is performed in the area of the external line along the axis and one injection in the middle of the cheek.

For raising the corners of the mouth, CO_2 injection must be at a distance of about 1 cm from the corner of the mouth. Two injections must be done into the nasolabial sulcus, in the middle of the nasolabial wrinkle, and above the corner of the mouth. The linear injection is CO_2 performed retrograde. For chin treatment, 1–2 injections are enough.

Carboxytherapy skin rejuvenation seems efficient in the treatment, and the therapeutic effect may be caused by vascular drainage, oxygenation, and collagen remodeling in the long run. CO_2 infusion can be done with a 30 G or 32 G needle with 15° angulation and 3 mm depth with a bevel border up, directly into the aged or wrinkled skin. For the periorbital hyperpigmentation treatment, injecting only 3 cc of the gas would be enough on each side. The bulging caused by CO_2 injection could be noticed by the naked eye, which guarantees the injection of the whole area. The treatment protocol consisted of 7–8 sessions at 7 days of intervals.

Carboxytherapy is an easy, safe, simple, and relatively effective method for facial rejuvenation with minimal downtime. Better results can be achieved when used in combination with a fractional CO_2 laser [8].

22.2.4 Psoriasis

Psoriasis is a chronic autoimmune skin disease characterized by the appearance of red, white, and gray papules, hyperkeratosis, cracks, and sometimes pustule.

Carboxytherapy is an additional therapy to treat small psoriatic plaques in the ulna, knee, and genital region. All injections of CO_2 are performed subcutaneously in two ways: the first-around plaque in a safe area of the skin; the second—once in the middle of the plaque. The volume of CO_2 per session is 20–40 mL. The angle of the needle inclination is 15°, dose 5 mL, needle length 30 G—6–12 mm, and the distance between injections is 2 cm. The recommended number of carboxytherapy sessions is 5–15, 1–2 times a week, and the number of procedures depends on the local status and patient health [9].

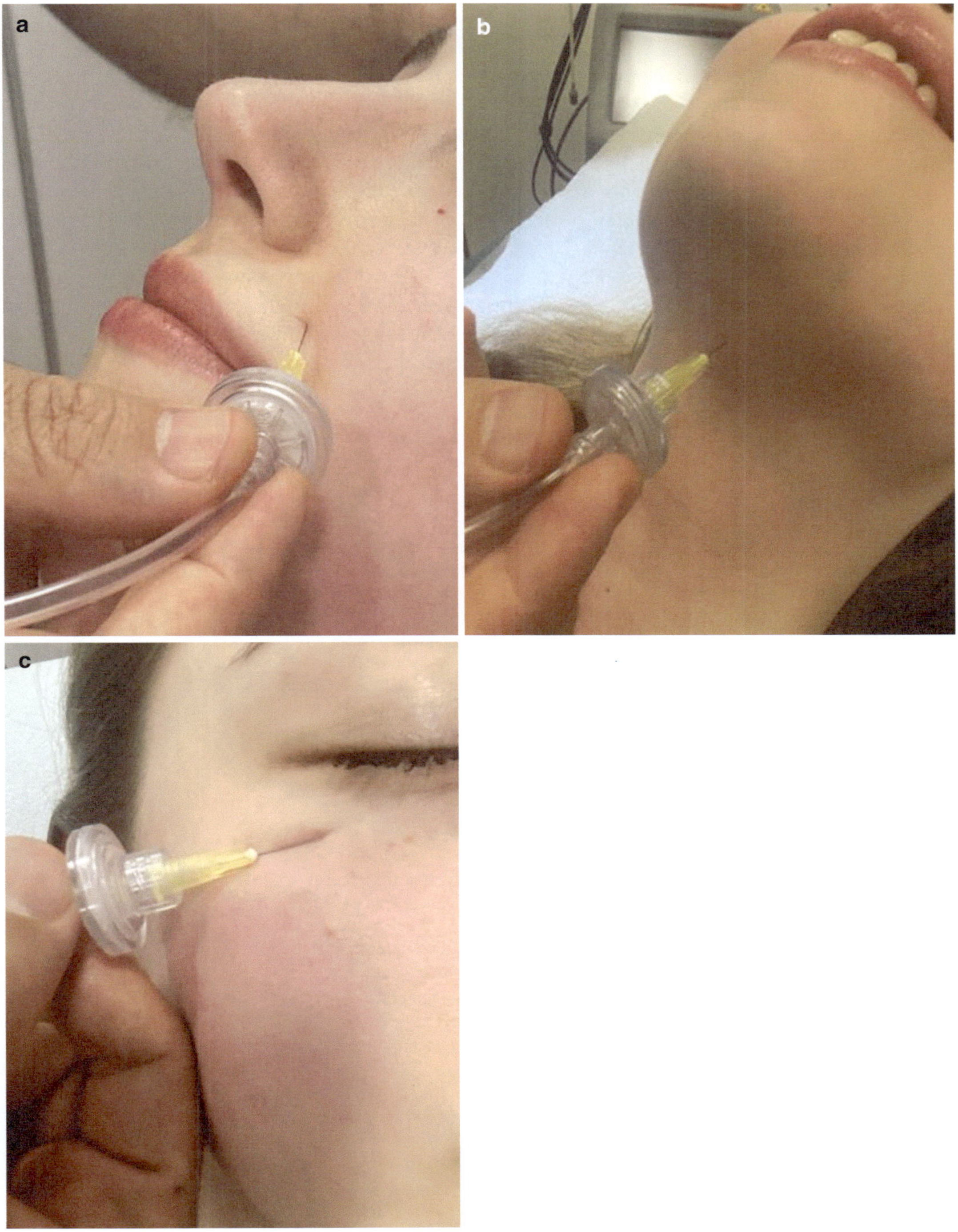

Fig. 22.1 Different applications of carboxytherapy for the face rejuvenation. Nasolabial sulcus (**a**), jowl (**b**), infraorbital (**c**)

22.2.5 Alopecia

Intradermal or subcutaneous applications of the gas can enhance the blood supply of hair follicles, oxygen and nutrients delivery to the hair bulb, and improve innervation [10].

The angle of needle inclination must be 15°; dose CO_2 is 5 mL, injection depth 1–2 mm, needle length 4–6 mm; the distance between injections is 1–2 cm (depends on the patient's sensitivity). After improving hair growth, the distance between injections must increase. The effect becomes noticeable after 3–4 sessions, and the final result will be achieved after injections.

CO_2 injections must be done 2 times per month, on average 6–8 injections. After hair growth begins, the intervals between procedures increase to 1 time a week or 10 days. The total number of procedures is 16–22 sessions. If there are no noticeable improvements within 2 months, it is recommended to stop the procedure.

Carboxytherapy in cosmetology and aesthetic medicine (Table 22.1), and carboxytherapy in dermatology (Table 22.2) managements are summarized below.

Table 22.1 Carboxytherapy in cosmetology and aesthetic medicine [11]

Area	Injection lines of CO_2	Needle length (mm)	Dose CO2 (mL)	Inclination angle
Upper and lower eyelid processing	2 injections are performed at a distance of 2 cm from each other in the direction of the lower eyelid. Each periorbital area is processed individually in a sequence: glabella, forehead, and cheek	4–6	5–10	15–30°
Forehead and glabella treatment	Injection in the forehead area is recommended to begin along the line 1–2 cm above the upper eyelid. In the glabella area, injection is performed over the wrinkle toward the nasal root	4–6	5–10	15–30°
Treatment of the cheek area	An antegrade method is used. Injections are performed in parallel along the line copying the shape of the face and lower jaw, the distance between injections is 3–4 cm	4–6	5–10	15–30°
Raising the "fallen" corners of the mouth	CO2 injections conduct at a distance of about 1 cm from the corner of the mouth. Two injections must be made into the nasolabial wrinkle: in the middle of the nasolabial wrinkle and above the corner of the mouth	4–6	1–5	15–30°
Dark circles under eyes treatment	The treatment begins with an internal angle of the eyes, about 1 cm under the edge of the lower eyelid, and continues in the direction of the external angle of the eye. The distance between injections is 1–1.5 cm, and the total number of lines is 2–3 at a distance of 1 cm from each other	4–6	5	15-30°
Neck and neckline treatment	Different methods are used depending on the place of treatment at the discretion of the doctor	4–6	5–10	15–30°
Double chin treatment	It is sufficient 2–4 injections, subcutaneous administration, by the antegrade method	12	5–10	45°
Sagging underarm skin treatment	Three lines are selected from the axillary fossa in the direction of the elbow. The distance between pricks and lines is 3–4 cm	12	5–10	45°
Treatment of the back of the hands to rejuvenate the skin	4–5 injections are performed: in the middle of the back of the hand and the wrist area	6–12	5–10	15–30°
Cellulite treatment	It is carried out 1–2 times a week, with the hip approximately divided into 6–8 zones—4 on the front side and 2–4 zones on the backside	12	10–20	45°

Table 22.1 (continued)

Area	Injection lines of CO_2	Needle length (mm)	Dose CO2 (mL)	Inclination angle
Fresh scars treatment	It is necessary to select a zone for processing, departing 1–2 cm from the scar. Twice a week	4–6	3–5	45°
Abdominal visceral fat treatment	It is necessary to divide the abdominal area into zones: two in the upper abdomen and four in the lower abdomen. Zones are processed simultaneously or with a one-week break	12	10–20	45°
Stretches and striae treatment	In the first stage, CO2 is injected directly into the stretches (smaller ones). In the second stage the linear method (more pronounced strings, wide and long stretches) and the zone is treated retrograde. The distance between injections depends on the length of the stretch	4–6	5–10	15–30°

Table 22.2 Carboxytherapy in dermatology [11]

Area	Injection lines of CO_2	Needle length (mm)	Dose CO_2 (mL)	Inclination angle
Alopecia	The distance between injections is 1–2 cm. At the beginning of the course of carboxytherapy, CO2 injections must be done 2 times a month, on average 6–8 injections. After hair growth begins, the intervals between procedures increase to 1 week or 10 days The total number of procedures is 16–22	4–6	5	15–30°
Psoriasis	CO2 injections must be done intracutaneously in two ways: the first, around the plaque in a safe area of the skin; the second, once in the middle of the plaque. The distance between injections is 2 cm	6–12	1–5	15–30°
Scleroderma	CO2 is injected intracutaneously directly into lesions	6–12	5	15–30°

22.3 Genital Indications

22.3.1 Genitourinary Syndrome of Menopause (GSM)

Genitourinary syndrome of menopause is one of the challenging problems encountered by gynecologists. It has genital, sexual, and urinary symptoms that harm the quality of life (as detailed in Chap. 16). These symptoms involve the vulvovaginal region, urethra, bladder, pelvic ligaments, and pelvic floor muscles due to a lack of estrogen and other sex steroids. Like other body parts, carboxytherapy in the genital area can also increase vascularization, angiogenesis, and collagen remodeling, providing better tissue oxygenation and rejuvenation. Thus, it can be performed primarily to treat burning, vaginal dryness, and dyspareunia symptoms of menopause. Vaginal moisture occurs not from the glands but from the increased blood flow in vaginal tissues. According to the best of our knowledge, both vulvar and vaginal applications of carboxytherapy have a positive effect on complaints of menopause depending on a lack of collagen, a decrease of extracellular matrix, poor hydration capacity, and vascularization. Furthermore, it is a quite easy, safe, and cost-effective method.

The intravaginal treatment protocol consisted of 6–8 sessions with an interval of 7 days. CO_2 infusion can be done with a 30 G needle and 15° angulation, very superficially, and 60–80 mL/min flow. The treatment takes only 5–10 min for the whole vulvovaginal region.

Especially for the patients who are not recommended to undergo estrogen treatments (breast cancer survivors, etc.), carbon dioxide gas insufflation can be a good choice as a conservative treatment method or combined with PRP, regenerative HA injection, laser, radiofrequency, and other energy-based devices.

22.3.2 Mons Pubis Reduction

Due to the lipolysis effect, carboxytherapy can be used as a non-surgical method for mons pubis reduction.

The treatment protocol consisted of 6-8 sessions with an interval of 7 days. CO_2 infusion is applied symmetrically for each part, with a 30 G needle and 90° angulation, 13 mm in depth, and 30–40 mL quantity/each point.

22.3.3 Vulvar Rejuvenation and Lichen Sclerosus Treatment

Like face rejuvenation, CO_2 gas therapy can treat laxity, scars, wrinkles, and collapses in majora and symptomatic treatment of lichen sclerosus disease. It increases skin tone and elasticity by improving angiogenesis, microcirculation, and collagen remodeling.

Vulvar treatment can be applied with a 30 G needle and 15° angulation, 13 mm depth, and 30–40 mL quantity/each point. The protocol consisted of 6–8 sessions with an interval of 7 days. In deeper injections, it can burn fat tissue and provide labia majora reduction. Periclitoral and anterior vaginal wall therapies may provide sexual enhancement by increasing blood flow, though yet to be verified.

22.4 Other Indications

Other indications include the treatments of:

- scar formation after surgery, burns, folliculitis, etc. (Fig. 22.2),
- chronic wounds (diabetic wounds, etc.) and ulcers,

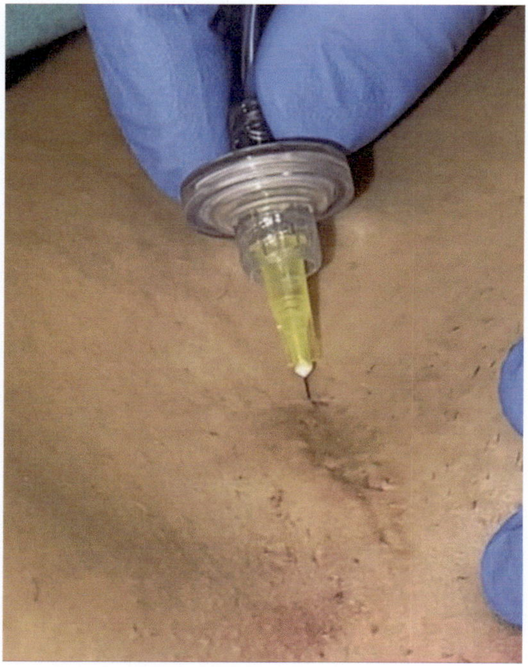

Fig. 22.2 Treatment of scars depending on genital folliculitis

- arterial diseases (atherosclerosis, Burger, Raynaud),
- scleroderma,
- lichen ruber hypertrophicus,
- erectile dysfunction due to vascular disorders.

CO_2 is used successfully and after plastic operations (liposuction or ultrasonic liposuction, facial tightening, blepharoplasty) as an effective rehabilitation and rapid skin tightening. Hypothetically, if applied before the autologous fat transfer, it can enhance fat survival.

22.4.1 Adverse Events

Before starting the injection, patients were informed about the resulting emphysema, which will resolve within 5 min. The inter-and postoperational adverse events are mild and transient, including erythema, pain, crepitation bubbles, and ecchymosis.

22.4.2 Combined Treatments

Genital carboxytherapy can be combined with energy-based devices, HA, mesotherapy, and PRP for aesthetic and medical indications. However, it is not recommended to be used in the same session because it changes the physiology and PH of the tissue and may affect the efficacy of the other procedures.

22.4.3 Post-procedure Term

Carboxytherapy is an easy, safe, non-allergic, non-toxic, simple, and relatively effective method for medical and aesthetic purposes. There is no downtime and no need for dressing or special care after the procedure.

Appendix

With the purchase of this book, you can use our "SN Flashcards" app to access questions free of charge in order to test your learning and check your understanding of the contents of the book.

To use the app, please follow the instructions below:

1. Go to https://flashcards.springernature.com/login
2. Create a user account by entering your e-mail address and assigning a password.
3. Use the following link to access your SN Flashcards set: ▶ https://sn.pub/tvlq7Q

If the link is missing or does not work, please send an e-mail with the subject "SN Flashcards" and the book title to customerservice@springernature.com.

References

1. Hexsel D, Mazzuco R. Cellulite. In: Tosti A, Hexsel D, editors. Update in cosmetic dermatology. Mumbai: Springer-Verlag; 2013. p. 21–32.
2. El-Domyati M, Hosam El-Din W, Medhat W, Ibrahim MR, Khaled Y. Carboxytherapy for striae distensae: a promising modality. J Cosmet Dermatol. 2021;20(2):546–53.
3. Lee GS. Carbon dioxide therapy in the treatment of cellulite: an audit of clinical practice. Aesthet Plast Surg. 2010;34:239–43.
4. Pianez LR, Custódio FS, Guidi RM, de Freitas JN, Sant'Ana E. Effectiveness of carboxytherapy in the treatment of cellulite in healthy women: a pilot study. Clin Cosmet Investig Dermatol. 2016;9:183–90.
5. Park JH, Wee SY, Chang J, Hong S, Lee JH, Cho KW, Choi CY. Carboxytherapy-induced fat loss is associated with VEGF-mediated vascularization. Aesthet Plast Surg. 2018;42(6):1681–8.
6. Michelle L, Pouldar Foulad D, Ekelem C, Saedi N, Mesinkovska NA. Treatments of periorbital hyperpigmentation: a systematic review. Dermatol Surg. 2021;47(1):70–4.
7. Mu YZ, Jiang L, Yang H. The efficacy of fractional ablative carbon dioxide laser combined with other therapies in acne scars. Dermatol Ther. 2019;32(6):e13084. https://doi.org/10.1111/dth.13084. Epub 2019 Oct 7. PMID: 31496020.
8. El-Domyati M, Hosam El-Din W, Medhat W, Ibrahim MR, Khaled Y. The use of Carboxytherapy alone or in combination with fractional CO_2 laser for facial rejuvenation: a split-face comparative study. J Cosmet Dermatol. 2020;19(7):1648–55.
9. Kamel AM, Abdelghani R. Carboxytherapy for treatment of localized chronic plaque psoriasis: Clinical and histopathologic evaluation. J Cosmet Dermatol. 2018;17(3):527–32. https://doi.org/10.1111/jocd.12494. Epub 2018 Jan 17. PMID: 29341446.
10. Doghaim NN, El-Tatawy RA, Neinaa YME, Abd El-Samd MM. Study of the efficacy of carboxytherapy in alopecia. J Cosmet Dermatol. 2018;17(6):1275–85.
11. Drogovoz S, Kononenko A, Syrona G, et al. Application of carboxytherapy in dermatology. PharmacologyOnLine. 2021;3:2075–98. https://pharmacologyonline.silae.it/front.

Regenerative Medicine 23

Width of life is more important than length of life.

Ibn-i Sina (Avicenna)

Regenerative medicine is a field of medicine working on regeneration and tissue engineering in order to regain human or animal cell or organ function. It generally includes stem cell and PRP treatments. The term "regenerative medicine" was first defined in 1992 by the US scientist and author Leland Kaiser. This term has become very popular with stem cell therapies [1].

There is a distinct difference between the word "regeneration" and the word "repair." Repair is used to refer to the reestablishment of tissue continuity and means incomplete recovery of morphological and functional aspects. For example, an organ with lost or damaged tissue after a trauma that has not been fully restored continues to function. However, regeneration describes the complete replacement of damaged tissue with new tissue not associated with scar tissue. For example, the endometrium regenerates itself regularly every month after its morphology deteriorates.

23.1 Regenerative Medicine Fields

Due to their regenerative properties, the usage areas of stem cells have shifted from chronic degenerative diseases to aesthetic medicine. Mesenchymal stem cells (MSC) have been preferred more often than embryonic and induced pluripotent stem cells (IPS) in tissue engineering due to their easy availability, their ability to differentiate into many cell types, and partly to avoid ethical issues.

Fat-originated autologous stem cells (ASC) are cells that can differentiate into vascular tissues. The mixture of cells obtained in adipose tissue aspiration is called the stromal vascular fraction (SVF) and contains multipotent MSC population cells. ASC are also effective cells for regeneration and wound healing. In recent studies, it has been shown that, in terms of cell numbers, SVF has much higher cell counts than cells obtained from bone marrow. Unlike bone marrow stem cells, ASC have advantages such as being able to be taken in large quantities with a standard simple liposuction, no need for culture, and low complication rates.

SVF is obtained by enzymatic separation of adipocytes and is a heterogeneous cocktail of stem cells, fibroblasts, endothelial cells, monocytes,

S. Eserdağ, *Aesthetic and Functional Female Genital Surgery*,
https://doi.org/10.1007/978-3-031-16019-6_23

macrophages, granulocytes, and lymphocytes. ASC can be isolated completely after separation from adipocytes and can be cultured to form fibroblast-like colonies. ASC applied with SVF or expanded in *in vitro* culture is the most commonly used MSC in aesthetic medicine. Since pure ASC requires *in vitro* expansion, SVF containing ASC is generally used. Both ASC and SVF contain molecules that increase vascularization and release growth factors [2]. These molecules are also responsible for increasing the survival of the fat graft. SVF containing ASC is also used in the treatment of necrosis after HA applied to the face.

Stem cell technologies are still in their infancy, and they carry risks such as tissue rejection, hyperimmune response, neoplasm, cross-contamination with other stem cell lines, and uncontrolled differentiation. Therefore, further research is required.

Currently, the only stem cell products that are FDA-approved for use in the US consist of hematopoietic progenitor cells that are derived from umbilical cord blood. These products are approved for use in patients with hematopoietic system disorders, but they are not approved for other uses. There are currently no FDA-approved exosome products.

23.2 Autologous Fat Treatments

Fat therapies can be performed in different ways according to the experience of the physician and the condition of the tissue. The procedures are called by different names because of the different preparation stages.

23.2.1 Macrofat Transfer

This is the transfer of fat with the classical liposuction technique with large, multiport cannulas. Although it is a good volumizing material, it contains risks such as granuloma formation, clumping of the skin, fat necrosis, and calcification. Due to the small amount of tissue remaining after the procedure, multiple applications may be required.

23.2.2 Microfat Transfer

Liposuction procedure is performed with small, multi-way cannulas. 20cc of syringe is preferred for not to distrupt regenerative cells. To have the tissue rich of stem cells, lipoaspiration should be performed superficially. Microfat grafting is mostly applied for volumizing purposes. Regeneration rate is slightly higher than with macrofat application. The risks are similar to macrofat application.

23.2.3 SEFFI (Superficial Enhanced Fluid Fat Injection) Transfer

This is the process of injection into the superficial tissue by adding PRP to fat removed via liposuction with small (0.8 mm and 0.5 mm diameter) multi-way cannulas. It contains viable adipocytes and the GF of PRP. It is thinner than Microfat, and it is used for both volumizing and rejuvenation [3].

23.2.4 M-SEFFI (Micro-SEFFI) Transfer

This is done to obtain thinner fat than SEFFI. In this process, PRP is added to the fat harvested by liposuction and then applied to the tissue with a very small (0.3 mm) multi-way cannula [4].

23.2.5 Nanofat Transfer

This is a regenerative method defined by Tonnard et al. in 2013 and patented by Tulip Medical Products. Since its introduction, Nanofat has been utilized for several different regenerative treatments such as scar improvement, burns, radiated tissue, and diabetic wounds. Nanofat is thought of as fat parcel sizes of 600 microns or less. The cellular composition of Nanofat has been shown to have a lower number of viable adipocytes when compared with that of larger parcel sizes such as macrofat, millifat, and microfat, yet in contrast contains a significant supply of SVF cells that could be injected through smaller gauge smaller needles. First, liposuction is made with special cannulas of 3 mm, multi-way, 1 mm diameter sharp holes on the sides and fat is harvested. Then, the method includes the steps of superficial injection of the highly thinned solution, which is then mechanically thinned, filtered, and separated, into the tissue with 27 G needles. It is used for rejuvenation purposes due to its ASC content and has limited volumizing effect. It can also be combined with macrofat graft to increase volume. Complication rates such as fat cysts and granulomas are very low [5].

The Tulip Nanotransfer™ protocol can be summarized as follows:

1. Tumescent infiltration to the area where fat will be harvested with Tulip cannula
2. Fat removal by lipoaspiration with the help of Tulip Carraway cannula
3. Loading the received lipoaspirate into the fat press (Fig. 23.1)
4. Adding equal volume of saline solution to the fat press
5. Fat and saline are mixed in the tube by shaking with linear movements
6. Transferring lipoaspirate from injector to injector 30 times from two injectors connected to a 2.4 mm diameter connector.
7. Repeating the same process 30 times with injectors connected to 1.2 mm diameter connectors.
8. Passing the aspirate through the filter one time with the nanotransfer device (Fig. 23.2).
9. Injecting the obtained solution (nanofat) into the superficial tissue with a 27 G needle.

23.2.6 SVF Transfer

The first use of SVF in aesthetics was performed in 2003 by Cohen and Holmes in a series of eight patients. Long-term improvement in wrinkles was observed in one patient 6 years after the study [6]. This is the process of removing the fat with lipoaspiration, separating it mechanically or enzymatically, and applying it to the tissue. It is called tSVF (tissue SVF) when it is obtained mechanically and cSVF (cellular SVF) when it is obtained enzymatically. cSVF contains cells with much more stem cell marker-positivity than tSVF in terms of cell number. In some cases where the main goal is to obtain ASC, using cSVF will speed up regeneration even more. Let's elaborate on this issue a little more.

Each tissue has a specific cell population that keeps its homeostasis self-regulating and stable. Histologically, the resident cells in the tissues consist of two main components, parenchyma and stroma. Parenchyma cells are specialized cell groups that provide specific cell functions, such

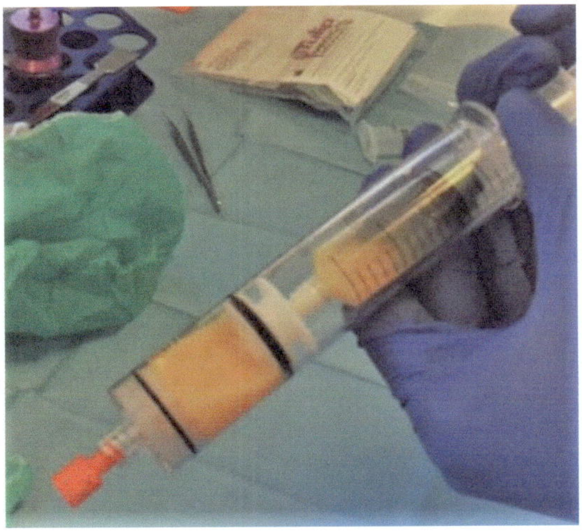

Fig. 23.1 Lipoaspirate is loaded into the press

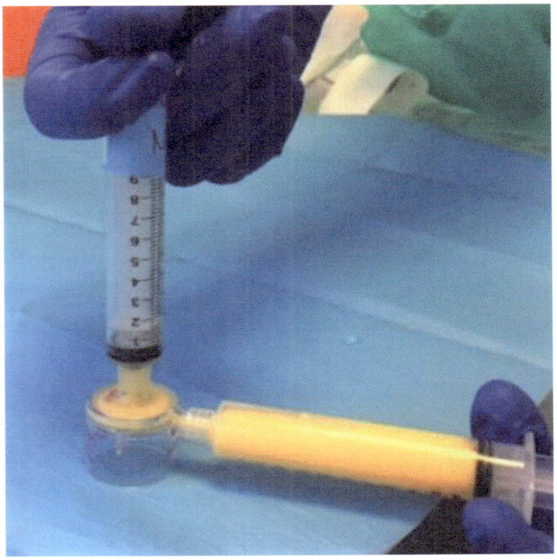

Fig. 23.2 Fat filtration

as cardiomyocytes in the heart, hepatocytes in the liver, or adipocytes in fat. Stroma, however, is responsible for supporting the parenchyma in physiological and pathological conditions and is a heterogeneous cell population that secretes growth factors and cytokines into the extracellular matrix environment for tissue repair and regeneration. In the event of tissue damage, stromal cells initiate a site-specific reparative response. This response includes the restructuring of the extracellular matrix (remodeling), increase in angiogenesis, modulation of the immune system, and cellular turnover.

Adipose tissue is one of the most suitable stromal cell sources with its properties such as easy and safe extraction and abundance in the adult body. The cellular components of adipose tissue consist of mature adipocytes forming the parenchyma and the supporting stroma, namely fibroblasts, endothelial cells, resident mononuclear cells, circulating blood-derived cells, and stromal cells containing progenitor cells.

In general, isolation of stromal cells is carried out by first enzymatic separation of lipoaspirate and then by centrifugation of mature adipocytes from stromal cells. Enzymatic application to stromal cells creates a heterogeneous, isolated cell population called stromal vascular fraction (SVF). However, enzymatic application is more expensive than mechanical application. Moreover, due to insufficient published information, its application in some countries has been limited [7].

Prepared SVF cocktail can be injected into skin lesions like lichen sclerosus (Fig. 23.3), or any part of skin for antiaging and regenerative purposes.

ASC can also be obtained from SVF by culture in a laboratory. However, the disadvantages of this procedure are that it is much more expensive, the patient waits for 2–3 weeks, and anesthesia is required again for the application.

Bone marrow is another source of mesenchymal stem cells. Mesenchymal stem cells and ASC obtained from bone marrow also have advanced regenerative potential like those obtained from adipose tissue. The only difference between them is that isolation from bone marrow is more traumatic and has a higher complication rate.

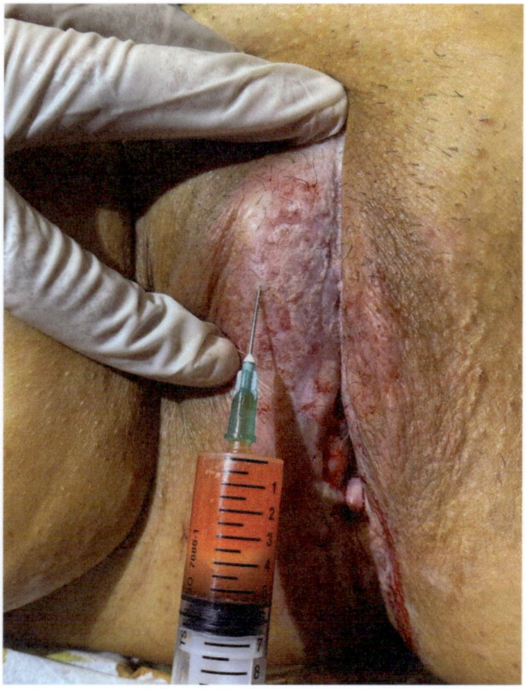

Fig. 23.3 Injection of SVF and PRP mixture solution in a patient with severe genital lichen sclerosus. Transfer can also be done through the cannula

Other sources of stem cells include amniotic fluid, umbilical cord blood, and Wharton's jelly. These cells have more proliferative and differentiation potential than those of fat and bone marrow origin. The disadvantages are that they are not easy to obtain.

23.2.7 Alternative Techniques

Currently we have different options to obtain nano-sized fat cells as well as SVF. Among them, Lipocube™ have a closed sterile system with patented specific structural geometry blades coupled with a flow pattern (Fig. 23.4). After the harvesting, the fat tissue is mechanically digested using the Lipocube™ and then incubated by mixing it with the Lipocube™ buffer solution, enhancing separation of regenerative cells from

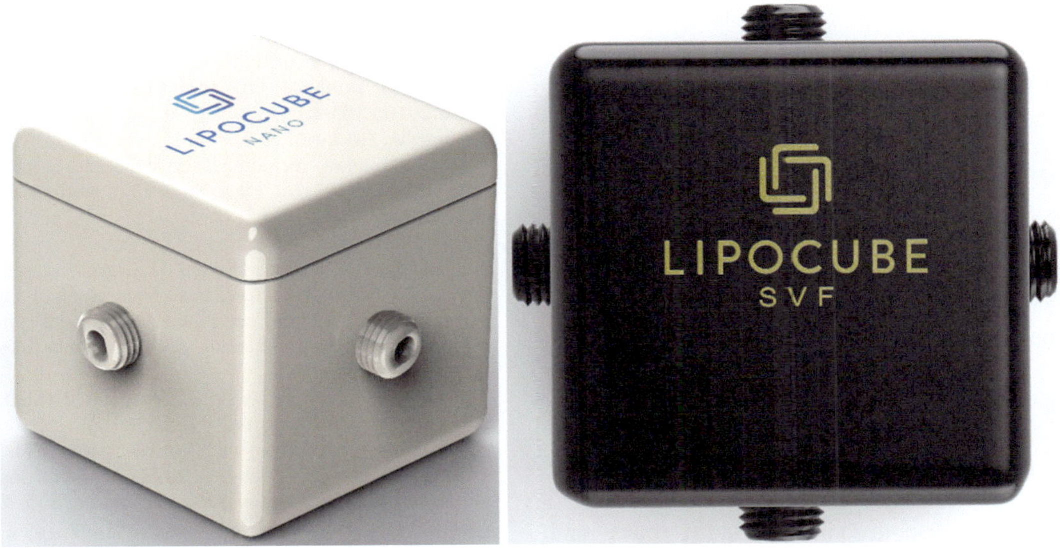

Fig. 23.4 Lipocube nano (left) and Lipocube SVF (right) cubes

fat tissue by molecular electrical charges. The resulting emulsion is processed in the specially designed Lipocube™ device named Cell-Drive™ within a predefined RCF spectrum, and the SVF is concentrated in a patented trap with a specific cell attracting coating and geometry. And then, the SVF is applied to the patient.

23.3 Exosomes

Exosomes are nano-sized biovesicles (generally with a size of 30-200 nm), and act as "intercellular messengers" released into surrounding body fluids upon fusion of multivesicular bodies and the plasma membrane. They are also named as "membranous vesicles" or "microvesicles", and enriched in selected proteins, lipids, nucleic acids, and glycoconjugates, and carry cell-specific cargos of proteins, lipids, and genetic materials. They can be selectively received by neighboring or distant cells, reprogramming the recipient cells upon their bioactive materials. Therefore, the regulated formation of exosomes, specific makeup of their cargo, cell-targeting specificity are of immense biological interest considering extremely high potential of exosomes as non-invasive diagnostic biomarkers, as well as therapeutic nanocarriers [8]. This intercellular communication plays important roles in many aspects of human health and disease, including development, immunity, tissue homeostasis, cancer, and neurodegenerative diseases [9]. They also remove unnecessary cellular proteins (e.g., during reticulocyte maturation). In addition, viruses co-opt exosome biogenesis pathways both for assembling infectious particles and for establishing host permissiveness.

Although exosome research is now in its infancy, they are being developed as new therapeutic agents in gynecology, dermatology, cosmetic surgery, and other disciplines. Especially adipose stem cell-derived exosomes (ASCE-Exo) have been found to have potent regenerative as well as anti-inflammatory effects for facial skin, scalp hair, and genitalia too. In the meantime, ongoing efforts have been to develop plant-derived exosomes for skin rejuvenation. For example, rose stem cell-derived exosomes are known to increase collagen and to lower melanin in human skin cells. These scientific discoveries are promising regenerative aesthetics currently available on the market. For instance, a product, named ASCE™/ExoSCRT™ (ExoCoBio Inc.), is based on purified exosomes to rejuvenate overall skin of our body involving scalp and vagina. In the near future, vaginal rejuvenation will see a paradigm shift created by exosomes.

Appendix

With the purchase of this book, you can use our "SN Flashcards" app to access questions free of charge in order to test your learning and check your understanding of the contents of the book.

To use the app, please follow the instructions below:

1. Go to https://flashcards.springernature.com/login
2. Create a user account by entering your e-mail address and assigning a password.
3. Use the following link to access your SN Flashcards set: ▶ https://sn.pub/tvlq7Q

If the link is missing or does not work, please send an e-mail with the subject "SN Flashcards" and the book title to customerservice@springernature.com.

References

1. Nowacki M, Pietkun K, Jundziłł A, Kloskowski T, Grzanka D, Skopinska-Wisniewska J, Scibior K, Gagat M, Pokrywczyńska M, Grzanka A, Zegarski W, Czajkowski R, Drewa T, Zegarska B. Use of adipose-derived stem cells to support topical skin adhesive for wound closure: a preliminary report from animal in vivo study. Biomed Res Int. 2016;2016:2505601.
2. Pourang A, Rockwell H, Karimi K. New Frontiers in skin rejuvenation, including stem cells and autologous therapies. Facial Plast Surg Clin North Am. 2020;28(1):101–17.
3. Bernardini FP, Gennai A, Izzo L, Zambelli A, Repaci E, Baldelli I, Fraternali-Orcioni G, Hartstein ME, Santi PL, Quarto R. Superficial enhanced fluid fat injection (SEFFI) to correct volume defects and skin aging of the face and periocular region. Aesthet Surg J. 2015;35(5):504–15.
4. Gennai A, Zambelli A, Repaci E, Quarto R, Baldelli I, Fraternali G, Bernardini FP. Skin rejuvenation and volume enhancement with the micro superficial enhanced fluid fat injection (M-SEFFI) for skin aging of the periocular and perioral regions. Aesthet Surg J. 2017;37(1):14–23.
5. Tonnard P, Verpaele A, Peeters G, Hamdi M, Cornelissen M, Declercq H. Nanofat grafting: basic research and clinical applications. Plast Reconstr Surg. 2013;132(4):1017–26.
6. Cohen SR, Tiryaki T, Womack HA, Canikyan S, Schlaudraff KU, Scheflan M. Cellular Optimization of Nanofat: Comparison of Two Nanofat Processing Devices in Terms of Cell Count and Viability. Aesthet Surg J Open Forum. 2019;1(4):ojz028.
7. Sesé B, Sanmartín JM, Ortega B, Matas-Palau A, Llull R. Nanofat cell aggregates: a nearly constitutive stromal cell inoculum for regenerative site-specific therapies. Plast Reconstr Surg. 2019;144(5):1079–88.
8. Zhang Y, Liu Y, Liu H, Tang WH. Exosomes: biogenesis, biologic function and clinical potential. Cell Biosci. 2019;9:19.
9. Pegtel DM, Gould SJ. Exosomes. Annu Rev Biochem. 2019;88:487–514.

Patient Consent Forms

Patient Consent Form for Female External Genital Organ Cosmetic Plastic Surgery (Vulvoplasty, Labiaplasty Operations)

Patient No:

Patient Name Surname:

Date of Birth:

Section:

Consent Date:

Dear patient/legally authorized representative,

To have information about your health condition/the health condition of your patient and all types of medical, surgical, or diagnostic procedures recommended to you/your patient and their alternatives, benefits, risks and even harms and to reject or accept all or some of them, you have the right to stop the operations to be carried out at any stage.

This document, which we want you to read and understand, has been prepared not to frighten you or to discourage you from medical practices, but to inform you and to take your approval in determining whether you will consent to these practices.

S. Eserdağ, *Aesthetic and Functional Female Genital Surgery*,
https://doi.org/10.1007/978-3-031-16019-6

Information About Genital Lip Aesthetics (Labiaplasty Operation)

In women, the lips in the genital area (labia minora and majora) may be structurally large, sagging, wrinkled, and/or asymmetrical (one larger than the other). The small lips being more prominent and sagging than the big lips can create different problems in terms of aesthetics as well as psychological, functional, sexual, and hygienic aspects. The first reason for performing the surgery is to have a better aesthetic appearance. In addition, sagging lips can cause problems such as frequent genital infections, itching, irritation while wearing trousers, bad odor, splashing of urine in different directions while urinating, and pain due to tension during intercourse. The operations performed to reduce the genital lips surgically and to improve them aesthetically and functionally are called labiaplasty operations.

Labiaplasty operations can be performed with local anesthesia (numbing the vaginal tissue with a needle), spinal anesthesia (numbing from the waist down), sedation (light sleep with intravenous injection), or general anesthesia (full sleep) according to the patient's tissue, general health condition, and wishes. Depending on the size of the operation area, the operation time is generally between 60 and 90 min. In general or sedation anesthesia, it is important to arrive without having consumed food and water for at least 6 h. The stitching threads used during the process are absorbed automatically after a certain period of time. Clitoral hoodoplasty (removal of excess skin above the clitoris) can be performed simultaneously with labiaplasty surgeries. In addition, vaginal anterior–posterior wall repair, rectocele (bowel prolapse) repair, perineum (between vagina and anus) repair, injection of the fat tissue taken from the person to the large genital lips (majora fat transfer), genital area bleaching, vaginal laser applications, and genital combined surgical and non-surgical operations such as PRP (Platelet-Rich Plasma) injection can also be performed simultaneously.

After the procedure, there may be edema, tension, itching, and tenderness in the operation area for a few weeks. In order to reduce these complaints, it is important to apply ice for the first 3 days and wash the area with warm water and regular dressings for 10 days. After the procedure, you should also use the antibiotics and pain medication we recommend.

Alternative Treatments

There is no alternative treatment for labial reduction.

Drugs You Use and Its Important Features

Please inform us about the medications you use (especially those such as aspirin and Coumadin-derivatives that reduce blood coagulation), your current or past important diseases, your previous surgeries, anesthesia methods used in your previous surgeries, and drug allergies. Painkillers and antibiotic derivatives will be administered in the post-procedure period. Use only the medications we recommend. In order to have a comfortable postoperative period, you should regularly do the dressings we have given and explained to you in writing.

Risks and Complications

The amount of skin to be removed in labiaplasty operations is determined by the condition of the patients' tissue and the patient's demands. Some patients request a slight correction, while others demand maximum tissue removal. The early risks and complications of labiaplasty include bleeding, hematoma (bleeding into the tissue), infection, syncope (fainting), wound dehiscence, late period risks after surgery, edema (swelling), stinging, itching, bleeding in the form of leakage, abscess, fistula formation, and stiffness in the operation area. If the perineum (between anus–vagina) correction is performed, problems such as pain during sexual intercourse depending on the tissue tension there, sensation changes, asymmetry (one lip stays different from the other), and scar formation may be observed (ACOG Bulletin, No: 378, 2017).

In addition, there are risks such as complications due to anesthesia, allergies to medicines used, shock, and death. When combined surgical or non-surgical operations are added, it should be known that each operation has an additional risk and complication rate specific to it. In all operations performed in the hospital or office, there are also the risks of contamination of epidemic infection, hospital infections, and COVID-19 (coronavirus) infection.

Information About the Probability of Success of the Process

There is no certainty in any surgical procedure. Although good results in both functional and aesthetic aspects are expected after the surgery, no guarantee or assurance can be given to patients about the results to be obtained. When undesirable results occur, additional/alternative treatment options can be offered to you.

Critical Lifestyle Suggestions for Your Health and Your Home Care

After labiaplasty operations, it is important to pay attention to your personal hygiene, to regularly dressing your wound area, to use the medicines prescribed by us regularly, and to come to the follow-up visits on the dates we recommend. What you need to do after the surgery will be given to you in writing and will be explained in detail. It is important that you change your dressings for 10 days as we recommend, apply ice for 3 days, and finish one box of antibiotics and pain medications. You should also stay away from heavy exercise, yoga, pilates, fitness, cycling, horse riding, heavy lifting, and sexual intercourse for four weeks. In order to facilitate wound healing, you should pay attention to your diet, especially by taking advantage of protein- and vitamin-rich foods. To avoid constipation, you should consume vegetables and fruits rich in fiber. If you have constipation problems despite the diet, please inform us so that we can recommend medication. Smoking is not recommended, as it interferes wound healing.

Informed Consent

I read the information described above and I was informed by the doctor who signed below. I learned about the purpose, risks, complications, and additional treatment options of the intervention. I consciously approve this intervention without being under any pressure or needing any additional explanation. Provided that my facial and personal information are kept confidential, I also allow my treatment-related information to be used as statistical data in scientific studies, permit the surgical team to take pre- and postoperative genital area photographs or video records and to use these records and information in scientific meetings, books, and scientific presentations when necessary. If I request to be discharged on the same day, I declare that I will stay in the city where I was operated on for at least one day after the surgery, due to the risk of fainting due to anesthesia and the early risks mentioned above.

Processing of personal data in this form in the physical or electronic environment in accordance with the legal and contractual obligations of the hospital and principles of patient–physician relationship in accordance with the data processing conditions stipulated in the legislation; domestic/foreign business partners, suppliers, etc. transferring it to persons due to the nature of the relationship and in order to be able to perform this form; I declare, accept, and undertake that I know that my rights that have been notified to me regarding these activities and that I can apply to the office/hospital that is the data controller at any time.

I authorize the person named .... to give consent and to receive all information about my treatment when I am unconscious or unable to give consent in any attempt to be made regarding my treatment (* The person authorized by the patient must sign as the patient's attorney/legally authorized representative).

.... (Please write "I understand that I read it, I accept it" with your hand writing.)

Patient Signature Date / Time Name-Surname (in handwriting)...

If the patient is unable to give consent:

Patient's attorney/legally authorized representative Signature

Date / Time

Name-Surname (in handwriting)...

Reason for the patient not to give consent (to be completed by the doctor):...

....

....

Sufficient and satisfactory information about the disease, the application to be performed, the reason for and benefits of this application, the care required after the application, the expected risks, the type of anesthesia to be applied for the application, and the risks and complications of anesthesia have been explained by me to the patient/patient's representative whose name is written above. The patient/patient's representative signed this consent form, confirming that he/she was adequately informed about the application.

Doctor **Signature**

Date/ Time

Name Surname :....................................

If the patient has a Language/Communication Issue:

I translated the statements made to the patient by the doctor. In my opinion, the information I translated was understood by the patient.

Translator **Signature**

Date/ Time

Name Surname (in handwriting) : ....

Patient Consent Form for Vaginal Tightening and Reconstruction Operations (Colporrhaphy Surgery)

Patient No:

Patient Name Surname:

Date of birth:

Episode:

Consent Date:

Dear patient/legally authorized representative,

To have information about your health condition/the health condition of your patient and all types of medical, surgical, or diagnostic procedures recommended to you/your patient and their alternatives, benefits, risks, and even harms and to reject or accept all or some of them, you have the right to stop the operations to be carried out at any stage.

This document, which we want you to read and understand, has been prepared not to frighten you or to discourage you from medical practices, but to inform you and to take your approval in determining whether you will consent to these practices.

Information About Vagina Tightening Operations

The vagina is the canal of sexual intercourse and can be enlarged, sagging, and numb, most often due to pregnancy, birth, aging, menopause, and weakness of connective tissue. Sometimes it can be structurally large (*Wide and Smooth Vagina*). Operations are performed to tighten the enlarged vagina; names such as vaginal tightening, vaginoplasty, or its medical name, colporrhaphy, are used. The most important purposes are to increase pleasure during sexual intercourse and to reduce sagging. Vaginal tightening operations can be performed with local anesthesia (numbing the vaginal tissue with a needle), spinal anesthesia (regional anesthesia from the waist down with a needle), sedation (light sleep with intravenous injection of anesthetics), or general anesthesia (full sleep with intubation) according to the patient's tissue, general health conditions, and wishes. Depending on the size of the operation area, the operation time is generally between 45 and 90 min. In general or sedation anesthesia, it is important to arrive without having consumed food and water for at least 6 h. Anterior vaginal wall repair, rectocele (bowel prolapse) repair, perineum (between vagina and anus) repair, labiaplasty (genital lip aesthetics), injection of fat tissue taken from the person to the large genital lips (majora fat transfer), genital area bleaching, and vaginal combined surgical and non-surgical interventions such as laser applications and genital platelet-rich plasma (PRP) injection can also be added simultaneously to vaginal tightening operations.

Alternative Treatments

In light of the current medical literature, the condition of your tissue, and your physician's experience in this field, surgical vaginal tightening is recommended to you. Among non-surgical alternatives to vaginal tightening operations, laser vaginal rejuvenation, radiofrequency vaginal tightening, and pelvic exercises, such as Kegel exercises can also provide certain benefits. However, surgical procedures are the first choice in patients with severe vaginal sagging or bladder or rectal prolapse.

Drugs to Be Used and Its Important Properties

Please inform us about the medications you use (especially those that reduce blood coagulation such as aspirin and Coumadin-derivatives), your current or past major diseases, your previous surgeries, anesthesia methods used in your surgeries, and drug allergies. Painkillers and antibiotic derivatives will be administered in the post-procedure period. Use only the medications we recommend. In order to have a comfortable post-operative period, you should regularly do the dressings we have given and explained to you in writing.

Risks And Complications

The pleasure felt in sexual intercourse may decrease due to many different reasons. Psychological factors related to oneself, biological reasons related to the genital area, compatibility with spouse, and marital problems are important factors affecting sexual pleasure (Bio-psycho-social Model Theory). Therefore, vaginal tightening surgeries may not have the expected effect in everyone. Additionally, vaginal tightening operations alone do not provide orgasm. The tightening to be performed in the operation is related to the width of the person's own vagina. For example, while a lot of tissue is removed and tightening is greater in those with a lot of enlargement due to many deliveries, less tissue is removed in patients with low number of births or none. Among the early risks and complications, bleeding, hematoma (bleeding into the tissue), infection, syncope (fainting state), wound dehiscence, bowel and bladder damage, late period risks, and complications include edema (swelling), stinging, itching, bleeding in the form of leakage, abscess, fistula formation, stiffness in the operation area, pain during sexual intercourse due to excessive tightening of the vagina, sensation changes, and scar formation may be observed (ACOG Bulletin, 2017). In addition, there are risks such as complications due to anesthesia, allergies to medicines used, shock, and death. When combined surgical or non-surgical procedures are added, each procedure has its own special risk and complication rate. In all operations performed in the hospital or office, epidemic infections, hospital infections, and COVID-19 (Coronavirus) infection contamination risks are also present.

Information About the Probability of Success of the Process

There is no certainty in any surgical procedure. Although good results in both functional and aesthetic aspects are expected after the surgery, no guarantee or assurance can be given to patients about the results to be obtained. When undesirable results occur, additional/alternative treatment options may be needed.

Critical Lifestyle Suggestions for Your Health and Your Home Care

After vaginal aesthetic surgeries, it is important to pay attention to your personal hygiene, to regularly dressing your stitches, to use the medicines prescribed by us regularly, and to come to the follow-up visits on the dates we recommend. What you need to do after the surgery will be given to you in writing and will be explained in detail. It is important that you change your dressings for 10 days as we recommend, apply ice for 3 days, and finish one box of antibiotics and pain medications. In addition, you should stay away from sports and physical activities such as heavy exercise, yoga, pilates, fitness, and heavy lifting for a month and sexual intercourse for 6–8 weeks. In order to facilitate wound healing, we recommend that you consume foods rich in protein and vitamins in your diet and vegetables and fruits rich in fiber to avoid constipation. If you have constipation despite diet, please inform us so that we can recommend medication. Smoking is not recommended, as it interferes wound healing.

Informed Consent

I read the information described above and was informed by the doctor who signed below. I learned about the purpose, risks, complications, and additional treatment attempts of the intervention. I consciously approve this intervention without being under any pressure or needing any additional explanation. Provided that my facial and personal information are kept confidential, I also allow my treatment-related information to be used as statistical data in scientific studies, permit the surgical team to take pre- and postoperative genital area photographs or video records, and to use these records and information in scientific meetings, books, and scientific presentations when necessary. If I request to be discharged on the same day, I declare that I will stay in the city where I was operated on for at least one day after the surgery, due to the state of fainting due to anesthesia and the early risks mentioned above.

Processing of personal data in this form in the physical or electronic environment in accordance with the legal and contractual obligations of the hospital and principles of patient–physician relationship in accordance with the data processing conditions stipulated in the legislation; domestic/foreign business partners, suppliers, etc. transferring it to persons due to the nature of the relationship and in order to be able to perform this form; I declare, accept, and undertake that I know that my rights have been notified to me regarding these activities and that I can apply to the office/hospital that is the data controller at any time.

I authorize the person named .... to give consent and to receive all information about my treatment when I am unconscious or unable to give consent in any attempt to be made regarding my treatment (* The person authorized by the patient must sign as the patient's attorney/legally authorized representative).

....

(Please write "I understand that I read it, and I accept it" with your hand writing.)

Patient **Signature**

Date / Time Name-Surname (in handwriting).................................

<u>If the patient is unable to give consent:</u>

Patient's attorney/legally authorized representative Signature

Date / Time

Name-Surname (in handwriting).......... ....

<u>Reason for the patient not to give consent (to be completed by the doctor):</u>.. ....
....
....

Sufficient and satisfactory information about the disease, the application to be performed, the reason and benefits of this application, the care required after the application, the expected risks, the type of anesthesia to be applied for the application, and the risks and complications of anesthesia have been explained by me to the patient/patient's representative whose name is written above. The patient/patient's representative signed this consent form, confirming that he/she was adequately informed about the application.

Doctor **Signature**

Date/ Time

Name Surname :...................................

If the patient has a Language/Communication Issue:

I translated the statements made to the patient by the doctor. In my opinion, the information I translated was understood by the patient.

Translator **Signature**

Date/ Time

Name Surname (in handwriting): ....

Patient Consent Form for Fat Injections to the Genital Region

Patient No:

Patient Name Surname:

Date of birth:

Episode:

Consent Date:

Dear patient/legally authorized representative,

To have information about your health condition/the health condition of your patient and all types of medical, surgical or diagnostic procedures recommended to you/your patient and their alternatives, benefits, risks, and even harms and to reject or accept all or some of them, you have the right to stop the operations to be carried out at any stage.

This document, which we want you to read and understand, has been prepared not to frighten you or to discourage you from medical practices, but to inform you and to take your approval in determining whether you will consent to these practices.

Information About Fat Injection to the Genital Area

One of the methods that can be used to increase volume and provide fullness in various parts of the face and body is fat injections. Fat transfer (lipofilling) can be applied to the cheeks, forehead, cheek-lip line, lips, chin tip, hip, and leg areas as well as large lips, mons pubis (lower groin area), and vagina.

Genital area fat transfer is usually performed in cases of collaps, wrinkles, and weaknesses in the external genital area that develop due to aging, rapid weight gain and loss, or weakening of the collagen tissue. Sometimes fat transfer is preferred to hide the appearance of the inner lips.

Another application area is to provide vaginal tightening. Sometimes it is also applied for correction of normal birth or cesarean scars. It can also be applied to reduce complaints in skin patients such as genital lichen sclerosus. Fat injections can be performed alone or simultaneously with vaginal tightening, labiaplasty, or different plastic and aesthetic operations. Since there are mesenchymal stem cells in adipose tissue, an anti-aging effect is also expected in the tissue in addition to fullness. There are two stages in fat transfers: fat harvesting and injection of the harvested fat. When choosing the area where the fat will be taken in fat injections, the regions where there is a lot of fat in the body are generally preferred. These areas are generally the abdomen, flanks, buttocks, or inner thighs. Generally, 30-60 mL of fat harvested by vacuum method (liposuction) is first subjected to some special processes such as washing, filtration, centrifugation, or thinning. Then, a small incision is made through the skin tissue, a thin tube (cannula) is passed through this incision, and fat is injected into the application area. Cold compression is started immediately after the procedure to reduce swelling. Cold compression is usually 15 minutes in every hour with gel or ice molds. It is important that the ice does not come into direct contact with the skin but rather is wrapped in a cloth before being applied to the area where the fat was given. During the procedure, depending on the patient's tissue, general health conditions, and wishes, local anesthesia (numbing the vaginal tissue with a needle), spinal anesthesia (local anesthesia with a needle from the waist), sedation (light sleep with intravenous injection), or general anesthesia (complete sleep with intubation) can be done. Operation time is generally between 30 and 50 min. After the procedure, swelling and bruises due to edema will decrease within a few weeks. Small pieces of tape placed at entry points for fat injection can be removed a few hours after the procedure or the next day. Finish one box each of the painkillers and antibiotics that we prescribe you. If the gradually decreasing edema increases at any stage or if there is an increase in sensitivity and temperature in the area, you should consult us or a doctor you can reach, as this may be a sign of an infection.

Alternative Treatments

In addition to fat, genital lip enlargement can be provided by HA (hyaluronic acid) injections. Most HA injections, which are usually performed under local anesthesia, are not permanent and require repetition.

Drugs to Be Used and Their Important Properties

Please inform us about the medications you use (especially those that reduce blood coagulation such as aspirin and Coumadin-derivatives), your current or past major diseases, your previous surgeries, anesthesia methods used in your surgeries, and drug allergies. Painkillers and antibiotic derivatives will be administered in the post-procedure period. Use only the medications we recommend. In order to have a comfortable postoperative period, you should regularly do the dressings we have given and explained to you in writing.

Risks and Complications

Early and late risks and complications of fat injections are as follows:

1. Infection (cellulitis) in the treated area: Since the substance used belongs to the body itself, the possibility of reaction is low and is very rare. Infection can only occur when an external contamination or fat injection disrupts the circulation in the application area. It manifests itself in the form of redness, increase in pain, excessive sensitivity, and increase in body temperature in the injection process area; it usually resolves quickly with the use of antibiotics. In the rare event of an abscess due to infection, drainage is provided with a small incision.
2. Another problem that will occur in the early and late periods is asymmetries. During the injection, the aim is to perform a similar procedure in symmetrical areas in both regions, and if there is already an asymmetry, different amounts of injections are applied to both sides

to balance this. Generally, the asymmetries in the early stages are due to edema. Although the same procedure is performed on all sides of the body, edema on both sides may be different. Asymmetries due to edema quickly resolve. However, permanent asymmetry may develop depending on the amount of fat tissue given or the rate of dissolution in that area. In this case, simple operations called revisions may be required.

3. Numbness or excessive sensitivity in the application area is a problem that we encounter rarely. Softening the area with massages can help improve the sensation more quickly.
4. Allergic reactions may occur depending on the anesthesia complications and the drugs used.
5. In all operations performed in the hospital or office, epidemic infections, hospital infections, and COVID-19 (coronavirus) infection contamination risks are also present.
6. Other risks include bleeding, bruises, infection, long-term degeneration; slight superficial fluctuations in the skin tissue are among the rare complications. Blunt-ended cannulas (thin tubes) are used during the fat delivery process. Therefore, the probability of vascular damage is extremely low. Very rarely, if fat passes into a vein, the fat inside the vein may move to organs such as the lung, eye, and brain and cause damage to these organs. Again, although extremely rare, fat cysts (lipoma) or palpable masses may occur with the accumulation of the given fat in one area. Its treatment is the use of massage and anti-inflammatory drugs. Although these masses are harmless, they can be permanent. Rare color changes have been reported in the application area.

Information About the Probability of Success of the Process

Six months after the procedure, the rate of fat tissue survival generally varies between 30% and 40%. In case of weight loss, the injected fat decreases. If desired, the process can be repeated at a later time. There is no certainty in medicine and surgery. Although good results are expected, as with any surgical procedure, no guarantee or assurance can be given about the results that can be achieved.

Critical Lifestyle Suggestions for Your Health and Your Home Care

It is important that you pay attention to your personal hygiene, change your dressings regularly, use the medicines prescribed by us regularly, and come to the follow-up visits on the dates we recommend after the process of fat removal and fat transfer. What you need to do after the surgery will be given to you in writing and will be explained in detail. It is important that you apply ice pack for the first three days and finish one box of antibiotics and pain medications. In addition, you should stay away from heavy exercise, yoga, pilates, fitness, thermal pool, steam bath, sauna, and sexual intercourse for 4 weeks. In order to facilitate wound healing, you should pay attention to your diet, especially by taking advantage of protein and vitamin-supported foods. We do not recommend smoking because it interferes wound healing and disrupts the nutrition of the adipose tissue.

Informed Consent

I read the information described above and was informed by the doctor who signed below. I learned about the purpose, risks, complications, and additional treatment attempts of the intervention. I consciously approve this intervention without being under any pressure or needing any additional explanation. Provided that my facial and personal information are kept confidential, I also allow my treatment-related information to be used as statistical data in scientific studies, permit the surgical team to take pre- and postoperative genital area photographs or video records, and to use these records and information in scientific meetings, books, and scientific presentations when necessary. If I request to be discharged on the same day, I declare that I will stay in the city where I was operated on for at least one day after the surgery, due to the state of fainting due to anesthesia and the early risks mentioned above.

Processing of personal data in this form in the physical or electronic environment in accordance with the legal and contractual obligations of the hospital and principles of patient–physician relationship in accordance with the data processing conditions stipulated in the legislation; domestic/foreign business partners, suppliers, etc. transferring it to persons due to the nature of the relationship and in order to be able to perform this form; I declare, accept, and undertake that I know that my rights have been notified to me regarding these activities and that I can apply to the office/hospital that is the data controller at any time.

I authorize the person named .... to give consent and to receive all information about my treatment when I am unconscious or unable to give consent in any attempt to be made regarding my treatment (* The person authorized by the patient must sign as the patient's attorney/legally authorized representative).

(Please write "I understand that I read it, and I accept it" with your hand writing.)

Patient **Signature**

Date/Time Name-Surname (in handwriting)... ....

<u>If the patient is unable to give consent:</u>

Patient's attorney/legally authorized representative Signature

Date/Time

Name-Surname (in handwriting)...

<u>Reason for the patient not to give consent (to be completed by the doctor):</u>..

....

....

Sufficient and satisfactory information about the disease, the application to be performed, the reason and benefits of this application, the care required after the application, the expected risks, the type of anesthesia to be applied for the application, and the risks and complications of anesthesia have been explained by me to the patient/patient's representative whose name is written above. The patient/patient's representative signed this consent form, confirming that he/she was adequately informed about the application.

Doctor **Signature**

Date/ Time

Name Surname :.....................................

If the patient has a Language/Communication Issue:

I translated the statements made to the patient by the doctor. In my opinion, the information I translated was understood by the patient.

Translator **Signature**

Date/ Time

Name Surname (in handwriting): ....

Patient Consent Form for Laser Vaginal Rejuvenation, Non-surgical Vaginal Tigtening, and Stress Urinary Incontinence Treatments

Detailed Information

Laser vaginal rejuvenation (LVR) is the process of regeneration and rejuvenation of the vaginal canal mucosa (skin) without surgery. It is most often applied to relieve the complaints of stress urinary incontinence (urinary incontinence during coughing, laughing, sneezing, weight lifting, and exercise), vaginal dryness, and atrophy (thinning of the skin tissue) that develop during menopause, to increase the sensation of the female and male partner during sexual intercourse, and to reduce pain during sexual intercourse. The thermal (heat-transmitting) and ablative (mildly destructive) effects of carbon dioxide lasers increase the production of collagen in the skin, strengthen the structure of the skin tissue, and eliminate gynecological complaints related to this. The procedure is not a surgical operation. It takes approximately 20 minutes performed manually and up to 3 minutes with a special robotic arm or accelerated mode. It is normal to have mild pain during the procedure and most of the time, no anesthesia method is applied. In women who have a fear of gynecological examination or who have a very low pain threshold, a mild sleep anesthesia (sedation) can be administered. In this case, there are risks that may develop due to anesthesia. If deemed necessary, LVR can be repeated once or twice with an average of 1–2 months intervals. In line with our recommendations, the process may need to be renewed every 2 years depending on the loss of collagen. After the procedure, there may be mild watery-bloody discharge that lasts for a few days, then plenty of clear discharge for 7–15 days, mild edema (swelling), and sometimes redness in the application area. On the day of the procedure, fever, sweating, mild pain in the vaginal area, pain complaints, weakness, and rarely fainting may occur. There may be complaints such as mild burning, stinging, itching, tingling, and pricking in the application area for up to 7–10 days. In general, sexual intercourse is not recommended for seven days. Since the development of laser-induced collagen connective tissue will take some time, the desired positive effects usually begin three weeks after the procedure. You may be asked by your doctor to use simple painkillers and antipyretic drugs for one or a few days after the procedure. If necessary, you may be recommended to use antibiotics. During the procedure, additional surgical or non-surgical operations such as labiaplasty, surgical vaginal tightening, genital area bleaching, and PRP (injection of plasma rich in platelets) to the genital area may be recommended to you in the same session. Each procedure has its own unique complication and possible risk rates. Vaginal rejuvenation with laser rarely involves risks such as bleeding, genital infection, and tissue allergy. In order to reduce the risk of infection, it is important to pay attention to genital hygiene as recommended after the procedure and avoid sexual intercourse for the specified period. It is not applied to those who have photosensitivity (allergy to sunlight) or in cases of pregnancy or suspicion of pregnancy.

If you have a menstrual delay, a blood pregnancy test should be performed to confirm that you are not pregnant. LVR is also not applied during your menstruation period. It is also not recommended for those who have cancer or premalignant cellular changes in the cervix or vagina. Therefore, you should inform us that your smear test is normal, especially within the last 1 year. The laser vaginal rejuvenation procedure can give different results from person to person, as in any genital cosmetic and surgical procedure. If the desired positive effect is not achieved, your physician may recommend different surgical operations, non-surgical procedures, or alternative treatment methods. For example, if the problem of urinary incontinence still persists despite laser application or if the desired results do not occur when performed for vaginal tightening, a surgical operation may be recommended. The laser procedure applied into the vagina does not cause infertility, does not affect sexual pleasure negatively, and does not change the menstrual cycle or the amount of bleeding. Additional sexual treatments and alternative methods may be recommended to increase sensations during sexual intercourse.

Informed Consent

My doctor gave me detailed information about all possible risks, complications (problems that may arise) related to the laser vaginal rejuvenation procedure, postoperative complaints, the success of the procedure, and the pricing. Apart from this written consent form, I was also verbally informed in great detail. I asked all the questions I wanted to ask and received their answers. I allow my information to be used in scientific studies, provided that my personal information is completely confidential. I have read and understood this form. I approve the medical procedure/procedures to be performed.

Name Surname and Signature:

Patient Consent Form for Genital Filler Applications

General Information

This form is intended to provide information about intradermal filler applications of hyaluronic acid (HA) or similar products and their possible risks and complications (undesirable consequences). Please read the form carefully. If you have questions or do not understand, please ask your doctor for help.

Fillers are used for purposes such as increasing the volume of any structure in the body (face, back of the hand, nose, genital area, etc.), filling wrinkles, regeneration, stimulating the production of connective tissue in the tissue, and increasing moistening due to its water-retaining feature. The duration of the fillers varies according to the product used and is an average of 4–12 months. There are also fillers containing synthetic material with longer durability. An anesthetic substance is applied by cream or injection method before the procedure. After waiting for a certain time, the skin is cleaned with antiseptic solutions, and the HA is applied by injection. More than one filler material can be used for the same patient, depending on the depth of the collapsed area. After the application, slight massage and ice compression can be performed.

Genital area fillers are made for aesthetic purposes to provide fullness to the large genital lips and mons pubis (lower groin area) in the external genital area and to improve wrinkles and collapses. At the same time, intravaginal injections can provide benefits in relieving the complaints of menopausal atrophy (thinning of the skin), vaginal dryness, vulvar vestibulitis (pain at the vaginal entrance during sexual intercourse), and lichen sclerosus disease. Volumizing genital fillers are not applied to the clitoral area, around the urethral orifice, and into the small genital lips (labia minora). Filling procedure can trigger a herpes outbreak in those with genital herpes. In some cases, a few weeks after the first application, an additional retouching application may be required. For reasons that are not fully understood, the permanence of fillers may be shorter than expected in some people. Therefore, no guarantee or assurance can be given regarding the results of the application.

Informed Consent

Important Issues to Be Considered Before Application

- When coming for the application, please come well rested and without consuming alcoholic beverages.
- If you are using any of the following, stop using at least three days before the procedure: ginkgo biloba, blood diluters, high-dose vitamin E, green tea, aspirin, and nonsteroidal anti-inflammatory (rheumatic) derivatives.

Side Effects That May Occur After Filler Application

- Redness, pain, tenderness, swelling, bruising, itching, infection, necrosis, abscess
- Allergic reactions, collapsed scar
- Palpable masses (granuloma), asymmetry, color change, embolism (clotting in organs such as lung, brain, heart, etc.)

Important Issues to Consider After Application

- Do not touch the application area.
- Do not massage the application area for at least 1 week.
- Avoid intense sports, cycling, or horse riding, sexual activity, and hot environments such as sauna, Jacuzzi for 1 week.
- If an unexpected effect develops, please contact your doctor.

Please fill out the form in writing YES or NO, and if YES, explain it.

Are you at risk of pregnancy?	Do you have an infection in the application area?
Are you breastfeeding?	Do you use cortisone?
Do you have diabetes mellitus?	Are you using any other medication?
Are you prone to bleeding?	Do you have allergies?
Do you have a systemic infectious disease?	Do you have an autoimmune disease?
Did you use aspirin or blood thinners before the application?	Do you have cold sores attacks?
Did you apply any cosmetic product to the application area?	Have you had a filler application before? If yes, did you encounter an allergy or an unexpected situation?
Do you have HbsAg, HCV, and/or HIV?	Do you have active skin disease?

I also accept that photo or video images can be taken of the application area, and that these images and file information can be used in educational meetings, books, and scientific studies, provided that my identifying information is kept confidential. I have been informed by my doctor about the procedures to be performed verbally and in writing in a language that I can understand, that all my questions have been answered, that I have obtained all the necessary information for me, and that I have read this information and consent form by signing the place where my name is written, and I declare that I allow my doctor to perform the filler application by my free will.

DATE:

Patient Name Surname and Signature:

Responsible Doctor and Signature:

After giving detailed information to the patient about the procedure, risks, and complications, she was awake and conscious and signed this form in my presence.

Consent Form for Laser Genital Bleaching Treatments

General Information

This form is for informing about the laser bleaching process and the possible risks and complications (unwanted results) of the procedure. Please read the form carefully. If you have questions or do not understand, please ask your doctor for help.

The laser we use in laser bleaching is a CO_2 (carbon dioxide) laser, which has an ablative (destructive) effect. Pigments that give the skin its color are located in the lower skin (dermis) and upper skin (epidermis) layers. With its ablative effect, the CO_2 laser acts on the epidermis and creates a peeling effect on the skin. Although 30–40% of the skin color is usually lightened after the procedure, the results may vary from person to person, depending on the pigment density, tissue conditions, and the person's skin color.

In the first few days after the procedure, the color of the skin in the area of application becomes darker, which is normal. Subsequently, bleaching will begin to occur along with peeling. If necessary, the process may need to be repeated after a while. In some patients, because of the characteristics of the person's skin color pigments, may not be the desired or expected level of bleaching.

Simultaneously with the laser procedure, some mesotherapy drugs with a bleaching effect can be injected into the skin. In addition, special bleaching solutions can be recommended when necessary.

The procedure can be performed with topical numbing cream or sedation anesthesia (light sleep). There may be complications related to anesthesia and unexpected allergic side effects due to any drug used.

Consent

Important Issues to Be Considered Before Application

- When coming for the application, please be well rested and without consuming alcoholic beverages.
- If you are using any of the following, stop using at least three days before the procedure: ginkgo biloba, blood thinners, high-dose vitamin E, green tea, aspirin, and nonsteroidal anti-inflammatory (rheumatic) derivatives.
- Do not apply anything (oil, cream, etc.) to the area to be bleached before the process.

Side Effects That May Develop After the Bleaching Process

- Redness
- Blistering (bulla)
- Infection
- Burn
- Flaking, scabbing
- Pain
- Sensitivity
- Darkening of color
- Allergy

Important Issues to Be Considered After Application

- Use the medicines we give properly. Avoid taking a shower for 24 hours, intense sports activities for 7 days, and use of sauna, pool, and Jacuzzi for 10 days. If there is no excessive burning or pain after the procedure, there is no prohibition on sexual intercourse.
- Avoid tight and synthetic underwear and tight pants to minimize complaints such as burning

and stinging. Choose cotton underwear, wide pants, and skirts.

- If an unexpected effect develops, please contact your doctor.

Please fill out the form in writing YES or NO, and if YES, explain it.

Are you at risk of pregnancy?	Do you have an infection in the application area?
Are you breastfeeding?	Do you use cortisone?
Do you have diabetes mellitus?	Are you using any other medication?
Are you prone to bleeding?	Do you have allergies?
Do you have a systemic infectious disease?	Do you have an autoimmune disease?
Did you use aspirin or blood thinners before the application?	Do you have cold sores attacks?
Did you apply any cosmetic product to the application area?	Have you had any filler application before? If yes, did you encounter an allergy or an unexpected situation?
Do you have HbsAg, HCV, and/or HIV?	Do you have active skin disease?

I also accept that photo or video images can be taken of the application area, and that these images and file information can be used in educational meetings, books, and scientific studies, provided that my identity information is kept confidential. I have been informed by my doctor about the procedures to be performed verbally and in writing in a language that I can understand, that all my questions have been answered, that I have obtained all the necessary information for me (Patient rights regulation, Official Gazette, date: 01.08.1998; number: 23420), and that I have read this information and consent form by signing the place where my name is written, and I declare that I allow my doctor to perform the filler application by my free will.

DATE:

Patient Name Surname and Signature:

Responsible Doctor and Signature

After giving detailed information to the patient about the procedure, risks, and complications, she was awake and conscious and signed this form in my presence.

MIX
Papier aus verantwortungsvollen Quellen
Paper from responsible sources
FSC® C105338

If you have any concerns about our products,
you can contact us on
ProductSafety@springernature.com

In case Publisher is established outside the EU,
the EU authorized representative is:
Springer Nature Customer Service Center GmbH
Europaplatz 3, 69115 Heidelberg, Germany

Printed by Libri Plureos GmbH
in Hamburg, Germany